What The Medical Establishment Won't Tell You That Could

SAVE YOUR LIFE

What The Medical Establishment
Won't Tell You That Could

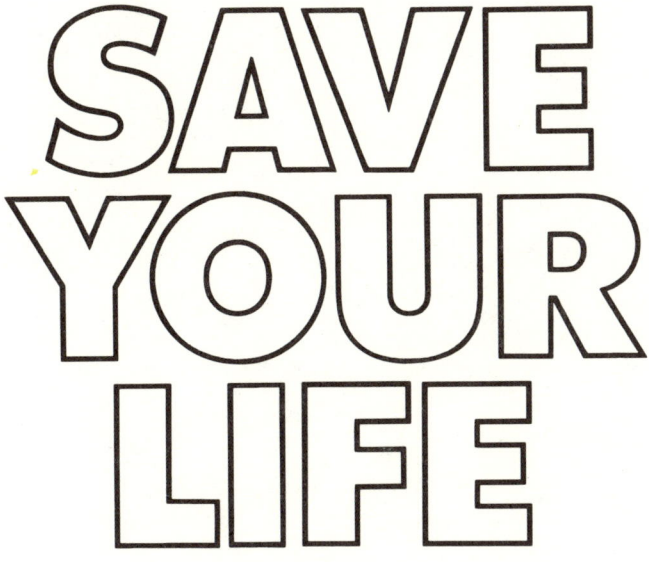

by
MICHAEL L. CULBERT

Foreword by
Robert Atkins, M.D.

Donning
Virginia Beach/Norfolk

Copyright © 1983 by Michael L. Culbert

All rights reserved, including the right to reproduce this work in any form whatsoever without permission in writing from the publisher, except for brief passages in connection with a review. For information, write:
The Donning Company/Publishers
5659 Virginia Beach Boulevard
Norfolk, Virginia 23502

Library of Congress Cataloging in Publication Data

Culbert, Michael L., 1937-
   What the medical establishment won't tell you that could save your life.

   Bibliography: p.
   1. Medical care—United States. I. Title.
[DNLM: 1. Delivery of health care—United States. W 84 AA1 C9m]
RA395.A3C89   1983   362.1'0973   82-9607
ISBN 0-89865-256-1

Printed in the United States of America

Contents

Foreword 1
Introduction 5
Chapter One
    The Medical Revolt 9
Chapter Two
    The Battle For Freedom of Choice 32
Chapter Three
    Rx: Murder—How Government and the AMA
    Stifle Innovation 71
Chapter Four
    The American Food Disaster—Culprit
    Number One 87
Chapter Five
    The Scandal of Cancergate 110
Chapter Six
    The ACS, the NCI and the War on "Unprovens" 143
Chapter Seven
    Modern Medicine's Magnificent Mavericks 180
Chapter Eight
    Vitamin B^{17} and Metabolic Therapy 210
Chapter Nine
    Suppressed Nutrients 245
Chapter Ten
    The Fight For Chelation 271
Chapter Eleven
    The Challenge of Promotive Health 286
Selected Bibliography 290

Foreword

Recently, before lecturing to a medical group, I had an opportunity to chat with several member-physicians.

I asked a dermatologist if he had ever used zinc or vitamin A in treating acne. He replied that he hadn't. "Nutrition has very little to do with skin diseases," he added.

Then, when I met a cardiovascular surgeon, I inquired whether he had considered chelation therapy as a technique for reversing arteriosclerosis. "Never heard of it," was the reply. "Anyway, arteriosclerosis is irreversible."

Frustrated, I engaged a rheumatologist in conversation. "Have you ever found vitamins B^6, B^3, PABA, or pantothenic acid useful in managing your arthritis?" I asked. "That's nonsense," was the rejoinder. "In fact, the Arthritis Foundation's official position is that no nutritional factor has ever been proven to be of benefit in arthritis."

I was almost too shaken to inquire of the psychiatrist if he had ever used megavitamin therapy in any of his schizophrenic patients, or even tried L-tryptophan to combat mild depression or anxiety. But I did get another strongly negative response.

Needless to say, when I asked a cancer specialist as diplomatically as I could whether he saw any promise in the nutritional-metabolic therapies in cancer, he bellowed, "You don't mean that quack remedy laetrile, do you?" He was about to launch into a tirade, at which point I thought it more prudent to change the subject.

You see, I am a nutrition-physician and I like to think (if the amount of time I spend in the medical library is any indication), a scholar on the subject of what nutrition can do in clinical, patient-oriented medicine. All the questions I asked were about nutritional treatments that have been studied, reported upon, and found effective. Yet none of the doctors used, or were even favorably disposed to try, any of them.

The question is: What does all this mean *to you?* When you become the patient, and seek help from doctors like these, the orthodox majority, what chance is there that some natural, non-toxic, health-directed life style change will be recommended, rather than an invasive pharmaceutical or surgical attack upon the "disease" he finds you to have? The answer is, not much.

At present, only a handful of America's doctors have the expertise, or even the willingness, to explore non-toxic therapies. But how did this come about? Why does your doctor believe, as he probably does, that nutrition, as a therapy, simply wouldn't work?

As you read Mike Culbert's book, you may learn some of the reasons for the anti-nutrition bias of the medical community. You certainly will be exposed to a wealth of factual information on this subject.

Part of the answer must be "pressure from the top." Your doctor is too much under the influence of his leadership. And *that* leadership, I strongly suspect, is too much under the influence of business interests. The powerful pharmaceutical industry has a very cozy thing going with the medical community. It is reaping the benefits of a full-time sales force over half-a-million strong—our doctors. Naturally, they do not want to lose the support of this sales force by encouraging the idea that illness can be prevented, and even treated, by natural, non-pharmaceutical techniques.

It is astounding, and a little frightening, to learn how little knowledge of nutrition most doctors have. All of their medical training has oriented them to respond automatically to illness with the question: What should I *prescribe* here? And all of the medical journals they read simply reinforce that attitude.

The net result is that, by and large, your doctor learns what the pharmaceutical industry wants him to learn. Contrary theories are not only not tolerated; they are actively discouraged. For instance, over fifty medical references are published each year about laetrile, appearing in just about every medical journal that is widely read. But these are not reports on scientific studies on its effectiveness or lack of it, or clinical data on its use. Rather, virtually every reference treats laetrile as outright quackery which is dangerous to a patient's health.

There is another reason for this bias, which is grounded in human nature. Most individuals, once having publicly rendered strong opinions, find it extremely difficult to reverse themselves. Many experts find themselves spending entire careers justifying ill-founded conclusions they reached, and broadcast, early in their careers. How many times I encounter "scientists" whose attitude is: "Don't bother me with facts; my mind is made up."

My own interest in this subject began in 1973 when, after

addressing a meeting of the *avant-garde* of nutrition-metabolic doctors, one took me aside and said, "Do you know that there are several *bona fide,* effective cancer treatments that are being squelched by the American Cancer Society?" Disbelieving, yet horrified, I asked, "Why would they *want* to do anything like that?"

For the past eleven years, I have pondered deeply on that question—why do leaders of medical orthodoxy *want* to perpetuate the very illnesses they have vowed to eradicate?

I still don't know the answer, I just know that they do. I have seen unreasonableness that simply could not emanate from an honest mind. I've seen it directed against a remarkable variety of effective treatments for cancer, as well as for mental disorders, cardiovascular conditions, arthritis, and, in fact, the entire spectrum of current ailments. And I know this firsthand, for I have borne the brunt of their closed-mindedness and intellectual dishonesty when they saw fit to attack the dietary principles I had worked out through painstaking observations on thousands of patients.

Mike Culbert's book provides you the information *you need* in order to interpret the bitter controversies that will continue to arise between medical orthodoxy and those medical researchers who have been forced to go "underground"—simply because they found a treatment that works, but that does not call for the pharmacological and surgical warfare that constitutes present-day medicine.

Culbert is right when he characterizes their efforts to suppress the many types of advances that have been made in conquering malignant disease as "Cancergate." But here the crime involves more than just the maintenance of political office—it involves a multitude of human lives, each with an untold degree of suffering.

Let me point out to you that I have never used laetrile in treating a patient, simply because the treatment of cancer is not my specialty. I don't even know whether it works. Yet I have seen patients treated with therapies directed toward strengthening the patient, rather than waging war against disease. They have been treated with a variety of diets, vitamins, vitamins C, A, B-complex, enzymes, and agents to stimulate their immune response—and they have, at least, improved.

I know simply this: as a practicing physician, I am interested in seeking techniques that can help my patients in their struggles, not in proving my previous learnings (or teachings) right. I fear that our medical leadership still has it the other way around.

If there is to be a medical revolution in America, it must be done by wresting those of that mentality from their positions of power. The book you are about to read will show you *why* that must be done.

ROBERT C. ATKINS, M.D.
New York City

Introduction

In January, 1982, the National Cancer Institute (NCI) released its long-awaited results of the so-called "laetrile clinical trial" at major cancer research facilities, a study which, it was said, would finally prove or disprove, once and for all, the efficacy of laetrile in treating cancer.

Just what had motivated NCI even to attempt such a trial was the greatest medical controversy in modern times. Not too surprising to the proponents of the controversial, damned, unwanted, overlooked and thwarted cancer remedy, the NCI "trial" turned out to be an example of what I call the Club—the vested medical, pharmaceutical, and government interests in American scientific orthodoxy—at its very worst.

In a scientifically meaningless exercise, a form of government-manufactured putative laetrile of an impure variety was utilized within a sloppily adhered-to "metabolic program" on a group of incurable cancer patients, two-thirds of whom had received (and failed on) prior "orthodox" therapy. Despite the fact that a remarkably large number of these incurable, expected-to-die patients remained "stable" while given injections even of degraded material, most of them had died by the time the "trial" had ended. The "trial," of course, was in the hands of "orthodox" scientists whose leaders were vocally hostile to, and doubtful about, laetrile. No raw data were available from the treatment centers involved and no laetrile-skilled physicians or researchers were allowed to be part of the program. The results, announced America's crippled medical orthodoxy, were said to be the final word: laetrile and/or its adjunctive metabolic therapy, were of no "substantive benefit" in the treatment of cancer.

I detail these outrageous shenanigans in Chapter Two. The

tests, again, meant nothing *scientifically*—for the patients were incurable and not expected to respond to any known form of therapy, and most of them had already been mistreated through earlier "orthodox" therapy. The results said nothing about pure amygdalin (the compound which should have been tested were the Club really interested in settling the dispute), or about metabolic therapy *per se,* about the prevention of cancer with vitamin B^{17} or the positive responses now scores of thousands of Americans (and many foreigners) have had due either to laetrile, or to laetrile with metabolic therapy, or to laetrile with standard therapies. The "trial" was carried out in the shadow of the overwhelming evidence, gathered from many countries by many doctors and scientists and by many thousands of patients, that laetrile is useful in both preventing and treating cancer.

Scientifically meaningless, yes, But not *propagandistically* so. Indeed, the NCI "trial," and other scattered tests in which test animals received large enough amounts of *oral* amygdalin so that cyanide poisoning occurred, were devastatingly effective in the public-relations war which American orthodoxy saw absolutely necessary to mount against laetrile or vitamin B^{17}.

It is the central thesis of this book that the Club must attack and destroy laetrile *at all costs*—and not so much because of laetrile's implied threat only to the $30-billion-per-year cancer industry, but because of what laetrile represents.

And what laetrile represents is nothing less than the holistic medical revolution which is now sweeping America—and, hopefully, the Western World.

Laetrile is, as I point out, the Marine Corps of that entire movement of alternative treatment and natural health ideology, which broadly can be described as promotive health, preventive medicine, holistic medicine, orthomolecular medicine, metabolic/ nutritional therapy, and the like. Not until the Laetrile War broke full-force upon the scene was this movement taken seriously. *It is now*—and therein lies the real merit of the whole laterile controversy.

Laetrile had to be fought tooth and nail by a crumbling, discredited medical and pharmaceutical establishment because, as the Marine Corps of the holistic movement, it had secured vital beachheads in the national consciousness and in medical practice. The notion of *preventing* degenerative disease, let alone the use of natural and potentially inexpensive substances to *treat* it, are the twin threats which face the Club.

The pressure of the entire holistic revolution is now obvious on all sides: whether it be legislative probes of the scandal-seared National Cancer Institute, curbs on the Food and Drug Administration (FDA), wholesale desertions of medical professionals from the American Medical Association (AMA), the quiet shift of interest by the American Cancer Society (ACS) away from radiation, chemotherapy and surgery to the sudden discovery of the merits of immunotherapy in cancer, the grudging acceptance by growing numbers of scientific researchers of vitamins, minerals and enzymes in the prevention and management of degenerative disease, the onrushing evidence linking lifestyle and polluted food to those very diseases, the proliferation of whole new medical organizations and alliances functioning outside the AMA and the whole allopathic school of medical thought, and the increasing number of practitioners of alternative therapy. It can be seen in the flourishing, rapidly growing vitamin/mineral supplements and "health food" industry and in the boom in self-help health and alternative medicine books and publications.

The Club, the medical/pharmaceutical/governmental axis, is responding in historic ways: hoked-up tests such as the incredible series of low blows aimed at laetrile; defamations of the character and credentials of major proponents of the new thought; the use of raw police power against dissenters; and marshaling of the pressures wrought by peer-review boards, insurance companies and licensing bureaus against practitioners who depart from holy doctrine; and, sad to say, the manipulation of the major media.

I say all of this by way of being, during most of my professional life, a journalist. Indeed, I entered the laetrile controversy first as a skeptical newsman, not as an impassioned advocate. I know from years of experience the ease with which established thought—and in this case, the Club—can get its message across. The handling by the major media of the alternative health movement in America has been, frankly, an abomination. Prostitutes of the pen and electronic media have been front-runners for the allopathic medical establishment and the real power behind it, the pharmaceutical industry. These same journalists, who clamor so much about their right to do what they do because of "the people's right to know," have been primary actors in a drama in which vast amounts of the American people, who depend on the media for informational guidance, have not been *allowed* to know about the onrushing health and medical revolution.

There have, of course, been outstanding exceptions to this general rule, and the names of several of these courageous and probing reporters appear in these pages. My hat is off to them almost as much as it is off to those incredible men and women of courage and fortitude who are forging the medical revolution in America—the doctors, scientists, researchers who have chosen to march to a different drummer.

My only *caveats* to the reader are these:

That you bear in mind that I am a journalist, not a physician, and that nothing I write here should be construed as diagnosing or suggesting treatment for a disease. As a writer, I will feel amply gratified if, in reading the following chapters, you have gained a new perspective on health and medicine as well as an appreciation of some of the forces which, perhaps unbeknownst to you, have helped shape your life.

Oakland, California
December 1982

Chapter One
The Medical Revolt

Steve McQueen and "Metabolic Therapy"

Never before have this nation's medical and media establishments given so much attention to the general story of "what are the quacks up to now?" Steven McQueen, at fifty years old a hero of hard-bitten cowboy and police movie roles, was actually being treated for cancer in one of "those" clinics south of the border. First, he had denied reports that he was suffering from terminal mesothelioma, a widespread malignancy of the lining of the chest which is usually fatal. Then he admitted it. *Then* he was discovered at the Plaza Santa Maria General Hospital, a fully licensed medical facility in Baja California, Mexico.

Not only that, McQueen made a television report to the Mexican nation, praising that country for allowing a hospital like Plaza Santa Maria to exist. He hailed its staff of Mexican, American, and German physicians—all trained in "alternative" cancer therapies—for giving him a new lease on life.

Then came the press reports, some garbled, some accurate. McQueen was being treated with a wide variety of "experimental" potions and approaches that had been widely condemned by American medical orthodoxy as unproven at best, and quackery at worst. The actor's treatment included dietary manipulation (stressing abstention from stimulants, animal fat and proteins, refined foods, and refined carbohydrates, and emphasizing in their place raw fruits and vegetables and their juices), live-cell therapy (injections of cells from animal tissues), a rigid detoxification program, an array of enzyme, mineral, and vitamin supplements, immune-stimulating substances including the Maruyama vaccine from Japan, and—most horrendous of all in the eyes of American orthodoxy—

laetrile, or amygdalin.*

Indeed, his treatment was an individualized version of a growing, if disorganized, discipline variously called "metabolic" or "nutritional" therapy, "holistic" medicine, and the like. In essence, it stresses a total life style change, particularly in eating habits and attitudes, and physically is concerned with nourishing the body with natural substances to shore up its internal defense mechanisms rather than providing single-shot attacks on tumors.

Why in the world would McQueen, at the pinnacle of a productive movie career in Hollywood, and *not* known as an anti-Establishment type, reject Establishment medicine and opt for something as seemingly bizarre as "metabolic therapy" at a Mexican-licensed clinic fifty miles south of the border?

The answer was simple. There was *nothing* American orthodoxy could do for him. While Cedars/Sinai Medical Center in Los Angeles remained tight-lipped about the McQueen case, admitting only that he had been there, the Hollywood star, now thin, emaciated, and looking *old,* said that at first he had been given two months to live, then just two weeks. (American officialdom replied that doctors don't "give" patients longevity spans, but it is clear that the semantics used by American oncologists and other cancer specialists do in fact include precisely the messages that patients perceive in them.) By all valid accounts, Steve McQueen was literally at death's door when he arrived at the Mexican treatment center on 31 July 1980.

I am aware of what actually occurred, and what did not, because at the time I was North American spokesman for Plaza Santa Maria General Hospital. As chairman of the board of the Committee for Freedom of Choice in Cancer Therapy, Inc., the nation's primary pro-laetrile organization, and an officer in American Biologics, a company specializing in metabolic pharmaceuticals, I had had a

---

*In this book, I use the terms "laetrile," "amygdalin," and "vitamin B^{17}" interchangeably. Biochemically, however, the so-called "laetrile" molecule is actually a biosynthesized product made from the cleavage of the natural compound amygdalin and its conversion to a *glucuronide.* The term "Laetrile" (with a capital "L"), a privately-created designation and trademark in the Merck Index, refers to a synthetic product. The proper scientific term for the compound under discussion, as it occurs in nature, and even in manufactured form (before it is broken down in the body), is *amygdalin.* Because of confusion over these terms, which developed earlier in laetrile's history, and also because of widespread media and statutory use ("laetriles" is used in California law in reference to the beta-cyanogenetic compounds amygdalin, prunasin, and substantially similar substances), as well as the political successes of the "laetrile movement," the public has accepted the word "laetrile" as virtually a household term. (Language is, after all, democratic.) The proponents of the vitamin B^{17} theory propose that all cyanide-bearing sugar compounds (beta-cyanogenetic glucosides, cyanogenic glycosides, *etc.),* also known as *nitrilosides,* be designated vitamin B^{17}.

lengthy relationship with Mexico's so-called "laetrile clinics" for years.

I at first urged the hospital to keep the fact that McQueen was under treatment there as quiet as possible, though I knew that sooner or later word would get out. Dr. Rodrigo Rodriguez, the young medical director at Plaza and a specialist in nuclear and nutritional medicine, completely agreed. Everyone involved knew that in a case as advanced as McQueen's—one that orthodox medicine said was terminal—every day, even every hour counted. Preliminary publicity about his therapy would not help matters.

Yet, incredibly, the initial word was good. By September, McQueen was not only still very much alive, but by his own words and deeds, he was responding very favorably to the "quack" program. American Biologics was instrumental in securing, for experimental use, a stabilized form of laetrile or amygdalin (Amygatrile), and this author, through the good graces of pioneering medic Chisato Maruyama in Tokyo, had been able to introduce experimental samples of Dr. Maruyama's vaccine for limited use at Plaza Santa Maria. The vaccine, while in use for fifteen years at the Nippon Medical School in Japan, had secured anti-cancer effects ranging from minimal to spectacular in almost 110,000 people. I considered it one of an array of non-specific, immune-system enhancing substances that might be useful in a total nutritional therapy.

By October, the rugged actor was able to swim in Plaza's Olympic-sized pool, make shopping sorties to Ensenada and Tijuana, and was on the way to recovering a considerable portion of his stamina and vitality. But his cancer persisted. Nobody at Plaza was making bets on his long-term survival. They *did* agree with what McQueen himself had told a Canadian newspaper, in one of his very few direct contacts with the press—he had already beaten the odds by better than six-to-one. He talked in terms of life-extension, even of possible recovery.

Television crews from all major networks, and journalists by the score, descended on Plaza Santa Maria, attempting to get inside information about the case. The news was flashed around the world—"McQueen Said Responding to 'Alternative' Therapy in Terminal Cancer."

The McQueen case went into a period of watchful waiting. Never before had so famous a personage openly admitted that he not only was being treated with "unproven" cancer therapies outside of the United States, but that he felt he *owed his life* to them. (Others who have acknowledged such treatments include actor Fred McMurray, who credited laetrile and a special diet, used as "backups" to radiation, for victory over throat cancer, and Alycia Buttons, the wife of Red Buttons, who credited a similar program for her victory over cancer.)

11

American medical orthodoxy was, as usual, apoplectic. This time it could not claim that the patient in question had been diagnosed outside the country and perhaps was thus being treated for a nonexistent disease. All it could do was to condemn the treatments being used—while admitting it had no effective therapy of its own for such advanced cases. One "television doctor" did make the claim that an experimental technique using chemotherapy (an injectable poison) might work against mesothelioma—sometime in the future. But the reality remained. At the time he was diagnosed as terminally ill, McQueen had nothing to lose, and everything to gain, by choosing an alternative approach.

Because McQueen had at first been referred to Plaza Santa Maria by orthodontist William Kelley, a longtime champion of alternative therapies whose dental license had been suspended because of his advocacy of alleged "unproved" remedies (though he had successfully tried them on his *own* cancer years ago), medical officialdom and the lap dog media turned on Kelley and his organization. Then, because laetrile was a part—but only a part—of the program, the Establishment increased its attack on the apricot kernel extract that had already kindled one of the biggest medical controversies of the century.

Nonetheless, with every passing day and week, McQueen continued to live and continued to improve. In fact, the actor decided that he was well enough to return to his ranch in southern California—a trip that turned out to be fatal.

After word got out that McQueen was indeed at Plaza Santa Maria and was responding favorably to the treatment there, controversy among partisans of various alternative therapies broke out over the nature of his treatment. To set the record straight, American Biologics and the Committee for Freedom of Choice in Cancer Therapy called a national press conference in San Francisco. Dr. Rodriguez was present, and answered questions from the press as best he could, without violating the doctor-patient relationship. At the press conference, Dr. Rodriguez confirmed that, yes, McQueen had indeed made substantial progress. His energy level was better, his tumefaction was reduced, his blood analyses showed that the progress of his cancer had been virtually halted. This did *not* mean, the Mexican physician was careful to point out, that McQueen was anywhere near full recovery. Battered with persistent demands to make a prediction in the case, Dr. Rodriguez stated flatly, "Doctors don't make predictions."

While Dr. Rodriguez was in San Francisco to explain the nature of McQueen's therapy, persons only indirectly connected with the case suggested to the actor that his recovery might be quicker if he underwent surgery to remove the existing tumors. Virtually all of the doctors who treated McQueen at Plaza, most definitely including Dr. Rodriguez, opposed the idea. They doubted whether his system was yet strong enough to withstand the surgery, and they argued that surgery was not presently necessary, even if he could survive it.

Steve McQueen did not heed the doctors who had brought him so far. The actor, whose rough-and-tumble life demonstrated a willingness to take chances, took another gamble. A few days later he was in another Mexican clinic, this one in Ciudad Juarez, below the Texas border. Following surgery on two sections of tumor, he developed an embolism. On the morning of 7 November 1980, he suffered a heart attack and died.

Cynical as it may sound, American medical orthodoxy could now breathe a sigh of relief. The actor who dared flee his own country for "unproven" treatments was dead at a clinic in Mexico. That was, in essence, how the major media treated the story.

Overlooked (as usual) were the awesome realities. McQueen fled American orthodoxy because he had no other option. He had shown a sustained, impressive response to the therapy, despite the fact that nobody had made any guarantees—and despite the fact that therapeutic response is not the equivalent of full recovery.

The McQueen case served a distinct purpose: it focused world attention on alternative therapies—those approaches "outside the pale" of American medical orthodoxy. At a time when the Western world is faced by the gravest cancer pandemic in its history, the publicity accorded Steve McQueen made it clear that there *are* other choices. Whether orthodoxy liked it or not, news of McQueen's death not only did not induce desperate, dying patients *away* from clinics practicing "alternative" therapies—it actually seemed to increase the number of patients. And why not? Under traditional, established, orthodox treatments, the United States is losing more than 1,180 citizens *per day* to cancer—one every 73 seconds.

Had Steve McQueen lived another six months, a year, or longer—which he may well have done had he avoided surgery— medical orthodoxy would have suffered acute embarrassment. But now it could ignore or cover up the positive facts and concentrate on the grim conclusion. The actor chose an "unproven" treatment and he was dead. The medical establishment reacted just as it had with two other celebrated cases, Joey Hofbauer and Chad Green, two children who were victims of both cancer *and* a venal cross-linkage of medical, pharmaceutical, and administrative establishments.

The "Medical Kidnappings" Of Cancer Patients

In October 1977 Joseph (Joey) Hofbauer, the eight-year-old son of John and Mary Hofbauer of Ballston Spa, New York, was found to be suffering from Hodgkin's disease, a form of lymphatic cancer, which had been diagnosed from a biopsy of a node on Joey's neck at St. Peter's Hospital in Albany. Well-meaning physicians told John Hofbauer, a Knights of Columbus insurance agent, that Joey should immediately be subjected to chemotherapy—the administration of highly toxic drugs, a "treatment of choice" for this form of cancer.

The Hofbauers had heard about the dreadful side effects of both chemotherapy and radiation treatments, and had also heard about the promising results of nutritional "metabolic therapy" at the Fairfield Medical Centre in Montego Bay, Jamaica, specializing in non-toxic modalities. They made a decision that was to affect their lives far more than they realized at the time. They dared to choose Jamaica, and the non-toxic as well as "unproven" remedies, over chemotherapy and radiation.

After all, as John Hofbauer told me months later, in the seesaw battle with medical orthodoxy and state bureaucrats that ensued, American cancer experts warned that the baseball-playing boy would have anywhere from two weeks to six months to live if he did not receive "standard" therapy. "It became more and more ludicrous to hear the so-called experts talk about when Joey was supposed to die—and they kept advancing the date," the practicing Catholic said.

Even so, by the Hofbauers' own account, Joey "prospered" in the balmy climes of Jamaica, where German and Jamaican cancer experts have pioneered a form of therapy emphasizing the use of natural fruits and vegetables and their juices, protein-digesting enzymes and vitamin supplements, including the use of the highly-controversial vitamin B^{17} (laetrile or amygdalin). In two weeks of treatment, his progress was quite visible.

Returning home to New York, the elated parents were astounded when, on 29 November 1977, two representatives of the Saratoga Department of Social Services, accompanied by a deputy sheriff, showed up with orders to place the child in the department's care because his parents had failed to provide "proper treatment" for him.

For days, Joey remained a virtual prisoner at St. Paul's Hospital. Luckily, local media exposed the seizure of the eight-year-old boy from his parents and the case began to make waves.

Orthodox cancer specialists wished to treat Joey with nitrogen mustard, the principal substance in a poison gas used in World War I. They also wanted to remove his spleen. This treatment, they claimed, has a "cure rate" of 75 to 90 percent. But the Hofbauers had already learned that cancer orthodoxy's cure rate means five years free of symptoms. A sudden return of cancer on the first day of the sixth year, and subsequent death therefrom, do not appear in such statistics.

A three-hour hearing before the Saratoga County Family Court ended in tears for the Hofbauers, as the case was postponed to a later date. John Hofbauer told the press:

> My child is a prisoner in the hospital. If I take him out of this hospital, I'm kidnapping—and if I lose at this hearing, they could keep my child

forever. The issue is whether I should have the right and freedom to obtain the therapy of my choice.

The Hofbauers' appeals to New York Gov. Hugh Carey fell on deaf ears. Twice Governor Carey vetoed "freedom of choice" bills allowing the use of laetrile, after the legislation had been approved by lopsided margins in both houses of the state legislature.

On 7 December Saratoga County Court Judge Loren N. Brown suspended the order that had granted the social services department temporary custody of the boy. He ruled that Joey could continue under the care of a metabolic therapist, psychiatrist Michael Schachter of Nyack, New York, for six months, with Dr. Schachter reporting to the court monthly on the progress of the case.

Partisans of metabolic/nutritional therapy throughout the country, already stirred to a fever pitch over the national controversy surrounding laetrile, were cheered by the lower court decision. Here, finally, would be an excellent case of metabolic therapy officially monitored and reported that could prove or disprove the effects of the broad-gauge "holistic" approach to degenerative disease against the gloomy prognostications of the nation's cancer establishment.

Dr. Schachter, no stranger to metabolic therapy and known as a medical innovator, fell immediately under attack. The New York State Health Department subpoenaed the records on all his patients to see to whom and under what conditions he was administering laetrile and another "unapproved" substance, MA-7, an immune system stimulant.

But the thirty-seven-year-old physcian refused to turn over his records and decided to fight the battle all the way up the court system. He was supported by his patients, who were outraged by the state's efforts to interfere with the privacy of the doctor-patient relationship. Attorney Henry Rothblatt said state authorities wanted twelve clerks and eighteen investigators to go over Dr. Schachter's records, a move which, if allowed, would render the physician "dead professionally."

In the meantime, Dr. Schachter continued to treat Joey, now surviving under an entirely metabolic program of vitamins A, C, and B^{17} (laetrile or amygdalin), enzymes, a special diet, and coffee enemas.

Looking back, the Hofbauers and Dr. Schachter recall that the attention he was getting, and the mounting problems for his parents, caused a great deal of tension for Joey Hofbauer, and undue stress is to be as much avoided in the intensive metabolic treatment of cancer as is animal protein. At one point, Joey had regressed to such a low level that Dr. Schachter seriously considered using radiation treatments. However, by changing dose levels of the metabolic program the physcian produced a 25 percent reduction in the size of Joey's neck nodes within a week.

But even as Joey once again bounced back and responded well to the treatment, New York had bad news for his parents. In March 1978 the Appellate Division of the New York Supreme Court granted the state departments of health and social services intervenor status in the Hofbauer case. This decision was critical. Fearing that the state would once again be allowed to seize their son and this time to force him into chemotherapy or radiation—or both—John Hofbauer took part of his family and fled New York to nearby New Jersey, a state that had already decriminalized the use of laetrile.

This move divided the family of seven. Before it was over, the Hofbauers had lived in five separate residences, with John, Mary, Joey and three-year-old Paul at one time living in a log cabin in a secret location, leaving the teenage children in upstate New York to finish their school terms.

For John Hofbauer, it meant six-hour daily commutes from New Jersey to his office in New York, a job strain that was to add to the worry of huge medical and legal fees that grew and grew as the devoted father fought to fend off the bureaucrats. For Mary Hofbauer, it meant the near disintegration of her family. "The family outings, 4-H, piano lessons, basically all of the home-type things all normal families enjoy, had to come to a halt," she said.

During spring 1978, both Dr. Schachter and the Hofbauers kept me personally informed of the progress of Joey under metabolic therapy. This was because I was national spokesman for the Committee for Freedom of Choice in Cancer Therapy, Inc., the major laetrile lobbying group in the country, and editor of its magazine, *The Choice*.

As a long-time chronicler of the amygdalin controversy and the growing battle for metabolic therapy/holistic medicine against the entrenched forces of the Establishment, I was particularly interested in the outcome of the Hofbauer case because it so well epitomized what the national conflict was all about. First, is metabolic or nutritional therapy a legitimate treatment for degenerative disease? Second, do parents and their physicians have freedom of choice in therapy despite what the educated best guesses of transitory science are? The freedom of choice issue had already become the major factor in the laetrile controversy.

While New York state officials said one thing about the six months of court-monitored metabolic therapy Joey was on, Dr. Schachter and the boy's parents said quite another.

On 18 May two state agencies filed affidavits that claimed that cancerous lymph nodes on Joey's neck "are now in other parts of the body, indicating a progression of the disease."

But Dr. Schachter, seconded by the Hofbauers, reported to me that Joey's progress under metabolic therapy was "fantastic" and that the affidavits represented "a deplorable attempt to discredit and demean me."

New York also ruled that even though the Hofbauers had fled the state, its agencies still had jurisdiction in Joey's case.

According to his father, Joey's condition was such that his swollen lymph nodes were not visible "unless he turns his neck a certain way," and his blood workups indicated a marked improvement in his condition.

By May, with the six-month court-monitored period due to end 9 June, Dr. Schachter had found that the boy's progress was so good that he had been able to cut back the dose levels of metabolic products by 75 percent. The original seven-centimeter tumor mass was all but gone, and Joey had returned to most normal activities. Best of all, not only was Joey healthy, but he had already survived longer than some of the doctors originally involved in his case had thought he would.

It was also determined that the Appellate Division of the state Supreme Court would begin open deliberations to determine whether, in fact, the state agencies would have the right to force standard therapy on Joey and whether the Hofbauers had been "neglectful parents" for having opted for unconventional treatment modalities. The court determined that the hearings should be held before Judge Brown.

Smarting from the brushfire successes of the national drive to decriminalize laetrile (vitamin B^{17}) and continuing federal court decisions in favor of freedom of choice in medicine, the massed forces of American medical orthodoxy sensed in the Hofbauer case a critical, landmark event. These same forces had been decisively set back by earlier rulings of the U.S. District Court of Appeals that the federal government had no right to interfere with the access of patients to laetrile. Moreover, several state rulings and opinions had made it clear that the federal Food, Drug and Cosmetic Act was never intended by Congress to interfere with the practice of medicine.

In hearing after hearing before state legislatures and various courts, spokesmen for the federal Food and Drug Administration, the American Cancer Society and state and local medical boards had argued in vain that, while orthodoxy has no known cure for cancer and no real agreement on what cancer is, citizens must be denied the right to seek "unorthodox" forms of treatment.

The Hofbauer case was seen as a showcase because of the embarrassing fact that the boy was doing so well on unorthodox therapy and was surviving well beyond the presumed target dates for his death. His continuing survival was, indeed, an implied insult to the hordes of highly paid cancer specialists and a shot in the arm to those schools of medical thought that the medical-government-pharmaceutical axis in this country had long written off as "quackery."

In short, the Hofbauer case *had* to be fought.

For that reason, a virtual "blue ribbon" group of spokesmen for medical orthodoxy dutifully trooped to New York to testify against metabolic/nutritional therapy in general and amygdalin in particular, even though amygdalin was only part of the program.

Dr. H. James Wallace, a Roswell Park Institute oncologist, was present to testify that a diagram he had seen of Joey's lymph nodes indicated "a definite progression in size and number" of such nodes. Dr. Daniel Martin, a New York cancer researcher noted for denouncing laetrile as a fraud and its proponents as liars, was present, as was Dr. Victor Herbert, chief of hematology and nutrition at Bronx Veterans Hospital, who has reserved his sharpest adjectives for laetrile.

Also present were, among others, Dr. Arthur F. Cohn, who had originally diagnosed Joey's condition and reported the refusal of his parents to subject him to standard treatment, and Dr. Anthony Tartaglia, chief of medicine at St. Peter's, who testified there had been "a very definite progression" of Hodgkin's disease during the time Joey was on the metabolic program.

But the Hofbauers, however seriously depleted their funds were, were not without expert counsel in the persons of National Health Federation attorney Kirkpatrick Dilling, a long-time battler on health issues, and Leslie Couch. These attorneys brought forth to do battle with the Establishment researchers and physicians, including representatives of the FDA, the biggest cannons the rapidly growing, laetrile-centered school of metabolic therapy could muster: Dean Burk, Ph.D. retired chief of cytochemistry at the federally funded National Cancer Institute, the seventy-four-year-old biochemist who for years had been the sole voice from within the Establishment demanding a fair trial for laetrile; Harold Manner, Ph.D. chief of the department of biology, Loyola University at Chicago, who stunned the American medical world in late 1977 with his disclosure that he and and a team of graduate students had secured 100 percent positive response and 89 percent complete regressions of breast cancer in mice with a program of amygdalin, emulsified vitamin A and proteolytic (protein-digesting) enzymes; Bruce Halstead, M.D. a veteran cancer researcher from California who has helped prove the nontoxicity and focal action of laetrile; and Tom Roberts, M.D. a metabolic physician from Virginia.

In his eventual ruling, Judge Brown took particular note of the fact that although Drs. Tartaglia and John Horton, chief of oncology at Albany Medical Center, had testified that after they examined Joey following the six-month treatment period they had found "numerous nodes" on the left side of his back, they had also found that he weighed sixty-two pounds—or up ten pounds—under the care of Dr. Schachter, that his color was good, that he complained of none of the symptoms that would normally indicate systemic involvement with Class B Hodgkin's disease, that his appetite was good, that he regularly played baseball, and that blood tests and urinalyses had come up with only a sedimentation rate of thirty as a "significant finding," one not specifically attributable to Hodgkin's disease. The best evidence, of course, was Joey himself—alive, happy, vigorous and even athletic.

Kirkpatrick Dilling scored points when he told the court that orthodoxy's concern over peeling skin on Joey's nose and back might have more to do with the fact he was playing baseball in the sun rather than being attributable to alleged overdoses of vitamin A!

On 28 June 1978, Judge Brown rendered his decision—a landmark, as it turned out, not for the Establishment, but for partisans of freedom of choice. Not only were the Hofbauers not "neglectful parents" for having their son treated metabolically, but, wrote the judge, "this court also finds that metabolic therapy has a place in our society, and, hopefully, its proponents are on the first rung of a ladder that will rid us of all forms of cancer." This ruling followed by days other court victories in which Dr. Schachter and his patients, in separate actions, won the right to continued doctor-patient privacy.

The state of New York wasted no time in appealing the Hofbauer decision, and ultimately lost. But an elated, if exhausted, John Hofbauer told me, "The testimony speaks for itself. The devastating effects of chemotherapy and radiation have been proved even by the proponents of conventional therapy." Still appalled that the state would not cease and desist in efforts to force orthodox therapy on his son, he added:

> All this constant harassment we have undergone has worked a severe strain on us, but we have kept fighting. Now, in the open, we have shown that all the things they did to us have helped drive the nails into their coffin.
>
> Through it all, I never said I would not go along with their orthodox therapy, but what they were really asking me to do was like asking me to throw my son out of a burning building, guaranteeing the breaking of every bone in his body, before I had a chance to look for the stairs and see if we could get out some other way. The state doesn't give you the right to look for the stairs—they ask you to throw your son out the window.
>
> Our family has been devastated and we have suffered terribly. The worst thing you can do to a mother is to take her from her children. New York state officials have done that to my wife. I don't choose to be a crusader with my son as a pawn. All I've ever done is react to what state and county officials have done to me.

The denouement of the Hofbauer case was tragic.

Suffering from the constant stress on the peripatetic family, Joey went through two relapses thereafter but bounced back both times. Every month he stayed alive *without* orthodox or standard therapy was a continuing insult to American medical and administrative officialdom.

He entered 1979 with more than a year of survival under unorthodoxy, a far cry from the "two weeks to six months" originally given him. Ultimately, the Hofbauers opted for an immunological-stimulating vaccine therapy under Lawrence Burton, Ph.D. in the Bahamas, and abandoned the metabolic diet and amygdalin altogether. There is no doubt that during most of that time, Joey looked—and *was*—healthy. The Hofbauers had some reason to believe that finally, with the stop in the Bahamas, their son might have won the final round.

It was not to be. As always, his ultimate demise on 10 July 1980, was blamed on quackery and unorthodox therapy. This is hardly the case. He had already survived upwards of three years, or far beyond all hopes of his success in this country, despite what "cancer experts" would *later* insist.

The Hofbauers' time in the Bahamas was also stressful. John Hofbauer told me that Bahamian medical authorities, pressured by the U.S., had not made them feel welcome. This feeling was heightened following a police raid on the Hofbauer apartment.

The death certificate for Joey read "Hodgkin's Disease," but as the elder Hofbauer explained, "That was the only way we could get his body off the island." He said the actual cause of Joey's death was pleurisy, pneumonia and the *possible* outbreak of the cancer process in his infected lungs.

"Joey had been fighting a lung infection for two weeks, but complications had arisen since a year ago when he suffered stress due to the raid. Then he had an abscess develop from an injection, a lung infection, pleurisy, and pneumonia. There were no local facilities in the Bahamas to treat the lung infection," John Hofbauer explained.

His father wrestled over the idea of an autopsy. One was performed. It showed "no trace of cancer in any of the tissues involved before—the spleen, liver and lymph nodes were normal," Hofbauer said. Later, Dr. Schachter, who had cared for Joey up until May 1979, told the press,

> "...The high level of stress on him and his family appeared to affect him adversely. The combination of this stress and the nature of his disease contributed to the impairment of his immune mechanism which resulted in his contracting a number of infections that aggravated his Hodgkin's

Disease....Preliminary findings by...the pathologist in Freeport who performed the examination revealed that most of the body was either free of Hodgkin's Disease or minimally involved. However, there was extensive involvement of the outer lining of the lungs, which apparently contributed to his death."

John Hofbauer said, "I'm sure that if Joey hadn't been under such harassment he would be alive and well today. He would be alive today if he had had the proper backup available to him."

But none of these observations and professional opinions slipped into the media. The only major media reports on the Hofbauer death were simply that his parents had refused him standard therapy, they had fled the state, they had been involved in bitter court battles, and now he was dead.

The Hofbauer case riveted national attention on an outrageous act, the kidnapping of a child by the state. But it was far from an isolated incident. In the period of 1976-78 five similar cases made news in the United States, and they helped fuel what for many was—and is—quickly becoming a revolt not only against established medicine in America, but a movement in favor of political reform to boot.

About the time the Hofbauers began their up-and-down battle to secure freedom of choice for Joey, the parents of a two-year-old leukemia patient in Massachusetts were beginning a similar odyssey. In August 1977, Chad Green was diagnosed in Omaha, Nebraska, with acute lymphocytic leukemia. Unlike Joey, he was treated with an orthodox modality—chemotherapy—and determined to be in remission after four weeks.

But because Nebraska doctors wanted to follow up the toxic drugs with brain irradiation as a "standard procedure," Chad's parents, Gerald and Diana, balked. Learning that therapists in Massachusetts would not use the procedure if the parents opposed it, the Greens left Nebraska for Scituate, Massachusetts.

In the meantime, Gerald's stepfather referred the Greens to literature concerning nutritional treatment, including laetrile. "We were overwhelmed with the knowledge and determined to help our son in these far more productive lines," Diana Green recalled. "Chad was immediately put on all-natural foods and supplements."

In Massachusetts, Chad "thrived" on the nutritional program, the Greens told me, adding he had more color, strength and energy than ever before. During this period they took Chad to Massachusetts General Hospital once a month for blood checks and a series of spinal injections, while opposing the use of radiation.

For three and a half months the boy did not receive prescribed oral chemotherapy treatments. During a checkup on 17 February,

Dr. John Truman determined that Chad had relapsed, but indicated he might still undergo a long remission if his parents restored the use of the tablets. The attempt to induce the Greens to return Chad to such a course of orthodox therapy went on daily, Diana Green told me, until the hospital at length threatened "possible legal action."

On 21 February, the Greens were informed that hospital attorneys would file a claim that the parents were "neglectful and abusive" in not continuing chemotherapy treatments. This was done, and Chad was forced back on chemotherapy. Immediately, the Greens said, he began suffering from a bloated abdomen, stomach pain, vomiting, slow motor activities, extreme irritability and hoarseness.

In March, the Greens, who are deeply religious, exulted that "God prevailed" as a district court judge dismissed the hospital's "care and protection" suit, thus giving Chad's parents the right to halt chemotherapy treatments, including the use of an experimental drug.

Their elation was short-lived. On 18 April Plymouth Superior court Judge Guy Volterra ruled that the Boston hospital had "legal custody" of the two-year-old even though his parents could retain "physical custody." While the parents desperately looked around for legal aid and moral support, their son was once again returned to chemotherapy treatments.

The Greens mapped plans to fight for freedom of choice all the way to the U.S. Supreme Court, with Gerald Green noting, "The kind of therapy isn't important. Our case is based on freedom of choice—whether we as Chad's parents have the right to choose or whether the court has the right."

The young couple, undergoing much the same strain and stress as that suffered by the Hofbauers, appealed the case to the Massachusetts Supreme Court and began involving Chad in a daily routine in which he received chemotherapy treatments in the morning and a nutritional program, later involving laetrile, in the evening.

On 9 July, the state Supreme Court ruled in favor of the hospital attorneys, listening to a spokesman who claimed that Chad was "energetic, and has been almost completely without any adverse side effects" from chemotherapy.

Diana Green told me, "I explained *why* Chad isn't having any side effects, *why* he is energetic. I told them about emulsified vitamin A, about vitamin C, the enzymes and the diet. But they're giving no credit to these things."

Incredibly, the State of Massachusetts was not about to let up on the Greens, and a pitched battle for custody raged over who ultimately should control the life of the elfin child.

In an expensive, two-week battle to regain full custody of Chad, the Greens, bereft of funds, brought in Drs. Burk, Halstead, and

Manner, among others, to argue on the safety of amygdalin-centered metabolic therapy for their son.

Brought in to testify against the Greens were New York hematologist Victor Herbert, who has since written off the B^{17} movement as "the cult of cyanide," and the FDA's Dr. Robert Young, among others. The experts charged that Chad might be suffering from "chronic cyanide poisoning" due to the amygdalin treatments.

On 22 January 1979, Judge Volterra forthwith ordered a cessation of the metabolic treatments and mandated that the boy be made a partial ward of the state.

"This was the last straw. They are playing with his life," Diana Green told me.

On the night of 24 January 1979, the Greens, flaunting possible contempt of court preceedings, fled Massachusetts for Tijuana, Mexico, to be able to continue their son on a mixed program of metabolic/nutritional therapy and chemotherapy at the famed Del Mar Medical Center of Dr. Ernesto Contreras.

There then began an incredible battle of propaganda waged through the media. Unlike the Hofbauer case, in which orthodox therapy never played a role, here was a situation in which contrasting forms of therapy were being utilized. Both sides could make equal claims given the outcome of the treatment. Truth to tell, both sides did.

I visited the Greens and Chad several times during 1979 in Tijuana. At all times he was bright, alert, and full of life.

There is a conflict between spokesmen for the Del Mar clinic and the Greens themselves as to the nature of Chad's treatment in Mexico, but it is known he went off of chemotherapy in August 1979, and continued at varying levels of metabolic therapy until the day he died, 12 October. He was also treated with the Hoxsey herbal therapy elsewhere in Mexico. Dr. Contreras believes the chemotherapy should have been continued.

"The chemotherapy regimen he received here was exactly the same as he had received in Massachusetts, except we added the metabolic therapy," Dr. Contreras told me. The Greens told the media they had taken the boy off chemotherapy tablets and had believed him under control. He was full of energy the day he died, when, they said, "He just closed his eyes. His heart stopped beating."

The Mexican and American doctors who performed an autopsy on the little body 15 October found no conclusive evidence of the cause of death, a reality made more complicated because the body was embalmed a day after the boy died. "This kind of sudden death is not usually associated with leukemia," Dr. Contreras said. Spokesmen close to the autopsy said no "heavy evidence" of leukemia was found even though some internal organs were enlarged, which *could* have been indicative of the disease.

(Indeed, on 5 January 1981, *Medical World News* reported: "Nor did University of California-San Diego forensic patholgist Dr. Frank Raasch observe enough leukemic cells to account for the child's death. Rather, he now attributes Chad's sudden death to 'very significant change in the conductive system of the heart, notably inflammation of the nerve cells in the sino-atrial node.' ")

Both the Greens and an American psychologist attached to the Contreras staff believed that stress and depression over Chad's deep desire to go home were highly significant factors in the child's demise. "In my opinion, the child is destroying himself because he wants to go home," the psychologist said a day before Chad died. There is no place for "broken heart" on a forensic report, of course.

Nonetheless, the Establishment media had a field day. "Laetrile Boy Dies in Tijuana," ran the accounts. Establishment medicine made we-told-you-so noises.

But the facts were somewhat more revealing. Chad fought cancer for twenty-five months, or well over half his young life. During the few months he was treated with chemotherapy alone, he lived as a tortured, frightened child. During the time he received either "mixed therapy" or metabolic therapy alone, he was happy, healthy, and living the life of a normal boy. This *quality of life* differential is the primary reason his parents knew then, and do now, that they did the right thing by bringing metabolic therapy into the treatment program.

It was immoral and obscene for the Establishment to claim, after the fact, that had Chad continued on barbarous chemotherapy alone he would have had anywhere from a 50 to 95 percent chance of "cure." We examine elsewhere the odd semantical trappings of "cure" used by American cancer orthodoxy.

But the Chad Green damage was done. When Establishment spokesmen were not darkly hinting that amygdalin itself killed Chad, at least they could point to a case in which metabolic/nutritional therapy had not "saved" the boy.

Both the Hofbauer and Green cases had national reverberations. Hundreds of thousands of Americans, watching both cases intently, simply could not believe that the government would actually kidnap children from their parents to enforce a given therapy on them, particularly when the nation's cancer establishment has long been forced to admit it knows neither the cause nor the cure of cancer.

The Hofbauer and Green cases are paradigms for the national furor over the plight of kidnapped child cancer victims—as well as the media's coverage of the same. They have to be contrasted with, for example, the case of Amanda Accardi, which happened after both the Hofbauer and Green events.

Unlike the other two cases, in which both children died at "alternative" clinics—single facts which helped to obscure the equally important realities that for long stretches of time they did fairly well on alternative forms of cancer therapy—Amanda Accardi not only showed distinct improvement while at an alternative clinic but left that clinic with a confirmation from American medical orthodoxy that her cancer was in remission.

But the outcome of the Accardi case while at the clinic, *unlike* the outcomes of the Green and Hofbauer cases, did not, for the most part, make front-page news. That is largely because orthodox spokesmen were not damning and condemning Amanda Accardi's death at the hands of the "quacks," as they had tried to do in the other two cases. Because Amanda did *not* die under alternative therapy she was simply less news than Joey Hofbauer and Chad Green. Sad but true—an Establishment-okayed viewpoint is simply "newsier" than a non-Establishment one—and, as a longtime journalist myself, I challenge editors and reporters of the major media to seriously dispute this, and to examine their handling of, say, press releases from the FDA, American Cancer Society, state health departments, and local medical boards as contrasted with their handling of press releases from alternative or non-Establishment health organizations.

The Accardi case ran this way: In July, 1981, 2½ year-old Amanda Accardi was diagnosed with acute lymphoblastic leukemia. The situation understandably panicked her parents, Michael, a twenty-six-year-old purchasing agent, and Katherine. They were even more disturbed when Children's Hospital (Los Angeles) doctors said the best they could do for the child was to place her on an experimental program of mixed chemotherapeutic drugs. Michael remembers doing a lot of reading about cancer and chemotherapy and soul-searching before reaching the conclusion that the drugs were so dangerous that he thought they constituted as great a risk as cancer. He refused to sign a consent form for the experimental program on July 11. He logically decided he needed a second opinion. "All I wanted was a second opinion. All I got was lies and deceit," he told me.

A spokesman for the hospital later told the media that although the hospital had arranged for a second opinion on Amanda's treatment with a doctor at another hospital, Children's was "reluctant" to let Accardi take Amanda from them because they doubted he would really seek out the second opinion. Accardi told me in an interview: "What second opinion? The other doctor was just a 'buddy' of the doctor to be in charge of Amanda's therapy."

When the hospital determined that the Accardis were not going to let Amanda be part of the chemotherapy program, it took legal steps to place the daughter technically under police custody pending a hearing on a restraining order filed in Superior Court against Michael after he became argumentative. And he had become argumentative when he learned about alternative methods of treatment.

"I knew the legal deck was stacked against me. I couldn't line up enough expert witnesses in that short time to be able to deal with what the hospital was saying," Michael Accardi recalls. So, in the early hours of July 16, when the hearing was to be held, Michael Accardi seized Amanda from her security guard-protected room, raced with her under his arm down four flights of stairs, kicked his way through an emergency exit, and even hid in the men's room of a nearby restaurant with the tiny girl as hospital personnel hunted for him in the general area. Then, by prearranged plan with Katherine, he drove with Amanda to Tijuana and admitted her to Dr. Ernesto Contreras's Del Mar Hospital.

Michael claimed that Amanda had already been treated with one chemotherapeutic agent against his permission and also said she underwent a spinal tap without his permission. The hospital denied the latter charge. But whatever happened or did not happen at the hospital, Accardi was convinced the hospital was asserting parental control over his child in order to subject her to a round of experimental therapy with poisonous drugs. "What I assumed was the ultimate parental responsibility," he said.

Almost from the first day under Contreras's program of mixed therapy, a regimen similar to that of Chad Green and involving low levels of chemotherapeutic agents along with laetrile, vitamins, enzymes, and dietary manipulation, Amanda started improving. Indeed, as had been noted by other proponents of mixed therapy, as long as amygdalin (laetrile) and the vitamin-enzymes-dietary approach were added, Amanda was able to undergo light chemotherapy without suffering side effects, a singular blessing in itself from "metabolic therapy."

Three weeks later, with Dr. Contreras himself exulting that "for the first time I'm really optimistic that Amanda will recover," Amanda was released from the hospital with her cancer in remission and plans to continue her on intermittent rounds of mixed therapy. Nobody talked of "cure." Because the Accardis were involved in legal snarls with Children's and the seizure of their daughter from the hospital, the young couple faced continued legal battles, but out of them came a court-ordered San Diego University Hospital assessment of what Dr. Contreras had earlier claimed—that Amanda's leukemia was in remission. A hospital spokesman described her as in "complete remission."

With childhood leukemia still a risky, tricky malady, nobody was predicting the final outcome. But the facts were that Amanda had done remarkably well under the mixed regimen and had been released in complete remission. The facts firmly showed what the judge had ruled earlier in the Hofbauer matter—that metabolic therapy has a place in cancer management, certainly a modest assessment of the controversy which should ordinarily not excite such impassioned debate. But as I intend to show, the orthodox medical establishment and its overlap of vested interests with the pharmaceutical industry and government bureaucracy, an alliance of interests I call "the Club," cannot allow even the *suggestion* of efficacy from "unapproved" methods—hence the cries of outrage in the Hofbauer, Green, and Accardi cases.

From a media standpoint, after it was determined that Amanda was doing well and was not going to die at the Contreras clinic, coverage of her plight quickly declined at the national level. (Regional media, truth to tell, *did* maintain interest in the case.) Many a cancer controversy-watcher by fall 1981 knew that Hofbauer and Green had died; almost none of them had heard that Amanda had survived.

Just prior to the Hofbauer and Green cases, "medical kidnappings" of child cancer patients had occurred in the matter of Nikki Decker of Florida, whose mother won a long, agonizing court battle to obtain the right of metabolic therapy for her leukemia-stricken four-year-old daughter, and of Kimberly Cox, a seven-year-old leukemia patient in Milwaukee.

In both these cases at least intermittent successes against the disease were attributed to the metabolic program, one hard enough to follow even when undisturbed by meddling orthodoxy. In the Florida case, Nikki's response to radiation and chemotherapy was that her appetite became so ravenous that she increased weight excessively while losing her hair.

When taken off the standard therapy, her overall health had shown a marked improvement. A county court had intervened to allow her to choose the nutritional/metabolic approach even as attorneys for the state argued that radiation and chemotherapy constituted the only "recognized" treatment for the disease.

In the Cox case, the seven-year-old Wisconsin girl had literally been held a prisoner in a Milwaukee hospital after she was removed from the custody of her parents, who had refused to let her undergo chemotherapy and radiation treatment. The family eventually fled their home state and won the right to provide their daughter with a metabolic/nutritional program.

In several "kidnapping" cases, the young patients on metabolic therapy showed only temporary responses, although they were usually dramatic. Their cancer histories were up-and-down struggles with orthodoxy and unconventionality interspersed with the undefinable element of extreme stress—both on themselves and their parents.

In September 1977, the Michael Benoits of New York, who had carefully followed the Hofbauer saga, became involved in a three-state cancer odyssey of their own. They had earlier allowed their nine-year-old son, Marc Garippa, to undergo chemotherapy treatments at the Albany, New York, Medical Center, but from the outset were disturbed by the side effects of the administration of toxic drugs.

Reading about the pitched battle of the Hofbauers, the Benoits took Marc and fled to Florida, where their son responded well to two months of nutritional therapy. But they were hounded both by officials in the Sunshine State and New York—who, just as in the Hofbauer case, claimed jurisdiction, even though the family had moved out of New York.

Michael Benoit was surprised when, back in New York finishing his work and closing down his home, state authorities showed up and accused him of child abuse. An Albany Medical Center physician claimed Marc would be dead in two weeks if chemotherapy were not resumed, Benoit recalled.

A hearing on the issue was not held until three weeks later. When it finally took place, New York failed to prove that the Benoits intended to stay there, so they had to let Benoit go. Even so, the long arm of New York bureaucracy reached to Florida and the latter state's social services department was notified that the Benoits were there—"wanted" parents who had committed the "crime" of fleeing one state to another to seek an alternative form of cancer therapy for their child.

So they fled again—this time to Arizona, where they had friends. Marc was put back on the nutritional program. His new doctor wrote to the original Albany physician seeking Marc's medical records. Instead of the records, the doctor received a visit from the Arizona Social Welfare Department, one of whose representatives flatly told the Benoits that she did not need a warrant—at least until forty-eight hours after she had seized their son on grounds of parental child abuse.

But at Good Samaritan Hospital in Phoenix, where Marc was taken, the Benoits were happy to discover a sympathetic physician in the person of Dr. Jesse Cohen, a hematologist. The hospital allowed them to continue Marc's administration of herbs, protein-digesting enzymes, natural vitamins, fresh vegetables, and coffee enemas.

Dr. Cohen found that chemotherapy would not ultimately be of any help to Marc. It was this professional's honest assessment that later helped Arizona Superior Court Judge Edward Rapp rule that the Benoits had the right to select the treatment of their choice for Marc.

But even this did not deter New York authorities. They denounced Dr. Cohen and promised further action against the Benoits, who went into seclusion. The father of Marc Garippa attributed his son's death in February 1979 to aspiration problems—not leukemia.

Testimonials To Alternative Therapy

In the raging battle between entrenched medicine and alternative therapy, propagandists for the Establishment side could point to the "losses" of metabolic or nutritional therapy—prominently, the McQueen, Green, and Hofbauer cases—as evidence that "unproven" remedies do not work.

Yet, while the deaths of such individuals made headlines across the country, with most of the media conveniently forgetting how the victims had all beaten the odds by big margins, the track record of orthodox treatments was far grimmer. For every McQueen, there was a chemotherapeutically deceased Hubert Humphrey; for every Chad Green, a dozen John Waynes; for every Joey Hofbauer, a score of Shahs of Iran. By any meaningful, visible, palpable understanding of cancer carnage, seekers of alternative therapies are clearly living longer and feeling better than those who undergo the route of surgery, chemotherapy, and radiation.

As a caveat here, let me point out that I am not arguing that because something is unorthodox it is automatically "good." Charlatanry and quackery *do* exist. The reality is simply that orthodoxy, up to now, has in the main worsened rather than improved the cancer picture—to the extent that, in a majority of cases, the refusal of *any* treatment might actually increase the odds of survival, compared to the use of standard cancer therapies.

While the McQueen case brought a brushfire of world-wide attention to the whole panoply of unorthodox therapies, and McQueen's death added we-told-you-so ammunition to the Establishment's arsenal, McQueen was not the only public figure who opted for another way.

Alycia Buttons, the wife of comedian Red Buttons, underwent an amygdalin-centered metabolic program for throat cancer under Dr. Hans Nieper in West Germany in the early 1970s. Red Buttons testified throughout the decade as to the apparent success of the program for his wife. Using the five-year survival rate as "cured"— which metabolic/nutritional therapists generally don't—Mrs. Buttons could be considered "cured."

Actor Fred McMurray has also attributed the Nieper treatment, involving "laetrile as a backup" and a metabolic diet, as well as radiation, for his recovery from throat cancer. As of 1981, his doctors told the actor the he was cancer-free.

Glen Rutherford, the Kansas salesman for whom the precedent-setting 1974 U.S. District Court case allowing "legal" laetrile into the country is named, by 1982 had more than ten years of full recovery from intestinal cancer. He has been a "star" patient at the Contreras clinic.

Orthodoxy has tried to claim that the electrical excision of Rutherford's tumor means that the Kansan's cancer was "cured" then and there. However, it brushes aside the clinical evidence that the primary tumor had shrunk drastically under amygdalin-centered therapy *before* the excision was attempted. Glen Rutherford's increased stamina and freedom from cancer since 1971 must be due to *something*—although orthodoxy won't hazard a guess as to what.

In the Philippines, Mrs. Carmen Gutierrez in 1982 had a "record" twenty years of survival under amygdalin-centered metabolic therapy, under the care of Dr. Manuel D. Navarro, M.D., Asia's primary vitamin B[17] pioneer.

Mrs. Gutierrez's case is particularly interesting in that her long, agonizing battle with metastasized breast cancer, first diagnosed in 1958, and her failure to respond to the entire range of orthodox treatment—surgery, radiation, and chemotherapy—before turning to Dr. Navarro made her one of the "special cases" selected for followup in 1961 by the Philippine Cancer Society. She was the only such case on metabolic/nutritional therapy. As of 1982, Mrs. Gutierrez remained free of all signs of cancer. All other patients in the original PCS survey were dead.

The Rev. Clifford Oden, a Texas minister, has been so exuberant about the change of health and life style wrought by metabolic/nutritional therapy in his own laetrile-treated case of colon cancer that he wrote a book about it called *Thank God I Have Cancer,* (New York, Arlington House: 1976).

Rev. Oden was diagnosed with adenocarcinoma in 1969. Routine surgery was performed, but then pathologists reported that the tumor had invaded the intestinal wall. Seven of the "experts" called in to study the case recommended a colostomy. Instead, he opted for the laetrile program. By 1982, he had been around to brag about the results for twelve years.

Under the closed-thought system of Establishment medicine, no amount of "anecdotes" are allowed to interfere with the officially sanctioned double-think of the day. Amygdalin, vitamins, minerals, enzymes, live-cell therapy, *etc., etc.,* are just too bizarre to work. Therefore, they *don't!*

But, aside from "name" cases like McQueen, it has not primarily been the evidence of survivors that has brought the matter of alternative therapy in cancer into the spotlight. It is the plight of caring parents and sick children, caught in the throes of the law, which has done so.

More than anything else, the battles of parents for the right to have their children treated as they saw fit helped bring home a concept that was already spreading with incredible velocity across the United States in the mid-1970s—the battle for freedom of choice in medicine. Involved was a complicated fusion of dissident scientific and political reformation that surfaced over the unlikely fight for the legalization of the apricot kernel derivative amygdalin or laetrile (vitamin B[17]). Not only has laetrile itself shaken the very foundations of Western science, but the political storm it touched off over the far broader issue of freedom of choice in medicine is bringing a political revolt to the fore. Indeed, in modern times nothing has compared, politically, with the success of the movement to legalize—or, more correctly, to decriminalize—laetrile. In twenty-four months' time it became an issue that ultimately wound up, in one form or another, before three dozen state legislatures, and to the outraged chagrin of the nation's bureaucratic-medical-pharmaceutical Establishment, it had been successful in twenty-four states by 1982. That is a record no other movement, from the Liberty Amendment to the ERA, has been able to match.

Chapter Two
The Battle For Freedom of Choice

**The Lowly Apricot Kernel
Inspires A Revolutionary Movement**

It is certain that the combination of forces I call the bureaucratic-medical-pharmaceutical Establishment—or "Club"—did not know what they were getting into the summer of 1972, when the State of California and the Alameda County District Attorney's office arrested an Albany, California, physician on charges of quackery for using laetrile in cancer therapy. After all, "unproven remedies" and "quack cancer cures" had been around before, had been vigorously harassed, and had been essentially suppressed. It took me, a newspaperman at the time, a long while to learn that just because the American Cancer Society, the American Medical Association, the Food and Drug Administration, and local medical boards list something as "unproven" doesn't necessarily mean it's also "quack."

There is a long and twisted history of the suppression of unwanted cancer treatments in this country, as I detail elsewhere, but up until 1972 the *modus operandi* of their removal from the scene had not varied: go after the credentials and/or licenses of the offending physician or scientist, drag him through as many court cases as possible, pillory him in the press, break him financially and in spirit, and then go home victorious.

These tactics had worked for several other unwanted, unproven remedies in the past, and there was no reason to expect they would not work again. The American Cancer Society continued to be the national propaganda front for orthodox cancer treatment, the Food and Drug Administration continued to be the policing arm for the complex of interests with a stake in contining the status quo, and the American Medical Association continued to be the Mosaic arbiter of all things medical, its pronouncements accepted as Gospel fact, the "learned journals" whose editorial boards it controlled or influenced serving as willing conduits.

But the arrest of John A. Richardson, M.D. changed everything.

In laetrile's up-and-down history, several physicians who had used the compound in the 1950s and 1960s had run afoul either of the law or of the pressure of medical orthodoxy. Interest in the substance (see my *Vitamin B^{17}: Forbidden Weapon Against Cancer,* New York: Arlington House, 1974, *Freedom from Cancer,* Atlanta: '76 Press, 1976, and New York: Pocket Books, 1977, for the amazing background history of the development and use of laetrile) was being maintained by only a handful of doctors in this country, a clinic in Mexico, a few scientific papers published outside the country and limited research and use in the Philippines, Japan, Italy, and West Germany. Laetrile had become "taboo," and the vast majority of physicians kept arm's length from anything which appeared on the ACS unapproved remedies list or which might interfere with their licensing or hospital privileges.

But unlike some, Dr. Richardson was a physician with no particular fear of licensing boards or legal loopholes. He fought back. An *ad hoc* group of Californians, mostly in the San Fransico Bay Area, set up a support group for Dr. Richardson, not because of any particular obsession with laetrile but because they saw a major political issue in the plight of the respected physician. They called themselves the Committee for Freedom of Choice in Cancer Therapy, Inc.

I did not join this movement as a journalist until 1975, and by then it had grown faster than a cancer metastasis. At its high point, in the mid-1970s, the national organization claimed 40,000 members in 500 chapters in this and several other countries. More than any other like-minded group, it eventually made laetrile a household word, and was usually described as the reason for its sweeping political success across the country.

From the beginning, the fight, first to defend Dr. Richardson's right to prescribe an unapproved substance and then to defend the rights of other physicians around the country, garnered support from a broad range of Americans, all of them alienated from, or by, the medical Establishment, either because that Establishment was well on the way to losing the vaunted "war on cancer" or because it had bruised these people one way or another.

Several tendencies were developing all at once, some from seeds planted in the 1960s, and they converged in the highly unlikely symbol of the apricot kernel. "Back-to-nature" young people, the disenchanted outcasts of the Vietnam War era, were incorporating self-diagnosis and unorthodox Eastern medical practices as part of their war with established conventions. A number of physicians and scientists were already well into aspects of preventive medicine and arguing that the future of medicine should be weighted toward prevention rather than treatment. Many of these mavericks had already grouped themselves into a number of organizations defending and using unapproved remedies that had already achieved therapeutic track records in other countries. Veteran health-oriented consumer groups, which had long fought for the validity of vitamins in disease prevention and treatment and espoused nontoxic therapies for degenerative disease, had already become anti-Establishment by having long been the object of the ire of the AMA and the interlock of forces foisting fluoridation upon the American people. And some physicians, orthodox in outlook but open of mind, were reaching out in desperation to the unorthodox because the orthodox ways were so obviously losing the war against degenerative diseases, particularly heart disease and cancer.

But it took the arrest of physicians for the use of laetrile, and the page-one plight of the criminalizing of desperate cancer patients, to bring matters to a head. This would not have been possible, I am sure, if what eventually developed out of all this—the interlinking of concepts of preventive medicine, nontoxic treatments, and holistic, or metabolic/nutritional therapy—had not rapidly developed a record of achievement in dealing with civilization's killer diseases.

Before the politicization of laetrile, the Establishment kept the unorthodox forces neutralized and isolated. They seldom made common cause, and because they usually did not deal directly with death-dealing *cancer,* long recognized as a word which conjures up the parallel term *death* in the minds of everybody, they had less of a sense of urgency, less need to organize, to become political.

Other promising unapproved cancer remedies—for example, Glyoxylide, Krebiozen, the Hoxsey herbal preparations—had briefly blossomed, then been to a large extent ground out of official existence because they had not become political issues. Laetrile was headed for the same bone yard. But it took a dramatic turn in 1972 when the Committee for Freedom of Choice in Cancer Therapy made freedom of choice a central issue. While the National Health Federation was winning its long fight to get the government out of the vitamin-control business, the committee launched efforts *not* so much to legalize laetrile (which, as a natural substance—or vitamin—should *itself* not need legalizing) but to protect the right of the physician and patient, *with the informed consent of both,* to have access to an alternative form of therapy. The concept was just that simple. And it took.

Neither flunked mouse tests, nor arguments about placebos, "false hope" and undercredentialed proponents, nor *New York Times* hatchet jobs on the major proponents of laetrile, nor a recitation of the number of John Birch Society members within the leadership of the movement, nor a recounting of the adventures and misadventures of Andrew McNaughton, a long-time laetrile backer, could keep people away from laetrile once the cat was out of the bag. And the cat was that laetrile or amygdalin *works*. That is, and given the degree of its use, *how* it is used, the degree and nature of a patients' prior treatment, and the degree and extent of damage from cancer, at the very least amygdalin *clearly* brings about both "objective" relief in terms understandable to American medical orthodoxy and widescale "subjective" relief. Not offered as a cure but at most as a *control* for cancer, laetrile became one of the hottest taboo items since bootleg booze in the 1920s and marijuana in the 1970s.

In what seemed to be the blind playing out of a Greek drama, all the characters performed their appointed roles. Proponents of laetrile, including physicians and patients, became martyrs to a cause and boldly pushed ahead; the police forces of the state ever bungled into more arrests, harassments, crackdowns, raids and the like, only inflaming onlookers who could hardly believe all this was going on; Establishment experts alternately treated laetrile with disdainful silence or haughty scorn, all in the hopes it would go away, or panicked into attention-getting and awkward overreactions.

True, the amygdalin movement did attract fly-by-night operators and an intermittently vast smuggling operation, or series of operations, all of them unfortunately necessary if Americans were to have access to the product form of vitamin B^{17} (a denomination opposed by officialdom, while generally admitting there was in fact no precise definition of the term *vitamin).* Although laetrile was statutorily illegal only in California, the federal Food and Drug Administration had treated the substance *as if it were* illegal since 1963, when the amendments to the Food, Drug and Cosmetic Act went into effect. Indeed, as the lengthy 1977 federal trial against four of sixteen defendants in "the international laetrile smuggling ring" in San Diego determined, the FDA had been banning interstate shipments of laetrile on the basis of informally written memoranda for fifteen years.

Were it not for notable success of laetrile-using patients, particularly those involved in a total metabolic program, laetrile could still not have achieved the successes it ultimately did. By the 1970s there were patients who had been surviving on laetrile for a decade or more. In Tijuana, Mexico, the Del Mar Clinic and, later, the Cydel Clinic, were amassing case histories by the thousands, and still more thousands were being assembled by such physicians as Drs. Richardson, E. Paul Wedel of Oregon, James Privitera and Stewart Jones of California, Philip Binzel, Jr., of Ohio, Helen Calvin of Indiana, and urologist Larry McDonald of Georgia, who went on to become a U.S. congressman.

From obscure medical beginnings in the 1950s, the use of laetrile in the hands of qualified physicians jumped dramatically. By 1978 the Committee for Freedom of Choice in Cancer Therapy could claim a medical mailing list of 5,000 doctors and medical personnel, including several hundred M.D.'s who were using amygdalin by itself, as part of a total metabolic program, or as adjunctive therapy to standard treatments. A whole new science—metabolic/nutritional therapy—was growing up to deal with cancer and the whole range of degenerative diseases and making common cause with the even broader field of holistic medicine, which brought mind-spirit ramifications to bear on the overall program.

If there were not surviving laetrile patients, admittedly only a handful, backed by many thousands more who had achieved temporary, positive benefits from the program, and many more still who had at least experienced pain relief or more subjective benefits, I am convinced laetrile would by now have gone the way of the dodo bird. American medical orthodoxy, in the main, just could not and would not believe what it was seeing—a medical revolution in the making.

Striking on all fronts, the Committee for Freedom of Choice in Cancer Therapy, sometimes alone, sometimes working with the original pro-laetrile group, IACVF (the International Association of Cancer Victims and Friends, originally organized as a support group primarily for Mexcio-bound cancer patients), the Cancer Control Society, the National Health Federation, and other organizations, took the battle for freedom of choice on the stump. There were mass rallies in state after state that resembled, sure enough, travelling medicine shows.

Public awareness and organizing the defense of physicians in the toils of the law was only half the original campaign. The other was to help train physicians in the burgeoning movement of metabolic therapy, one drawing on the "orthomolecular" champions of megavitamins, the more vintage health-food proponents, the maverick preventive medicine advocates, and specialists in one or more "unproven" or accepted therapies available in other countries but frowned upon here, most noticeably chelation therapy for heart disease.

At the political level, the results were stupendous. Beginning with Alaska in 1975, Freedom of Choice chapters banded together to draft, beat the drums for, and ultimately pass laws *not* legalizing laetrile *per se,* but protecting physicans from official punishment should they dispense it or allow its use in their clinics. Alaska achieved this first "decriminalization," in the face of warnings from the FDA and the Cancer Society, in 1976. For a time, the Establishment regarded Alaska as some kind of fluke, while the FDA stepped up its campaign of harassment, seizure and surveillance on a scale unmatched in modern history for a nontoxic substance.

In 1977, Indiana, whose forces were also organized and led by local Freedom of Choice chapters, fell. Amygdalin proponents sang songs in the visitors' gallery and stayed until the last minute of the legislative session was ticked off to make sure the Indiana vote for freedom of choice was approved over the veto of the state's governor, who had knuckled under to the furor of anti-laetrile propaganda unleashed by the Establishment. And then came Florida. And Texas. And Nevada. And the battle was on in earnest.

Caught with their bridges blown and airplanes on the field, Establishment forces in 1977 awakened to the reality that they were dealing with a phenomenon far more vast than a squabble over a "quack cancer cure." For the first time, the massed forces of medical and bureaucratic orthodoxy and elitism were not only being opposed, they were being *successfully* opposed by an unlikely coalition of common people held together both by the reality of cancer in their families and their distrust of—and, at times, rage against—an Establishment forcing Americans either into the underground for a taboo cancer treatment, or to foreign lands to procure it, or simply left to die by "approved" methods.

Intimately familiar with—and a vital part of—this state-by-state campaign, I saw the same scenarios unreel in one statehouse after another: for the Establishment, the well-dressed and usually mild-mannered, almost *blasé* academicians of the state or local AMA board, the regional ACS representative, and a bevy of experts flown in by the FDA. Whether the federal level was directly represented and how many "experts" were present usually depended on just how important the established forces perceived the state in question to be. But all of these gentlemen, and occasionally ladies, repeated the now hoary and usually incorrect claims about laetrile. Their central argument was that the material *itself* was not dangerous, but the fact it might keep patients away from an approved remedy made it a social peril. This argument simply did not wash with the businessmen, farmers, lawyers, housewives, and shopkeepers who traditionally make up local legislatures. In most states where laetrile bills were actually allowed to get to a full floor debate, they passed hands down and by whopping majorities.

For laetrile, one or more spokesmen of the proponent organizations and scores, even hundreds, of cancer patients, either with direct experience of laetrile or in a seething rage over what was being done to them by what I came to style the "cut-burn-and-poison" school of orthodox cancer therapy. It was these cancer patients, brought in by the busload—as in Florida and Kansas—or simply jamming the hearing chambers—as in Wisconsin, Alabama, and so many other states—who made the difference. The loss of such key states as Texas and Florida traumatized the Establishment. It updated its attack on laetrile with new assaults on the credentials of the proponents, and unearthed more laboratory experiments in which laetrile had ostensibly failed to shrink tumors (a point of only secondary interest to metabolic therapists, who argue that vitamin B^{17} is a vitamin to nourish the body, not a drug to shrink a tumor, and that tumors are only symptoms, not the disease itself—which they see as chronic, systemic and metabolic in nature). Then, as we shall see, the Establishment gambled most heavily—and desperately—on "toxicity."

It is no coincidence that the "laetrile smuggling ring" trial was the lengthiest federal trial in the history of that particular San Diego jurisdiction, or that federal and state agencies went to extraordinary lengths to put the distributors of "bitter food tablets" and the laetrile-containing food products Aprikern and Bee Seventeen out of business, or that they confiscated apricot kernels by the ton in Florida and Tennessee, and involved apricot-kernel-selling health food stores in litigation in many states. But each new thrust and parry in the laetrile war only heightened public awareness about what was going on and turned laetrile into a widely recognized term.

Common, everyday people simply did not *believe* that the corner was about to be turned in the "war on cancer"—a conflict fraught with semantics redolent of the recent military disaster in Southeast Asia. They were unimpressed by multiple doctorates, silk suits, polysyllabic—and evasive—pontifications about consumer protection, and recitations of mouse-test failures. All they were interested in, I learned in state after state, were the answers to two questions: "Will laetrile hurt me?" and "If not, why can't I have it?"

The court victories won by partisans of freedom of choice also flushed the moral bankruptcy of the opposition into the open, and once again proved that the American Republic, however tattered, is still well-served by a court system underpinned by a Constitution whose framers were awesomely sensitive to individual rights and deeply distrustful of government. When a U.S. district court in Oklahoma City ruled in favor of surviving cancer patient Glen Rutherford of Kansas in 1975, a whole new area of attack was opened up. The Rutherford decision was widened to a class action involving all "terminal" cancer patients. By 1978 a series of court skirmishes, in which the proponents of laetrile, dwelling on the freedom of choice issue far more than the efficacy of amygdalin, beat back the entire federal legal establishment, and opened the door for legal importation of amygdalin for cancer patients.

As state-by-state decriminalization of amygdalin continued and the U.S. District Court-approved affidavit process for legally importing foreign amygdalin prospered, the substance headed for Supreme Court hearings. The fact that laetrile ultimately wound up before the high court not once but twice was another historic first— something the critics within the Establishment would later call "the political success of a scientific failure."

The published accounts of desperate, dying cancer patients attempting to secure their laetrile through court order, and the delays and heartache this involved, ever brought the questions of laetrile and freedom of choice to the fore. The accounts of frustration, then temporary elation, then heartbreak became legion.

As a particularly illustrative case in point, ponder the plight of Mrs. Sydelle Woronoff's fight against cancer. Similar cases were to be reported by the hundreds as the laetrile revolution swept across America, but I select hers as synoptic of what was happening, and also because it did so much to decriminalize vitamin B^{17} in New Jersey. Mrs. Woronoff was diagnosed with widespread cancer in April of 1977. When she underwent an exploratory operation, a temporary colostomy was performed and she was placed on the hormone Prednisone for three weeks. In May her spleen was removed and a biopsy taken of her liver. It proved to be malignant.

Not until 5 July was another exploratory operation performed. Mrs. Woronoff's attending surgeon reported that her small intestine was "seeded" with cancer, and the eighty-year-old woman was declared "terminal." The surgeon said that chemotherapy would be the only hope, an outside hope, but it could not be used unless the intestine began to heal.

Mrs. Woronoff was confined to bed in a New Jersey hospital in severe pain and was usually comatose. Demerol and morphine were routinely given, as was a hyperalimentated solution of intravenous glucose, since she could no longer eat. Hospital officials were frankly simply waiting for her to die—the usual scenario in cancer wards.

But then an interesting turn of events occurred. Mrs. Woronoff's daughter, Mimi Alperin, and her husband Irving were flying from their home in Atlanta, Georgia, to New Jersey to visit the dying patient. Before they boarded the plane, they chanced on a paperback copy of *Laetrile Case Histories,* a popular book detailing the clinical experience of the embattled Dr. John Richardson in California. (By this time, the state had stripped Dr. Richardson of his license, but his Richardson Center, staffed by three M.D.'s and ample backup personnel was still expanding its clientele.) The Alperins found they could not put the book down. While the medical establishment has bitterly pooh-poohed the Richardson cases as incomplete, unillustrative, and occasionally unsubstantiated, the book remains a treasure trove of case histories of terminal patients responding in one or more ways to laetrile, particularly when given as part of a metabolic therapy program.

The Alperins immediately contacted the office of Georgia Congressman Larry McDonald, a supporter of laetrile and freedom of choice and a legislative consultant to the Committee for Freedom of Choice in Cancer Therapy. His office in turn referred them to Greg Kaye, the state chairman of the Committees for Freedom of Choice in New Jersey and a prime mover in the fight to decriminalize vitamin B^{17} in that state.

On Friday, 8 July, the Alperins met with Kaye, who quickly warned them that, despite what the opposition was saying about the proponents' claims for laetrile, the substance was not a "miracle cure" and that a terminal patient should not expect a miraculous recovery. If, in the Woronoff case, it only provided surcease from pain and the chance for the woman to die with dignity, it would have proved itself. The Alperins agreed.

Kaye asked if Mrs. Woronoff's personal physician was willing to administer the injections. Mrs. Alperin explained that the doctor "never used laetrile, did not believe it is effective in cancer therapy, but is willing to administer it simply because nothing else can be done." That is to say, the physician, unlike many, was willing to live up to his Hippocratic Oath despite what local medical boards and the federal government might say. And the first commandment of that oath is "Do no harm."

At the time, there was a laetrile drought on the East Coast, one of those intermittent tragedies brought about by government interference both with shipments available through court order and the still-flourishing underground network of the material. It usually came from Mexico, which by that time was producing both vials and tablets from two laboratories, both legally—if just barely—operating under Mexican government guidelines. Irvin Alperin decided that the only way to get a supply was to fly to Mexico and pick it up.

He flew to Tijuana on Sunday, 10 July, leaving Mimi behind for a bedside vigil with her mother, whose death appeared imminent. The next day, armed with a court-ordered affidavit, Irving crossed the border from Tijuana to San Ysidro, California, bringing 100 three-gram vials of laetrile with him, a right that had been won by the lengthy *Rutherford et al.* vs. *U.S.* case in the Oklahoma district court.

Upon declaring his merchandise, as Alperin later told Kaye, he was incensed to hear a customs official exclaim in glee, "We've got another one." Alperin was taken aside, his affidavit examined, and he was forced to pay a five-percent duty on the material. A year before, even this would have been impossible. As late as 1977 the great majority of cancer patients were still being forced to smuggle in their own life-sustaining materials from Mexico in scene after scene of agony and frustration. Some, of course, went through the extreme despair of having spent their last few hundred dollars grasping at straws only to see customs officials confiscate their precious goods from them at the border.

But now, Alperin's laetrile was suddenly "legal." He had been forced, by government edict, *not* law, to purchase a roundtrip airplane ticket and undergo additional expenses to visit a foreign country to pick up apricot kernel extract in order to provide some relief, if perhaps only psychological, for a cancer patient on whom medical orthodoxy had already given up. This was exactly the situation of literally thousands of cancer patients at the time.

Back in New Jersey, it was determined that, since Mrs. Woronoff was comatose and unable to ingest food, the only way to bolster the amygdalin injections with a partial metabolic program was to enrich the glucose solution with ten grams of vitamin C and other vitamin supplements. If she improved enough to swallow, other supplements could then be taken orally.

On Tuesday, 12 July, with Mrs. Woronoff, still comatose and in severe pain, her personal physician administered the first twelve-gram injection of laetrile, and the vitamin-enriched glucose solution was hooked to her arm. Early on Friday, 15 July, Mimi Alperin excitedly called Kaye. She said that, rather than expiring as her doctors expected, Mrs. Woronoff not only was suddenly free of pain, but that she had experienced passage through her colostomy for the first time, was talking coherently, had been able to walk to the bathroom, and was hungry. She had taken her first meal of chicken broth and had even asked her daughter to bring sheet music to the hospital since she was thinking in terms of being released and beginning a career in show business as a vocalist and musician. Needless to say, Mrs. Alperin was ecstatic.

The joy did not last long, as Kaye later recounted it in *The Choice*. That same afternoon she called back, this time in tears. The hospital bureaucracy had found out that her personal physician had committed the mortal sin of administering an "unproven remedy" to his patient on the sacrosanct grounds of the hospital. The medical staff president threatened suspension of and sanctions against the physician if he did not cease and desist at once. When the Alperins tried to intervene on his behalf, they were called "smugglers" by hospital spokesmen.

By Saturday, 16 July, the attending physician was faced with a tough decision. He and his nurses had witnessed tremendous improvement in Mrs. Woronoff since the injections began. Should he be true to his Hippocratic Oath or yield to the hospital bureaucracy? He courageously chose the former course.

After the fifth injection of laetrile was administered, a nurse informed on him. He was immediately suspended from the staff and banned from the hospital.

The individual involved was hardly an upstart. He had been on the hospital staff for twenty-six years, was chairman of the hospital's "formulary committee," was chairman of the county board of drug abuse services, held several teaching positons in the hospital, and was a former president of his local medical society. This is to say, he was an impeccably credentialed Establishment physician. Now his career was in jeopardy because he had bucked that very Establishment.

Luckily, hearings had already begun on the New Jersey freedom of choice bill, one of many such sessions being held in statehouses across the country. As usual, representatives of the bureaucratic-medical-pharmaceutical Establishment, many of them appearing at taxpayer expense, had been brought in to render hours of testimony about the perils of amygdalin, the profiteers in the Laetrile underground, the quack nature of the substance, and so on. But, also as usual, amygdalin users, surviving patients, and relatives and friends of surviving patients—the "little people"—were on hand to tell the other side. Mimi Alperin was there, too, tearfully telling about the plight of her mother.

Happily, the media jumped onto the story with a vengeance. By this time, the nation's major newspapers and wire services were being fairly objective in dealing with laetrile, following a quarter-century of noninvestigative reporting and the customary printing and airing of handouts from the FDA, American Cancer Society and AMA. The human interest angle of hundreds of cancer patients showing up at state legislative hearings across the country was simply too much for honest journalists. They saw, as I had been fortunate to see several years before when the laetrile story broke in the San Francisco Bay area, that there was "something to laetrile."

Wire services carried an account of the Woronoff case and the situation of the attending physician. To escape media and public resentment and possibly to avoid law suits, the hospital in question quickly reinstated the banned physician, but he still faced disciplinary action. His reinstatement carried the caveat that he should never again administer an unproven remedy within the hallowed halls of the hospital.

By this time, Mrs. Woronoff had gone four days without her amygdalin and other vitamins. She was in terrible pain again and back on Demerol and other analgesics, all of which failed as they had in the past. The Alperins now went to the courts out of desperation.

On 22 July they appeared before Superior Court Judge Thomas Yaccarino of the Chancery Division, Monmouth County Court, and sought a restraining and show-cause order against the hospital involved. Judge Yaccarino wasted little time in granting it. The order immediately allowed any licensed physician in the state of New Jersey to administer laetrile to Mrs. Woronoff in the defendant's hospital, without penalty, punishment or disciplinary action. The hospital was ordered to show cause why it had acted as it had. The decision, instantly opposed by the FDA, the American Cancer Society, and hospital lawyers, was a landmark for freedom of choice, one of dozens throughout the country.

But although the freedom of choice movement gained, the patient ultimately lost, as was often the case. For Mrs. Woronoff had been deprived of her metabolic therapy for ten days. She died one day before the hospital was supposed to show cause for its actions. Official reason: death from intestinal cancer. Suspected reason: heart failure.

Mrs. Woronoff did not die in vain. Many thousands of New Jersey citizens were incensed over the tableau: bureaucracy and orthodoxy barring a dying cancer patient from something, whether it worked or not. In this case, the reality had been a dramatic, if transient, effect. How *could* anyone deny such help? Months later,

New Jersey became the fourteenth state to decriminalize the use of laetrile. What carried the day was not so much the efficacy of laetrile, but rather the freedom of choice of physican and patient to have *access* to it, particularly when the patient was already "terminal."

In July 1977, as the furor over state freedom of choice bills unavoidably hit the media practically everywhere, the Lou Harris Poll surveyed 1,600 Americans on laetrile-connected issues and came up with these findings:

• Americans opposed the FDA ban on interstate shipment and sale of laetrile by 53 percent to 23 percent.

• They supported their own state legislatures' legalization of laetrile by 68 percent to 13 percent.

• Some 73 percent of college-educated Americans—versus 54 percent of non-college-educated Americans—shared the view that laetrile should be permitted. (Harris found this a "significant finding," inasmuch as the Establishment pitch was that proponents of laetrile and unorthodox therapies were the uneducated gullible.)

After being exposed to all the arguments for and against laetrile, people—by 5 to 1—"would like to see the drug legalized in their own states, even if the FDA continues its ban nationally," pollster Harris assessed. He added:

> The key to the public's attitude on Laetrile can be found in the fact that nearly 8 out of 10 persons agree that "since we don't know how to cure cancer, if Laetrile is harmless, people ought to be able to buy it if they want to use it."
>
> Reinforcing this view are public doubts about the FDA and other government health agencies. These doubts were triggered by what the public feels was poor handling of the swine-flu vaccine program and the lack of a satisfactory explanation of the deaths of American Legion members following their convention in Philadelphia last year.

In spring 1978, the Roper Poll came up with similar findings. Fifty-eight percent of adult Americans believed the sale of laetrile should be legalized, according to Roper's survey of 2,000 Americans. Wrote Burns Roper, "Not only do a majority of all Americans favor the legalization of Laetrile, but every one of the forty subgroups we have analyzed separately has more people in favor of its legalization than opposed." He added that only subgroups thought of as being composed of the "comparatively ignorant and gullible" turned in less than absolute majorities in favor of legal laetrile.

Clearly, despite multi-million-dollar efforts by the FDA and the American Cancer Society, which admitted in 1977 that one of its primary propaganda objectives was opposition to the laetrile movement, Americans were balking. The FDA put up "Laetrile Warning" posters in every post office and federal medical and pharmaceutical facility in the country. In many cases, proponents responded by tacking up over them "FDA Warning" posters of exactly the same size, paper texture, color, and type as the government originals.

In state after state, as in a special two-day hearing of the FDA in Kansas City, Missouri (brought about by the Oklahoma district court's order to the FDA to develop an "administrative record" to explain its decade-and-a-half ban on laetrile), proponents of the government side and established medicine were booed down and jeered as they issued the standard arguments against laetrile specifically, and unproven remedies in general. Americans simply were not buying the standard line.

For the first time in modern American medical history, that combination of vested interests and undergirding ideology that I call the Club began to show signs of schism when faced not only by the lowly apricot kernel but by legions of its champions and an even greater multitude of Americans ever more suspicious of government pronouncements in general.

Always before, in-house discipline and the iron curtain of disdainful silence had been the Establishment's way out of unpleasant realities, as it suppressed substances and medicines developed outside the pale of "Mother Church"—which, in this instance, could be perceived as the theory and practice of allopathic (conventional) medicine bolstered by the international drug cartel, invested with state power by the FDA and officially and professionally sanctioned by the AMA, with the food processing industry lurking close by. The hoary tactics of neutralization, isolation and elimination had not worked against laetrile. Clearly, the Establishment side, with billions of dollars at stake, was losing.

I write "billions of dollars at stake" advisedly. By 1982, the combined national health bill, usually referred to euphemistically as the bill for "health-care delivery," was in excess of $300 billion a year, even though the total costs in terms of lost man-hours and hidden expenses are always hard to pin down. With medical costs skyrocketing much faster than inflation, and with $300-a-day hospital beds commonplace, the prospects are the nation's health tab will approach $350 billion in 1983. And when it is seen that a good 80 percent of this figure is a consequence of degenerative disease—*not* bone-settings, whooping cough, TB, general infections, and parasites—the scope and nature of what is at stake become clear.

The *prevention* of degenerative disease, as advocated for years by the health food industry, naturopaths, and assorted medical mavericks, is an outright threat to the need for *treatment* of these ills. The backup pharmaceutical industry which grows fat off the production of the toxic drugs involved in treatment, and a rapidly growing industry of electronic software and hardware switched from warfare to health, have invested billions of dollars gambling on the *poor health* of the nation. The drug company "detail man" is actually the chief professor in the physician's postgraduate training—not because the physician is a venal dolt, but because he cannot possibly keep up with all the "advances" in medicine. He is inundated monthly by new drug preparations, and must rely on the integrity and honesty of the drug companies, and of the FDA which supposedly monitors them. As we shall see in the next chapter, this may be a vain reliance indeed.

I also write "Club" advisedly, since it is not my contention, nor is it the contention of most people who have labored in the freedom of choice movement, that most physicians, most bureaucrats, and most drug developers are dishonest. Not at all. But history has decisively shown that when giant vested interests get together, they alter and color the flow of information to those on the firing line, and eventually become the controllers and educators of those firing-line soldiers, who in this case are physicians. If allopathic medicine, the drug cartel, and their interlock with government agencies and powerful pressure groups like the ACS wish to say white is black, it is not the fault of the workaday physician if he believes it, particularly when he reads it over and over again in "learned journals" endorsed by the AMA.

So, by 1977 the Club had to do something. It had to defend its earlier positions and yet open the door a crack toward tolerance and the capacity to articulate, however slowly, awkwardly, and woefully, that most feared of all human admissions, "Perhaps I was wrong."

Already such a bastion of Establishment thought as the *New York Times* had editoralized gently in favor of freedom of choice, while remaining schizophrenic in its overall coverage of laetrile. It had allowed an outrageous yellow-jouranlism-style attack on the proponents of laetrile while ignoring, for months, the scandalous story of the coverup of positive laetrile results at the nearby Sloan-Kettering cancer complex.

But then came the very Establishment and medically respectable *New England Journal of Medicine (NEJM)*, practically a Sunday School workbook to accompany the Holy Writ of Mother Church as enshrined in the *Journal of the American Medical Association*. NEJM editor Franz Ingelfinger, himself a cancer victim and heatedly anti-laetrile, editorialized in the 20 May 1977, issue:

> As a cancer patient myself, I would not take laetrile under any circumstances....If I were still in practice, I would not recommend it to my patients. Yet, perhaps there are some situations in which rational medical science should yield and make some concessions....If any patient had what I thought was hopelessly advanced cancer, and if he

asked for laetrile, I should like to be able to give the substance to him to assuage his mental anguish, just as I would give him morphine without stint to relieve his physical suffering.

Dr. Ingelfinger didn't back off one inch from his assertion that laetrile is "another one of those quack cures that sweep relentlessly through our volatile society," but he correctly saw that the medical Establishment was only increasing laetrile's popularity by continuing to denounce it, particularly without any meaningful human tests on the substance. He suggested "two years of trials" for amygdalin, if only to gather the documented evidence that would ultimately bury it as a failure.

His was the first major voice in an Establishment-aligned journal calling for what laetrile advocates had asked for for the better part of a quarter century—actual human trials of the substance, even though, as the metabolic therapy revolt gained speed in the 1970s, *not* as a drug to shrink a tumor but as a natural nutrient to shore up the body against cancer.

A number of other respected cancer researchers, including some at Sloan-Kettering who were honest enough to stick by their guns and admit at least a "shred of evidence" for laetrile had been seen in highly controversial mouse tests, adopted a similar stance.

Striking like a bolt of lightning was the call, also through the *NEJM,* this time in January 1978 by Dr. Charles Moertel of the Mayo Clinic, for a "controlled clinical trial"—that is, a human test—of the substance. Dr. Moertel's voice was particularly influential, not only because of his vocal opposition of laetrile.

After noting with considerable candor that "the simple fact is that laetrile has never been properly studied in the hands of those competent to make such a judgement," Dr. Moertel added that the accomplishments from relying on certain animal tumor systems for the development of chemotherapeutic agents of substantive value had been "less than spectacular." Hence, "it must be questioned whether we are justified in placing absolute and total reliance upon them for bringing forth all future cancer therapy, especially to the point of declaring any alternative approach unethical."

Then he assessed:

> Laetrile is clearly a major medical and social problem in this country. It can no longer be swept under the rug and ignored as just another quack medicine.
>
> ...Such legislative and judicial decisions (on its decriminalization) have been criticized as irrational responses to a vocal minority, but clearly this charge is not true. They have been rendered in

response to the will of the overwhelming majority of the American people....Past experience has demonstrated that our rhetoric of damnation and indignation is not effective and, indeed, can be counterproductive.

And, in an extremely careful use of semantics, Dr. Moertel widened the credibility door, just a crack, to that "perhaps I was wrong" possibility:

> Perhaps an even more compelling reason for clinical trial is the lingering doubt, which must be harbored by any scientific mind, that perhaps the overwhelming public acceptance of this therapy could reflect some element of therapeutic effectiveness. Certainly the results in our artificial and contrived animal-tumor-model systems are not proof positive against this possibility.

Just as the potent Moertel analysis was coming out, the National Cancer Institute, conduit of the federal funds for the badly botched war on cancer (see chapter five) made an electrifying announcement at its Bethesda, Maryland, headquarters. Breaking step with the Club, the NCI would undertake the gathering of 200 to 300 "laetrile case histories" from physicians and patients reporting some kind of benefit to see if there were any reason to design a human trial of the substance. The NCI went to great lengths to explain that the results of such a "retrospective analysis" could not be expected to prove or disprove laetrile efficacy, and could only serve as guidelines for a possible future trial. In addition, the NCI almost agonizingly reassured Americans that the records would be confidential, that they would not be turned over to the FDA for future prosecution, and that no litigation of any kind would result from the survey.

"Laetrilists" had to be shown. Antigovernment to the point of near paranoia, many individual proponents and most proponent organizations had developed an automatic fail-safe mechanism of disbelieving whatever the government had to say about laetrile. After all, the FDA's campaign of harassment and verbal venom was continuing unabated, as was the propaganda machinery of the ACS. While the anti-laetrile rhetoric of both the NCI and the AMA had significantly mellowed in the preceding twenty-four months, the continuing assaults by the FDA-ACS combine could hardly stir glimmerings of trust among proponents of laetrile.

However, both the Committee for Freedom of Choice in Cancer Therapy and I, as the spokesman for it at the time, had already established a record of not running away from a laetrile debate with the Establishment, even when we knew in advance that the deck was stacked. This tack had already proved effective in a propaganda kind of way during the 1977 hearings of Sen. Edward Kennedy's Senate Health Subcommittee, when laetrile proponents were called to testify at the last minute. I had urged that our spokesmen appear before Senator Kennedy, and I also urged collaboration of the committee with the NCI's "retrospective analysis."

In the Kennedy hearings, every effort had been made to orchestrate an anti-laetrile propaganda barrage in time to dominate that day's news. For two hours, the same panel of Club spokesmen representing the FDA, the ACS, the NCI, and cancer researchers were allowed to deliver a withering blast of anti-laetrile pronouncements, some of it based on outrageously doctored material. Then, California prosecutors were brought in to testify about the alleged profiteering by the "international laetrile smuggling ring," as ostensibly captained by former Stanford University engineer Robert W. Bradford, founder-president of the Committee for Freedom of Choice.

Two hours were to elapse before proponents got their "day in court." But in advance, by noon, the bulk of the Washington media already had enough grist for afternoon dailies and the six o'clock news. Luckily, however, some media representatives lingered to hear the other side, including physician-cancer researcher Bruce Halstead's statistical destruction of the "laetrile toxicity" issue and important insertions into the record by Bradford, Dr. Richardson and laetrile's primary pioneer, San Francisco biochemist Ernst T. Krebs, Jr. The ultimate result was partially balanced coverage, not the one-sided putdown that would have taken place if laetrile proponents, as many pro-laetrile people wanted, had decided to stay away from the hearing.

Both the Committee for Freedom of Choice and I knew we were taking a calculated risk in announcing cooperation with the NCI's case-gathering survey. An effort to license and test laetrile by the McNaughton Foundation had suspiciously failed in 1970, and the entire behavior of the Establishment before and since then hardly provided much reason for optimism. Nonetheless, I took note of the fact that, unlike our predecessors in the unproven remedy field, never before had there been the scientific research, vast abundance of users and practitioners, and now the political clout, of laetrile. The muted rhetoric from some quarters was reason enough to assume an at least mostly fair effort by the NCI, which had already covered its bets by announcing in advance that the survey wouldn't prove anything definitely one way or the other.

We did not agree on the test parameters to be used, inasmuch as they called solely for consideration of reduction of tumor masses in cases of thirty-day prior use of amygdalin with or without accompanying metabolic therapy. Nonetheless, I had wrested a verbally awkward crypto-assurance from the NCI that even a survey of patients' well-being might be grounds for future interest by the NCI, even if laetrile failed the tumor test. Having interviewed or been in touch with hundreds of amygdalin users since I began investigating the substance in 1971, I was reasonably certain that even under the NCI's tumor-obsession guidelines, we would have *some* positive results as long as the analyses were fair.

It is true that laetrile users stayed away in droves. We had already calculated that at least 75,000 North Americans had used the substance either for therapy or prevention over the previous few years. We arrived at this figure by examining the monthly caseloads at the two major Tijuana clinics and estimating the caseloads of the major American laetrile-using doctors. Of course, there was *no* way to estimate how many people were using such natural sources of amygdalin as apricot and peach kernels for prevention.

In the meantime, the Committee for Freedom of Choice continued to hold physicians' workshops on amygdalin, metabolic therapy, and cancer. At these gatherings, we learned a lot from metabolic therapists in the field. They in turn traded information, and they then educated hundreds of interested medical personnel, some of whom actually came into our meetings incognito and/or with bogus names to avoid the embarrassment, and possible medical-board action, of even being *seen* among medical pariahs. NCI researchers were invited to attend these sessions, and young Dr. Neil Ellison, who was coordinating the NCI laetrile record-gathering, attended one.

We were all delighted when, in September 1978, the NCI released its results. True, only ninety-three case records were submitted. All were either from physicians or patients who had some reason to believe they had seen or received positive benefits either from laetrile alone or laetrile in combination with a total metabolic program (usually meaning vitamins A, C, E, B^{15}, proteolytic enzymes, detoxification and a special, mostly vegetarian, diet). And, true, the orthodoxy-bound review panel, "blinded" so that it could not determine which cases before it were laetrile cases and which were cases of individuals treated with toxic chemotherapy, ultimately wrote off all but twenty-five of sixty-seven potentially "evaluable" cases as not falling within the NCI's strict guidlines for complete evaluation. Nonetheless, six of the remaining cases showed definite antitumor effects, including two instances that the NCI described as complete disappearance of "all evidence of cancer." In three other cases, direct antitumor effects were not noted, but life extension far beyond the norm had occurred in the varieties of cancer classified.

That is to say, the NCI, through its own parameters and definitions of what cancer is and how to treat it, all at variance with the nation's metabolic therapists, had come up with nine cases highly suggestive of laetrile efficacy. This was the first time, ever, in America that orthodoxy and officialdom had dared to admit even a whisper of an insinuation of phrases used by Establishment spokesmen about there "having never once been observed" either a "shred of evidence" or a "valid sign of efficacy" in the use of laetrile. The NCI findings were even more vital than the discovery over the preceding years of the positive—if suppressed—results on laboratory mice in tests conducted at Sloan-Kettering.

The NCI stuck to its original premise that such results could not in themselves prove the efficacy or lack of same for laetrile. But, in what we could only take as backhanded support for the general metabolic, or holistic, program against cancer, the report contained this intriguing paragraph:

> The patients treated with Laetrile were almost always given concomitant metabolic therapy, including substances that might be regarded as immune stimulants, as well as general supportive care measures such as improved diet, psychological support, and the unmeasurable degree of hope. This fact makes it difficult to attribute any tumor responses to Laetrile alone.

(Interestingly enough, at about the same time Establishment spokesmen were busily describing just such a regimen, for Joey Hofbauer, as "primitive," "barbaric," and "bizarre.")

The NCI also admitted that while the two total remissions it confirmed might well be "spontaneous remissions"—the disappearance of symptoms for no known medical reason—*at the time there were actually only 176 such documented cases on record!*

Quickly, the NCI turned over the case-review results to its "decision network committee," a panel of specialists who make decisions on whether the federal agency will go into testing of a particular substance. We had been hearing for months that the NCI was deeply troubled over what to do about laetrile, and that with the installation of Dr. Arthur Upton as its new director, some degree of change was in the wind. The vote of the network panel bolstered these reports. It split fourteen to eleven *in favor* of going ahead with human tests.

Now, for the first time, and about a quarter of a century late, medical orthodoxy was going to take an official look at laetrile.

The clinical trials did not get started until 1980, both because the FDA would not at first release an investigational new drug license (IND) to the NCI and also because NCI experts were not of one mind as to how to proceed.

From their inception, the trials, targeted for the Mayo Clinic, Memorial Sloan-Kettering Cancer Center, the University of Arizona, and the University of California at Los Angeles, became mired in controversy.

Robert W. Bradford, who was a cofounder of the Committee for Freedom of Choice in Cancer Therapy, and who went on to establish American Biologics, a distributor of amygdalin and other metabolic products, as well as the educational/research organizations bearing his name, collaborated with the Mayo Clinic's Dr. Moertel in attempting to set up general metabolic protocols for amygdalin use.

Bradford was already in ideological trouble with part of the "laetrile movement" for even agreeing to cooperate with the government in amygdalin trials in the first place, and now he stuck his neck out a country mile. His own independent research, mostly aided and abetted by biochemist Henry W. Allen of California, showed, he said, that most injectable commerical amygdalins on the market were contaminated, decomposed products due not so much to malice on the part of manufacturers but because the art of manufacturing *stabilized* injectable amygdalin had seemingly vanished since the early 1950s. Moreover, he said his company's own product, produced in Italy, was indeed purified, natural, stabilized amygdalin in aqueous solution.

Assailed on all sides as an opportunist wanting to sell his own product, Bradford persisted nonetheless and offered NCI free of charge enough of his own material to service up to 300 patients. NCI ignored the offer and also ignored what Bradford said were agreements to trade information.

Utilizing both the Freedom of Information Act and contacts within the government, Bradford claimed in early 1980 that what the government was about to test in its laetrile trials was not actually amygdalin at all but a degraded or decomposed form of it. The proof of the pudding, as attested to by outside expert opinion, was that at least one version of the test material revealed no cyanide under infrared spectroscopy—that is, the material could not be amygdalin.

Bradford was also certain that the contractual arrangements between the NCI and chemical companies enlisted to produce government laetrile constituted an "old boy" network of former employees of a defunct pharmaceutical company, charges never dealt with by the government. Feeling that we all might have been deceived by this umpteenth chapter in the anti-laetrile conspiracy, I joined Bradford, for the Committee for Freedom of Choice in Cancer Therapy, Inc., and Dr. Bruce Halstead in a suit to force the government to cease and desist in the amygdalin trials until and unless it demonstrated that what it was testing was pure amygdalin. Our suit got nowhere, but doubts about the outcome had been raised through the media.

It was thought that the clinical trial, which ultimately cost taxpayers upwards of $500,000, or twice the projected original cost, would take about two years. Both sides questioned whether such a trial could ultimately totally prove or disprove anything. What finally developed turned out to be a showcase example of the Club at its trickiest worst. Since I was among the only proponents in favor of a clinical trial, however limited it might be, I was privy to at least part of the inside workings of what occurred.

It was not until the "last word" in the trials was finally published, in the 28 January 1982, *New England Journal of Medicine* under the signature of Dr. Moertel *et al,* that at least our suspicions about the material were confirmed. The material was, indeed, a goverment-directed attempted carbon copy of material said to duplicate that "of the major Mexican manufacturerer," which was confirmed to me as meaning CytoPharma de Mexico. The material was not pure, stabilized amygdalin but in fact a "racemic" mixture of the compound, which—as the Bradford and other outside, independent research clearly demonstrated—tended to break down or decompose into any of 100 or more compounds, none of them being pure amygdalin. The government, however, could claim it was testing a copy, or at least an attempted copy, of a product sold as "laetrile" and still be telling the truth.

We may never know whether the attempted carbon copy was of the contaminated material seized by the FDA in 1977 or simply an attempt to duplicate non-contaminated CytoPharma material. Government spokesmen, badgered by a few of the informed media about the nature of the material, when asked why the federal side had not simply bought a supply of CytoPharma material, fell back on the "contamination" argument. This left the implied message that Mexican material was essentially contaminated and hence dangerous. While this argument was true from time to time, it begs the question. From the beginning of the Contreras clinic in the 1960s until the present day, and including the full caseloads of the Cydel and Plaza clinics, why were not hundreds, if not thousands, of cancer patients dying from contaminated material? Even a Moertel study, produced during an early part of the NCI-conducted clinical trial, pointed out that laetrile or amygdalin in medical hands was essentially non-toxic, and the government had only a handful of cases (all of them from misuses of the product) to point to in the running battle against the few cases of toxicity attributable to laetrile. (I cover the full range of the Establishment's "dirty tricks" against laetrile later.)

Too, the government side could justifiably claim that laetrile proponents had been sellling and advocating the CytoPharma product before. (Bradford had in fact been a quality-control adviser to CytoPharma at a time when the plant was by far the biggest distributor of laetrile products, none of which are known to have been the direct cause of anybody's death, particularly when correctly administered and monitored by physicians.) This was true. But it was also true that until advanced research on newer and better laetrile products was seriously renewed in the late 1970s, Americans who sought laetrile or amygdalin routinely *had* to rely on the Mexican products. Several European products at the time were not much better, and some of them were worse.

At any rate, what the government side admitted testing was an attempted copy of a Mexican product which itself was a mixture of forms of amygdalin, *isomers,* which at least at some point may not have been amygdalin at all. Even so, as proponents had pointed out and still do, even degraded and decomposed forms of amygdalin or amygdalin-*like* products could indeed produce, as they historically have, both transitory and partial antineoplastic effects and analgesia if only because of the release of benzaldehyde or benzoic acid.

We were of course not at all happy with the way in which patients were to be selected for the clinical trial at the several cancer centers. It is interesting to note how the government side variously described the patients. At the unexpectedly early release of preliminary data on the tests at a press conference 30 April 1981, the patients who were selected for the study were variously said to be those who had "proven cancer beyond any hope of cure of therapy known to extend life expectancy," and/or were patients "for whom no other treatment had been effective, or for whom no proven treatment existed" and who were "at least one month past any previous surgery, radiation or chemotherapy." In the final *NEJM* article, the patients are said to have been those other than "patients for whom standard therapy is known to hold a curative potential or to extend life expectancy" but also patients who were not in the "terminal episode" in that they were not "totally disabled or in preterminal condition."

The only translation of these various descriptions that can be logically synthesized is this: incurable or inoperable patients who were in good enough condition to enter the program but who were not expected to live and on most of whom orthodox therapy had been tried and failed. A more succinct definition of this from poker parlance would be *a stacked deck.* The laetrile controversy was to be decided by the course of trestment on 178 of the "walking dead," many of whom could reasonably be expected to have immune systems already brutalized by previous therapy. Two-thirds had received prior orthodox treatment.

For the Committee for Freedom of Choice in Cancer Therapy, Inc., I vainly sought the release of raw data on a per-patient basis, even with their anonymities guaranteed, to be able to determine exactly what kind of patients were to be on the program—and to confirm the rumors we were hearing that several patients were turned away simply because they were not "far enough gone"! No such raw data were forthcoming, even when I invoked the Freedom of Information Act.

We were also distressed that not a single metabolic physician or laetrile practitioner would be directly involved in the treatments.

Nobody skilled in this form of therapy, let alone anyone viewing cancer as a systemic, chronic, metabolic dysfunction rather than a mass of tumors, would be part of the treatment program. We would have to rely on what orthodox clinicians said and did—a clear case of the fox sent to guard the henhouse.

We also recognized that an oral agreement to exchange information between the NCI side and ourselves was never implemented. The NCI, in effect, took our points of view and suggestions but offered nothing of substance in return. For all of these reasons, and now very much smelling a rat, we persisted in the federal suit, but were successfully challenged by the government side as to a "lack of standing." Indeed, as one government attorney told the media, *nobody,* save a patient in the program himself, had the "standing" to stop a federal testing program *even if* the outcome of the test were known in advance!

The press conference of 30 April 1981, before the American Society of Clinical Oncology, turned out to be a surprise on several fronts. It occurred just as a serious congressional review of the NCI's full range of activities, several of them highly questionable, was getting under way; it occurred far earlier than the conclusion of the clinical trial was expected; and it was novel that a scientific finding on a major medical controversy would be aired in the form of a slide-presentation and a press packet handout *in lieu of* a published paper with all the data, which was said to be "months away."

The media was informed at this most incredible press conference that "within one month of beginning Laetrile treatment, 50 percent of the patients showed evidence of disease progression and 90 percent had progressed within three months. Fifty percent...died before five months and only 20 percent were alive by eight months."

The conclusion was that amygdalin or laetrile and a backup of metabolic therapy (the following of lower dosage levels of vitamins and enzymes and a modest adherence, if any, to the diet) "does not produce any substantive benefit in terms of cure or improvement of cancer per se, slowing the advance of cancer, improving symptoms or general condition of the cancer patient, or in terms of extension of life span."

The numbers referred to by NCI may very well have been genuine. However, during the slide presentation, the NCI flashed on the wall an intriguing graph, which it passed over virtually without comment, and which did *not* appear in the press packet distributed that day. It was called "Objective Response Rates" and clearly showed that 70 percent of patients were listed as "stable" at the end of three weeks. *After* that time, "stable" patients rapidly declined in number.

Why the disparity? Well, for *most* patients, as was later pointed out to me by Dr. Moertel, the three-week period essentially covered the 21-day period in which the patients received *injections. After* that time they were placed on tablets and oral supplements. That is to say, most patients most of the time were listed as "stable" as long as they were on injections, even of degraded or decomposed material! "Stable," as I was told by the NCI investigators themselves, meant what one might expect—that the patients were neither improved nor worsened. There was a clear statistical correlation between the number of "stable" patients and the period in which they received injections. But the media, in general, were not apprised of this.

Between the press conference and the publication in 1982 of the final results, we, as plaintiffs in the U.S. District Court and as major proponents, made much of the stability factor, the single statistic which—aside from the fact only the patients who were expected to die anyway were allowed into the program—cast considerable doubt on the trial, which was said not to be completely finished.

During the interim, Moertel and others, asked to explain why injections had ceased after 21 days, defended themselves by saying that they were following by "chapter and verse" the instructions of metabolic practitioners and theorists, most certainly including Bradford and the treatment regimen he and I outlined in *Now That You Have Cancer*. Yet NCI chose to ignore, as part of the ongoing correspondence between ourselves and them, the all-important letter of 13 December 1978, which detailed the general "laetrile program" as basically followed at that time. In that letter, Bradford clearly stated: "The daily intravenous regimen should not *suddenly be abandoned* for the oral route, but there should be a period of *an additional 21 days* in which 9 grams are given IV three times a week with 500 mg tablets three times a day before meals...." (emphasis mine).

That is, the government side was able to pick and choose the information it wanted from proponents, then "hang" them with that information if need be. We found the injection-period cutoff to be among the most ethically questionable practices within the entire trial.

Not until the *NEJM* article was published was the semantical meaning of "progressive" disease more narrowly defined. Intriguingly, the initial 70 percent "stable" diagram was missing from the "finished" paper, as were, of course, all raw data on the patients themselves. The words "progressed," "stable" and "objective response" become of utterly vital importance in wending one's way through the semantical thicket of the *NEJM* report, whose summation did indeed capture the media and deliver the most punishing propaganda attack on the forces of laetrile and metabolic therapy to date. As Moertel *et al* point out, *only* reductions in tumefactions and liver distentions (in leukemia patients, for example) and the lack of new metastases met the criteria for "objective response," and only "objective response"—in the main—was being looked for in these not-expected-to-live inoperable or incurable cancer patients provided degraded amygdalin and moderate adherence to an across-the-board, non-individualized metabolic/nutritional program. And, within even "objective response," the parameters are clear: 50 percent or more decrease in the largest tumor mass, at least 30 percent decrease in the sum of liver distention, and no increase in the number or size of metastases. The other way to say that is that a decrease in tumefaction of 40 percent, or of liver distention by 20 percent, however dramatic it might be, would not count. Technically, a patient might remain "stable" even though there were considerable changes in his tumefactions—not enough increase to be determined to be in "progressed" disease, or enough decrease to fall under "objective response." All of this, of course, is almost entirely meaningless to the concept that cancer is a chronic, systemic, metabolic dysfunction in which tumors (which in many cases may be composed of a good deal of *normal* tissue) are only symptoms, not the disease itself. There is no statistical accounting of how many patients actually showed improvements that were not great enough to be called that, and of course nothing to indicate just how the patients *felt*.

In *NEJM,* it was said that "ninety-five patients (54 percent) had measurable progression of malignant disease at the termination of their courses of intravenous amygdalin (sic)." This is a considerable departure from the earlier slide that showed 70 percent "stable" during roughly the same time frame. However, and despite what set of semantics one is using, during the time period corresponding to the injectable part of the treatment, *either* a majority of patients (70 percent) or a large minority of them (46 percent) were either stable or without signs of progressive disease! Can *this* be considered a test which absolutely—as the *NEJM* editor railed—"closes the books on Laetrile?" Hardly.

Hence, what the taxpayer-funded study (which should have been entitled "A Government-Funded Study of a Government-Produced Attempted Copy of a Form of Decomposed Amygdalin Sold as 'Laetrile' on 178 Patients Previously Treated Without Success by Orthodox Medicine and/or Who Were Inoperable or Incurable or Otherwise Not Expected to Live") showed was that a minimal metabolic program and prematurely ended injections of degraded or decomposed amygdalin failed to save the lives of most of a group of 178 patients who were expected to die anyway.

This was deceit of a high order, but it accomplished its task beautifully for the Club. "Laetrile Worthless, Study Shows," ran headlines across the country. *The New York Times,* so adept at earlier missing the story of the coverup of positive amygdalin tests at nearby Sloan—Kettering Institute, weighed in with another editorial apparently to put the last nail in the coffin.

Too, the *NEJM* "final word" report provided more ammunition for the media to continue the "cyanide toxicity scare" tactic earlier arrayed against amygdalin or laetrile.

The Moertel study referred to a handful of cases of elevated blood cyanide levels and toxic symptoms from *oral* misuses of the product, and then added the warning that laetrile-using patients ran a cyanide risk in using the product, adding that proponents did not adequately warn patients about this danger.

This gratuitous swipe was particularly enraging to proponents, particularly the Bradford interests, since the caveats about over-ingesting the *oral* product had been in broad circulation for years (a maximum 1.5 grams per day range). The toxicity cases referred to in the report called into question just how carefully the NCI researchers monitored their own patients and raised more questions of ethics.

References to amygdalin toxicity (the cyanide issue is dealt with more extensively elsewhere) contradicted the earlier studies by Moertel on amygdalin toxicity alone as well as the earlier statement from the preliminary findings that "overall, according to the methods and safeguards of our study, amygdalin (*sic*) was safe and reasonably tolerable."

Moertel, the other NCI researchers and informed scientists know very well that injectable laetrile (provided up to as many as 72 grams IV per day) is among the most non-toxic of cancer modalities in existence and that even the oral product is far safer than any other recognized chemotherapeutic agent for cancer.

Nonetheless, by combining the failure of amygdalin or laetrile in this hoked-up study with fresh fears about cyanide toxicity, the NCI provided sufficient fuel for a field-day attack on metabolic and nutritional therapy.

But nobody who carefully read the whole paper, or who was even minimally privy to the facts, believed for a minute that the NCI clinical trial could be the death of either laetrile or metabolic therapy. The reality was that far too many people, including patients and doctors, had seen far too many successes and benefits from amygdalin and nutritional management to be other than irritated by this latest low blow from the Club.

Historically, the mere fact that NCI had been maneuvered into a position where it had *had* to "test laetrile" was the great success. And the findings of laetrile efficacy, however minimal, in the documentation which went into the NCI's original decision to test the compound, let alone that area of efficacy suggested within the study itself, were landmark events in the history of suppression of useful cancer remedies by the Club. The clinical trial would never have come about were not a medical revolution against drug-based medicine-as-usual clearly on the move.

The grudging acceptance of the laetrile reality had been best articulated by a California internist, Phil R. Alper, M.D., when he wrote in the 10 July 1978 *Medical Economics,* "If laetrile were running in an election, it would win by a landslide.... Considering its background, and the forces opposing it, laetrile *has* won by a landslide. Its use has been legalized by almost one third of the states....Public opinion polls support its legalization by wide margins. Patients go to extraordinary lengths—and expense—to obtain it. And there are some doctors—not all of them necessarily quacks—who have a measure of faith in laetrile." *Sic!*

"No ordinary here-today-and-gone-tomorrow quack cancer cure, amygdalin—as it's called chemically—has been kicking around since 1920," Dr. Alper wrote. "And if so far no one has clearly demonstrated its effectiveness, neither has anyone conclusively shown it to be ineffective in humans." So saying, Dr. Alper went on to make a case for government and medical orthodoxy to allow physicians to use laetrile on terminally ill cancer patients or to use it adjunctively with standard modalities.

So successful had laetrile become politically that no less than five papers on "the laetrile phenomenon" were submitted for the January 1979 meeting of the American Association for the Advancement of Science (AAAS)—a milestone in the history of cancer's "unproven methods."

Setting the stage for five papers, arranged by Gerald E. Markle and James C. Petersen, respectively an associate and an assistant professor of sociology at Western Michigan University, the organizers told AAAS members:

> At no time in American history has there been a more effective challenge mounted to medical expertise and authority than that mounted by the contemporary laetrile movement. Despite opposition from the FDA, the American Medical Association, the American Cancer Society, and virtually all of the American medical community, support for this purported cancer cure continues to grow....The first paper takes a case-study approach and focuses on the recent laetrile controversy at the Memorial Sloan-Kettering Cancer Center illustrating the richness and complexity of the dispute. The next paper provides an historical context to the recent success of the movement. The third paper examines the conceptualization of the laetrile problem and attempts to explain a variety of legal issues, including the right of privacy; the rights of physicians, informed consent, and government control, are considered. The final paper examines the social context of the controversy and attempts to answer the following question: Why has the laetrile movement been so successful in the late 1970s?

By 1982, anti-laetrile forces had won at least some time for regrouping through two separate Supreme Court actions. These in effect upheld the FDA's right to treat laetrile or amygdalin as any other "unlicensed new drug" and kept the substance within the meaning of the Food, Drug and Cosmetic Act; that is, it is not "grandfathered," as argued by earlier U.S. District Court decisions.

However, the 1980 presidential elections had brought into office more representatives who by nature are freedom-of-choicers. With the court battles having gone about as far as they could go, it became obvious that the final political victories for B^{17} and metabolic therapy would have to be achieved through the legislative route.

But whatever the route chosen, the ultimate victory of alternative medicine is on the way to vindication—an idea whose time has come.

Medical Miasma:
Orthodoxy Losing The Battle of Degenerative Disease

It is the general premise of this book that laetrile's political and scientific victories are the battering ram for medical revolution in America, that the apricot kernel derivative laetrile is bringing with it the vindication of that whole nebulous area we awkwardly call holistic medicine or metabolic/nutritional therapy, and that it would not have been possible without politics.

But it also would not have been possible without a parallel central truth. The "old medicine," which must give way to a "new medicine," has lost the battle against degenerative disease, not only in this country but in the entire Western world, the "civilized" world of industrial technological societies, with their polluted water and air, and an awesomely polluted and synthetic food supply.

Going into this decade, the National Center for Health Statistics revealed that the sum total of deaths from cardiovascular and arteriosclerosis problems—"heart disease," in short—was a little less than a million a year. This figure was actually a slight improvement over prior years. Cancer, however, was estimated in 1982 to be the cause of 430,000 deaths, a figure which keeps rising annually above the predictions of most health planners. If figures from heart disease, diabetes, cirrhosis and other degenerative diseases are added to cancer, they account for well over 1.5 million fatalities annually, with heart disease the cause of 51 percent of all deaths.

Despite the near-pandemicity of these degenerative diseases, it is cancer which constitutes the biggest of the "growth" industries in terms of the total health picture, for both its incidence and fatalities continue to grow beyond predictions despite the alleged best efforts of the "old medicine." In the American Cancer Society's *Cancer Facts and Figures 1982,* the annually updated version of the ACS' grab bag of mostly bad news on the cancer front, we find that 835,000

Americans will be diagnosed with cancer. But that is only part of the story: the National Cancer Institute (NCI) differentiates between non-melanoma skin cancer and the other forms. There being an estimated 400,000 new cases of the former annually, the yearly cancer-incidence rate is ripping along at about 1,235,000 new cases per year.

There are several ways to look at that incredible statistic. One is to balance it against a barrage of end-of-year figures put forth by the embattled NCI in the late 1981 attempting to vindicate standard medicine against an ever-growing "database" of cancer incidence: one out of three people now destined to get cancer (up from one in four) while one out of six (down from one out of five) are expected to die from it. The ACS pre-1982 assessment was that 58 million Americans now living are destined to get cancer in their lifetimes (by statistical juggling and given the seemingly exponential rise in cancer incidence, this is probably conservative). It is now killing 1,180 Americans per day, or one every 73 seconds. It hits two out of every three families and is the major killer of children under fourteen and middle-aged women.

The reason cancer, which kills one out of every three patients, is held in greater terror than is heart disease, which is the cause of slightly over half of all fatalities from all diseases, is that the word cancer is associated—appropriately—in the average mind with *death,* whereas heart disease is not. The population has been weaned to believe that heart disease is almost a normal part of the aging process, and to articulate the very phrase conjures up visions of hospitals and doctors with stethoscopes. Cancer, however, the bringer of great agony and suffering, may strike seemingly out of the clear blue sky with virtually no prior signs of ill-being, and may cut down a youth today, a middle-aged mother tomorrow. The fatalities from cancer constitute the equivalent of a new Vietnam War for Americans every six weeks or so, yet millions of protesters do not jam the streets pleading for the government to "do something" about it.

Going into the present decade, a conservative estimate was that at least 35 million Americans had hypertension, 4.3 million had coronary heart disease, 1.9 million rheumatic heart disease, and about an equal number had suffered strokes. Somewhere between a third and a half of the entire population suffer from the earliest warning sign of degenerative diseases, low blood sugar (hypoglycemia)—whose last stop is usually diabetes—but only a fraction of the sufferers are aware of the problem and only a minority of physicians can adequately diagnose it (Harold W. Harper, M.D., and I called attention to this growing problem in *How You Can Beat the Killer Diseases.* New Rochelle, N.Y: Arlington House, 1977). Since both hypertension and hypoglycemia are silent, precursor states indicating serious degenerative disease problems to come, it is safe to estimate that far over half the population is affected by degenerative disease at this time—and that even *this* figure is almost certainly conservative.

The American Heart Association estimated in 1981 that the annual cost of cardiovascular—"heart" disease in direct terms—was $46.2 billion. The cancer watchers are warier, and take great pains to separate out costs of hospital stays, drugs and direct treatment from indirect costs such as man-hours lost. Even in 1982, ACS was still parroting the estimate of *Consumer Reports* that an average cancer bill was $20,000. That figure is actually much higher—$30,000 is more realistic—with cancer treatments in six figures far from uncommon. If we exclude the fairly manageable skin cancers from the annual figures and estimate the remaining diagnosed cancers at a compromise figure of $25,000, we have, in terms of *treatment* cost alone, a formidable $27 billion—a figure which can hardly begin to account for the damage to the nation caused by cancer overall. When proponents of alternative therapy throughout the 1970s railed against the "cancer industry," they were not just shooting from the lip: the total treatment and research/development figures for cancer make that industry well in excess of $30 billion a year.

While heart disease and cancer gained plenty of attention in the post-World War II era, a group of diseases frequently best known by their abbreviations kept creeping up to wreak havoc at ever greater numbers—we started hearing more and more about MS (multiple sclerosis), considered by orthodoxy to be incurable; MD (muscular dystrophy), CF (cystic fibrosis), and such cripplers as lupus. Along the way, arthritis jumped into a position of ominous strength as it became clearer that this malady, also mistakenly thought to be exclusively a problem of the aged, cropped up in younger and younger Americans. By 1980, it was estimated that 31 million Americans were afflicted by any of the one hundred forms of this painful malady, and that its cost to the nation directly and indirectly was $14 billion annually.

With more than $10 billion in federal funds alone already misspent on the "war on cancer," which has made no appreciable dent in either the incidence of or fatality levels from the disease, and with more Americans than ever being cut down by cardiovascular involvements at earlier ages, it doesn't take a triple-Ph.D. mentality to know that something is dreadfully wrong. The situation reaches dimensions weighty enough to lead a pastor to blasphemy when it is realized that medical research in this country along promising avenues of therapy for both cancer *and* heart disease is being stymied by an interlock of vested interest, bureaucratic arrogance, and medical tyranny. As we will detail later, nontoxic, nonsurgical chelation therapy *is* available as a prevention for and treatment of heart disease. Yet not one in 100 Americans has ever heard about it, there are fewer physicians around who know anything about it, and most Americans face the likelihood of expensive, mutilating surgery and/or the use of toxic substances in their losing battle against cardiovascular diseases of all kinds.

Aside from laetrile, immune-system-stimulating agents (only partially "approved" in the U.S.), protein-digesting enzymes, and vitamin A therapy are routinely available in the Germanies for cancer treatment, but Americans must go underground to get them or find metabolic physicians who will risk getting in hot water for administering them.

It is another major premise of this book that the nation's food processing industry, which helped get us into the degenerative disease crisis, and the major pharmaceutical trusts, which prepare expensive drugs allegedly to help "solve" the crisis, are perfectly contented with the way things are. Indeed, the extent of the war against laetrile cannot be explained *only* by laetrile's threat to arrogant psyches with a vested ego interest in not being caught in lies, or even by the threat of natural substances to the cancer industry, one worth, as we have seen, a conservative $30 billion a year.

Hardly. The panicky reactions to laetrile constitute only the tip of the iceberg. If it can be seen that laetrile, a natural substance, and the whole regimen of natural substances of which laetrile is one element, are essentially nontoxic, potentially inexpensive and useful treatment for an excruciatingly expensive disease, and that they probably play roles in *preventing* that disease; and if it can be seen that the degenerative diseases, of which cancer is only one, are interlocked, then the realization, perhaps at times only subconscious, that degenerative disease can be *prevented*, let alone *treated* with inexpensive simplicity, strikes fear into the hearts of the *status quo* merchants.

Laetrile has to be fought because of what it *represents*—a frontal assault on medicine as usual—and fought with every dirty trick in the book, the last-ditch one being "toxicity," a subject we will deal with in another chapter. As cancer falls to amygdalin and metabolic therapy, so does the entire allopathic house of cards and the drug interests, food processing, and federal controllers with it. Only in this light can the extraordinary measures against "unproven remedies" of all kinds be understood.

Americans and their legislative representatives are not to be faulted for asking: *Why* is the battle against degenerative disease being lost, *if*—as we are constantly told—we have the best health care in the world? Twenty years ago there were two hospital employees for every patient; by 1976 there were three. Between 1965 and 1976 the total number of people—physicians, nurses, paramedics, hospital employees—in the "health-care-delivery industry" jumped from 3.3 million to 4.4 million. In twenty years medical care cost zoomed 133 percent while the consumer price index rose only 74 percent. What have we received for our money? Certainly not an increase in life expectancy, which has hardly changed in a quarter-century. And certainly no decrease in the killer diseases; indeed, they are blossoming as never before.

The Doping of America

In the meantime, it's a field day not only for practitioners of medicine as usual, whose paragon is the white-smocked surgeon, that elite, best-paid member of the medical team, but for the producers of drugs, both major and minor, that are dumped by the trillions of tablets and capsules per year on a population for whom they may serve as little more than symptom-maskers of the early signs of degenerative disease. It has become a ritual. If we feel bad, we pop a pill. If we're out of sorts, there is a bottle of processed chemicals handy. By failing to take responsibility for our *own* health, we have left it up to the ornate clinics and sumptuous hospital edifices, those sanctuaries of an arcane medical language, complicated, almost extraterrestrail equipment, and a white-uniformed army of physicians, nurses, and orderlies to take care of us. But for the vast bulk of our medical problems, most of the time, "relief" is supposed to be only a tablet away.

The American Enterprise Institute for Public Policy Research reported as early as 1970 that the pharmaceutical industry in the United States had grown by 100 percent in the twentieth century. And in 1973 the Consumer Union noted that in the United States 20,000 tons of aspirin were consumed every year, or about 225 tablets per person. *Scientific American* revealed in 1973 that the central-nervous-system-affecting agents were the fastest-growing sector of the drug business, accounting for 31 percent of total sales.

In 1974, the National Commission on Marijuana and Drug Abuse reported that dependence on prescription tranquilizers had risen 200 percent since 1962, while per capita consumption of liquor was up only 23 percent and the intake of illegal opiates had gone up by 50 percent. As of 1970, 762 *million* prescriptions worth $2.5 billion were being written for nonhospitalized patients every single year.

For more than a decade, drug industry profits have outranked those of all other manufacturing industries listed on the New York Stock Exchange. And why not? Drug prices are often controlled and manipulated, and what may cost one dollar a bottle abroad might cost ten dollars here. And, as was determined in 1978 as drug companies fought the drive to allow the substitution of generic products for brand names in medical preparations, the same substance can cost two to five times less if its generic name is used.

In 1982, despite the ravages of economic recession, the U.S. drug industry was doing just fine, thank you, with projected earnings estimated to be 20 percent over those in 1981, when the industry pulled in $12 *billion*. Part of the boom in profits, truth to tell, was a change in the wind at the FDA which, by 1980, was taking up to ten years for approval of new drugs. Final-stage testing requirements are now cutting the last clinical testing period from an average of thirty-five months to as little as a year or less.

A key example of a drug on which America almost literally depends is Valium, one of the tranquilizers most often prescribed and routinely recommended for complaints both major and minor. As Dr. Harper and I argued in *Killer Diseases*, it is oh-so-easy for a physician to dash off a prescription for Valium in just a few seconds as he listens to a hypoglycemic reel off a list of vague symptoms—especially when it would be oh-so-time-consuming to subject the patient to a six-hour-long glucose tolerance test, the only way the real nature of his complaints might be determined.

The markup of Valium was estimated in 1974 to be from $50 per kilogram when it is produced in Switzerland to $75,000 per kilo in the United States before it is ready for sale as tablets. It was dispensed 22.5 million times in 1974, at an average of sixty tablets per prescription. And in 1979 the Senate Health Subcommittee was told that some 68 million prescriptions for Valium, Librium, and other substances of the benzodiazepine family had been written in the U.S.A. in 1978, with a wholesale market value of $360 million. This included *44 million* prescriptions for Valium alone, or about twice the 1974 level!

Worse, the Congressmen learned, addiction to Valium can cause withdrawal symptoms more prolonged and severe than those from heroin. Other serious side effects have been reported from Valium use, and yet Valium somehow made it through the FDA's screening and monitoring process, the apparatus the medical/pharmaceutical industries tell us is the best and safest in the world.

Intriguingly enough, the June 1980 edition of *The Journal of the American Medical Association*, the American medical monopoly's repository of sacred writ, devoted four full-color pages to advertising for Valium.

As Ivan Illich has recorded in his excellent *Medical Nemesis* (Random House, N.Y., 1976), Valium's producers, Hoffman-LaRoche, spent $200 million over ten years and commissioned 200 doctors a year to produce favorable scientific articles about Valium properties. Meanwhile, the drug industry—in 1973—was spending about $4,500 on each practicing physician for advertising and promotion of drugs, at the time nearly equivalent to the cost of a year in medical school.

In April 1976, Chairman Gaylord Nelson of the Senate Select Committee on Small Business reported that "the almost complete takeover by the [drug] industry of post-graduate medical 'education' is cause for alarm." Nelson's committee also heard from the FDA's Richard Crout that the drug industry selects and pays for "the bulk of educational information provided to the practicing physician."

It is quite true that some major drug companies also produce vitamin preparations, with a tidy profit in mind. But vitamins as an industry (vitamin supplements and "health foods") hardly constitute anything like the overlapping profits of the drug cartel. Hence, it is still unwelcome news to the pharmaceutical industry in general than an adequate use of vitamin supplements may be the best prevention of, let alone treatment for, a whole range of disorders and problems for which synthetic drugs are recommended. It is even more horrifying, of course, to realize that proper eating habits—and proper food—would eventually eliminate or greatly reduce the need for vitamin preparations.

American Medicine: Unsafe at Any Cost?

A frightening parallel reality to the doping of America under the present status quo, as well as orthodoxy's losing the battle against degenerative disease, is the health problem *caused* by modern medicine. This situation became known as the "iatrogenic"— literally, doctor-caused—disease factor in the 1970s. It is not so much doctors themselves, but the drugs and procedures they are using, that are suspect in bringing iatrogenic disease into the forefront of the nation's major health problems. By 1976 it was estimated that adverse drug reactions probably total at least *three million* a year, with estimates of hospital deaths due to drugs hitting as high as 140,000 a year. Even using conservative figures from the Boston Collaborative Drug Study, adverse-reaction deaths would rank as the eleventh most deadly killer in the United States. About 300,000 people are admitted to American hospitals annually because of *prescribed* drugs, at an added hospital care cost of $4.5 billion a year. If this were not in itself tragic, ponder the parallel reality that in a typical year 10 to 20 percent of all prescription medications may not "work," anyway—a shocking finding disclosed in 1981 by Dr. Sidney Wolfe's Public Citizens Health Research Group (*Pills that Don't Work,* Farrar, Straus, Giroux, 1981). The research group listed 600 prescription drugs, many of them widely used, for which "benefits are either zero or close to zero," and some of which have such bad side effects that they may actually constitute a case of the cure being worse than the disease!

In 1979 it was reported that the chances of a patient picking up a *new* infection by visiting the hospital are about one in twenty—a conservative estimate—and that about 15,000 people die in the United States annually from hospital-acquired infections alone. The *Southern Medical Journal* reported in May 1967 that one out of every five patients admitted to a typical research hospital acquired a *new*—that is, iatrogenic—disease caused by the therapy he was receiving! Half of these were due to complications in drug therapy, ten percent from diagnostic procedures. The percentage of Americans who die in hospitals was estimated to have increased by a third between 1955 and 1967. Little change for the current era is expected since the "need" to die in hospitals and clinics has virtually become a ritualistic part of American culture. Resisting treatment and "care in our last days" within the gleaming alabaster and marble womb of a mighty, Blue Cross-approved medical temple is regarded as old-fashioned.

Indeed, self-confessed "medical heretic" Robert S. Mendelsohn, M.D. has described modern American medicine as a "church" complete with rituals and incantations—and a thought system which goes with it, beginning with the act of birth (described as a medical operation) and proceeding right through the act of death, usually conducted in a temple of dying (that is, a hospital).

In his incisive *Confessions of a Medical Heretic* (New York: Warner Books, 1979), Dr. Mendelsohn decries the propaganda whereby Americans are sent dutifully marching off for their annual checkups:

> Without the ritual of the checkup, internists would have trouble paying office rent! How else can the doctor ensure a steady supply of sacrificial victims for the Church's other sacraments without the examination? The Gospel said many were called and few were chosen, but the Church of Modern Medicine has gone that one better. *All* are called and *most* are chosen.

Under what its critics now call "fragmented" medicine, the "old medicine," by emphasizing the surgeon and the speed with which a patient—or victim—is rushed into the operating room as soon as he or relatives sign a consent form (and by no means always *with* a consent form) is not without its geometrically spiralling problems. A congressional committee report indicated in 1974 that some 2.4 million surgeries on Americans which cost $4 billion and took 12,000 lives were unnecessary in the first place! And, in 1981, a poll taken of registered nurses by their magazine, *RN,* found that almost half those responding believed three out of every ten operations are unnecessary. Furthermore, Dr. G. Thomas Shires, president of the American College of Surgeons, told the professional cutters' organization the same year that nearly 30 percent of all doctors performing surgery are "untrained and unqualified." This does not disturb the cut-burn-and-poison brigade, however. "Heroic" surgery, toxic drugs, and tissue-blasting radiation remain their "treatments of choice" for cancer. For coronary heart disease, they choose coronary bypass, at up to $30,000 a whack, even though the figures on its use fail to indicate it results in much long-term benefit. Dr. Alexander Leaf of Harvard Medical School (as mentioned by George Leonard in "The Holistic Health Revolution," *New West,* 10 May, 1976) pointed to a study of a group of forty patients admitted with ruptured aortic aneurysms. The combined hospital bills of these patients came to more than $1 million, or an average cost of $25,000 per patient. Only one of them came out of the hospital alive. And the Harvard School of Public Health released a study in 1981 finding that, despite the fact that 110,000 American were spending $1.8 billion a year on coronary bypass surgery, most people with clogged arteries can be treated successfully enough with medicine so that the operation is simply not necessary.

That doctors and hospitals seem intimately linked *to* death, rather than rescuing patients *from* it, has several times become embarrassingly obvious:

Dr. Mendelsohn has reported that the death rate in Los Angeles County dropped eighteen percent in 1978 when doctors went on strike to protest hikes in malpractice insurance premiums. UCLA's Dr. Milton Roemer, professor of health care administration, in surveying 17 major hospitals disclosed that sixty percent fewer operations had been performed. When the strike ended, the death rate was back to "normal" in Los Angeles County.

Elsewhere, as in Colombia, whose medicine is patterned after that of the U.S.A., the death rate in the country dropped thirty-five percent during the fifty-two day period in 1976 in which all doctors except those in emergency care went on strike.

There will never be a way to assess the full damage of medicine as usual to patients of degenerative disease because such damage may be hidden by statistics. I learned this over and over again while pursuing the laetrile controversy. If a cancer patient dies while on the laetrile program, he may be said to have died "from laetrile" or "while on laetrile." But if he dies from the brutal side-effects of chemotherapy and radiation, which so pulverize the body's immune system that it cannot combat even simple infections, it is *never* stated that he died from radiation, or 5-FU, or Vincristine. No, it is either from the cancer itself or a complication of it—but it is never mentioned that the "complication" that arose might have been from the treatment itself. This fact was confirmed to me again in 1982 by a California pathologist who said that half the cadavers he had autopsied in his professional career were of cancer victims—and that half of these had obviously died of *chemotherapy*. "No, you may not use my name when you quote this," he added.

As the modern medical mavericks note, American—indeed Western—medicine has become fragmented, overspecialized, and, worst of all, impersonal. The idea of the visiting family physician with the pleasant bedside manner, an art which was usually half the "cure" in those warmer days of yore, has been replaced by the modern reality of assembly-line medicine. Pity the poor hypoglycemic, who may be bounced from the G.P. to the internist to the neurosurgeon to the psychiatrist in an ever-more-expensive revolving door of frustration before the real nature of his complaints has been responsibly diagnosed—if it ever is.

A lower-tract complaint may bring the aggrieved first to the walnut-paneled office of a proctologist. But, as Dr. Edgar Berman so well put it in *The Solid Gold Stethoscope,* the proctologist's area of expertise is limited to a single square inch of puckered tissue, beyond which gastroenterologists have more or less marked a "thou shalt not pass" line. This means a visit to yet another specialist, and before anything is determined, another round of specialists, probes, and clinic visits will ultimately occur. The patient may not sense an immediate flight of funds from his pocket, but the cost of medical insurance under his group plan will rise just the same.

Fragmented, impersonal medicine fraught with the perils of needless surgery and delayed negative reactions from drugs, all at a prohibitive ballooning in cost—is this to be the future of American medicine?

Medical Revolution in America

More and more, both fully accredited physicians and legions of patients and healthy people think not. Health conventions and seminars emphasizing offbeat approaches to self-help in medicine and disease prevention are drawing more participants than ever before. Homeopathy and naturopathy are having a comeback, and the orthomolecular theories of megavitamin use in disease have made inroads into many areas of the old medicine. In California alone there are hundreds of centers in which holistic medicine of one variety or another is practiced in one way or another. A number of holistic clinics emphasizing metabolic therapy are now functioning in several states, usually staffed by orthodox M.D.'s as well as such unorthodox folks as the friendly neighborhood acupuncturist and an expert in mental visualization techniques.

Prevention-minded physicians have tended to cluster in such groups as the International Association of Preventive Medicine (IAPM) and the American Holistic Medical Association (AHMA). Defenders and practitioners of chelation therapy have closed ranks in the American Academy of Medical Preventics (AAMP). Numerous other organizations, all spurning the wisdom and advice of the American Medical Association, continue to sprout up.

Increasingly, both physicians and patients have turned to the courts to secure their birthright to freedom of choice in medical treatment.

The victory by laetrile proponents and patients in the in the U.S. District Court for Western Oklahoma, providing access to vitamin B[17] was only the first assault in the battle for freedoms eroded by the growth of the federal government. As we shall see, Dr. Ray Evers and his patients went to court and won the right to use and be treated with chelating agents in degenerative disease, and this was but one of a series of important victorious court battles in 1978.

When the medical boards of New Jersey and Pennsylvania stripped innovative physician Peter DeMarco of his license to practice medicine, concerted action by his patients helped restore his Pennsylvania license.

Vitamin distributors Steven Michaelis and Douglas Heinsohn won important court battles to allow them to distribute apricot kernels and to bar the government from confiscating their merchandise by overstepping search-and-seizure regulations.

Michaelis, a pharmacist, and Heinsohn, a salesman, are not physicians but are nonetheless champions of metabolic/nutritional therapy. DeMarco is a medical innovator, as is Ray Evers, a long time exponent of total metabolic therapy. These and many other courageous men and women have been in the toils of the law because they went against the grain.

If there is a single, undergirding concept that links all these rising factions pointing to a new medicine, it is the *holistic* one—the belief that man is the sum of his parts, and perhaps more, and that everything in him and about him is interconnected. Therapeutically, this means that a skin disease is not a separate problem, but the manifestation of a holistic one. Cancer is no more lump-and-bump disease than syphilis and smallpox are skin lesions.

The movement is one of bringing the body back into natural balance under the theory that the abnormal conditions of modern technological society have provided a threat to human metabolism for which it is simply not prepared. Noting that man has moved *away* from natural eating habits and the intake of minerals, vitamins, and enzymes those habits included, the new medicine is insisting that we restore those habits, whenever and however possible. But the physical harmony of the body is usually seen as only part of the picture. Bringing the influence of the mind and the tranquility of the spirit to bear on the process is perceived by many to be as important as, if not ultimately more important than, the sum total of all the physical aspects of a holistic program.

As the new medicine moves away from the old forms of fragmented medicine, allopathy, and dependence on surgery, harmful drugs and radiation, it will make many mistakes. Fresh ground is broken almost daily in the theory and practice of preventive medicine and metabolic therapy. But if the growing forces of the movement have at their disposal just a fraction of the billions of dollars of research money available to *status quo* medicine, all the questions posed by this new wave of thought will ultimately be answered.

Until they are, there will be increasing numbers of Hofbauers and Greens and Accardis demanding the right to have their children placed under "alternative" forms of therapy, and there will be flourishing black markets in medicines and substances the Establishment continues to ban and damn. The tidal wave of change is bound to be successful simply because it is energized by a medical idea whose time has come.

Thomas Kuhn forcefully argued in *The Structure of Scientific Revolutions* that every dominant science eventually oversteps itself— that its very successes force it into extreme positions and practices that speed its demise. In its death throes, its nostrums do not work and things simply don't make sense. No better description befits the old medicine as it grapples with the realities of the degenerative disease pandemic now sweeping across the Western world. Its nostrums do not work and things simply don't make sense.

In the following chapters we will examine factors in both the suppression and advancement of the medical revolution, one whose victory is assured—a victory which is simply a matter of time, place, and manner.

Chapter Three
Rx: Murder—How Government and the AMA Stifle Innovation

The FDA Is Dangerous To Your Health
For years American cancer patients routinely have been fleeing to Mexico, Jamaica, West Germany, and several other countries where they could be treated with substances not yet approved by American medical orthodoxy. Their plight grabbed most of the headlines: stretcher cases arriving in San Diego for the dusty trip to any of five "alternative therapy" clinics in Tijuana; just barely ambulatory East Coasters making it to the Fairfield Medical Centre in Jamaica for the enzyme-based metabolic therapy there; the more affluent—if castoff—Americans dumping thousands into round trip flights and lengthy stays in Western Europe for treatment at any of several spas.

Yet cancer sufferers are far from being the only victims of American orthodoxy, governmental bungling and bureaucratic blindness. In October 1978 *Newsweek* reported the situation of Diantha Ain of Simi Valley, California, who suffered so much pain from a ruptured spinal disk that she was scarcely able to walk. In the U.S., the only way out for her would have been a drastic, four-hour operation to remove the disk and fuse her spine into position using pieces of bone removed from her pelvis. Luckily, a physician put her onto an unorthodox approach and she went to Vancouver, Canada, for an injection of chymopapain to shrink the ruptured disk. She was able to walk out of the hospital the next day. She could not get chymopapain injections in the United States because the substance was not "approved." (See *Note,* page 86.)

Bernard S. Abrams, a Columbus, Ohio physicist, flew his six-year-old daughter Felice to England in 1977 to receive sodium valproate, the only medication that could control her epileptic seizures. Abrams then successfully campaigned on behalf of epilepsy victims to get the drug onto the U.S. market, where it had long been banned by the Food and Drug Administration.

The FDA has also blocked the introduction of beclomethasone, a revolutionary asthma remedy, readily available in other countries. The same was true for bethanidine, minoxodil and oral diazoxide for severe hypertension, a host of substances for crippling rheumatoid arthritis, chenodeoxycholic acid for gallstones, verapimil for heart disease, lactulose for liver disease, and carbenoxolone for ulcers. To say nothing of the all-out efforts to bar chelating agents in the treatment of heart disease (see chapter ten) and certain vitamin preparations.

Drugs for high blood pressure, asthma, arthritis, tuberculosis, and many other ailments have been available in other countries for as many as nine years before being okayed for use in the United States. Says Los Angeles cardiologist Dr. Melvyn Ellestad, "It's a national scandal that our patients are deprived of lifesaving drugs available elsewhere in the world."

So great has the gap become between the introduction of needed medicines in America and those available elsewhere, particularly in Europe, that Congress and the FDA are hearing a great deal about the "drug lag"—now manifest in these figures: the average number of "new chemical entities" approved annually by the FDA was forty-three before 1962; since then it has sagged to sixteen. As an example, four times as many drugs were introduced in the decade 1962-1972 in Great Britain as in the United States. The average cost to drug-producing companies to comply with paperwork on each new "chemical entity" ballooned from $1.2 million before 1962 to $12 million thereafter. And the average amount of paperwork required for each new "entity" has likewise increased considerably, from about seventy-five pages to 75,000—with some reports of up to 200,000 now occurring—this amount of verbiage literally delivered by the truckload to FDA officials.

The Pharmaceutical Manufacturers Association estimates that it takes approximately $55 million and about five years to get a new drug developed and approved by the FDA, a statistic which, more than any other, explains why only the giant drug companies, often linked in an international pharmaceutical cartel, bother to make the attempt. And pity the backers of a substance, such as the abundant chemical amygdalin (laetrile), on whose extract there is no meaningful patent, no meaningful way, through the profits inherent in patent ownership, of recovering the enormous investment in time and money for product development.

The average annual percentage of such entities approved by the FDA coming from non-American sources soared from 30 percent before 1962 to 63 percent since. The average time required for the FDA to act on a new drug application has also zoomed, from seven months to twenty-seven months, with the total often being many years.

The reason for all this, of course, is the Food, Drug and Cosmetic Act as amended in 1962. Enacted on the heels of the thalidomide scare, the 1962 amendments specified that all drugs could no longer be marketed simply after being proved safe; they must also be described as effective—something normally done only on the basis of extensive animal and limited, controlled human tests. The Food and Drug Act also carries with it such a plethora of red tape and complications that physicians around the country have found themselves in bureaucratic hot water if they use a medicine for something other than that specified in its "package insert."

Most observers of the U.S. drug scene note that had penicillin, aspirin, insulin, and digitalis been introduced after 1962, they would still be waiting to clear the FDA regulations. What it all amounts to is a serious drug lag, one in which Americans are denied the substances they need and, unable to finance treatment abroad, are destined to suffer and die at home. This is such a shameful state of affairs that the FDA and its enabling legislation are now under severe congressional scrutiny.

The direct effects of the Food, Drug and Cosmetic Act have been the elimination of medical competition from the marketplace, the notorious drug lag, and an increase in the operations of the FDA—which now cost taxpayers about $1 billion a year—and a geometric increase in suffering and death. It has been estimated that twenty-four times the number of Americans who died in Vietnam expired at home because of the amended food and drug law.

The President's Biomedical Research Panel, which convened in 1974 to report on the National Institutes of Health, concluded, "There is a different kind of hazard to public health, posed by the prolonged delays and great costs of developing new and potentially useful drugs which the FDA's own protective system has imposed. In some respects, the agency has become a formidable roadblock."

For example, according to the *Congressional Record* for 21 July 1976, a man from Louisiana

> devised a product which is useful in filling decayed and abscessed teeth. According to dentists using the product, they would have been unable to save the teeth without the product. Because the cost of obtaining an NDA [New Drug Application] approval was too great for this single innovator, he reached an agreement with a nearby dental school to have their researchers conduct the testing. However, FDA refused to grant this innovator an IND [Investigational New Drug application] despite the clinical data he had been able to obtain. Without the IND, the dental school will not touch the product. The

upshot of this is that the product will be manufactured and marketed overseas. Americans will have to do without it, perhaps indefinitely.

In the same *Congressional Record,* Idaho's then Rep. Steve Symms, the author of key legislation to reform the FDA, bared the plight of a small drug company in Georgia:

> They manufacture heparin sodium injection, which is an anticoagulant that has been on the market since the mid-1930's. The major use of the drug now is for open heart surgery and in maintaining life for kidney dialysis patients. All companies manufacturing the product had to submit new drug application data.
> They [the companies] were not able to pool their resources for a combined NDA. This small firm had to cough up $10,000 to, in their words, "tell the FDA officials, most of them completely inept, what the drug did, how it worked, and why it was safe. Now this is something that people in pharmacy, medicine and nursing already know, and we found it difficult to translate the information to the officials of the FDA."

Not only that, but simply to comply with red tape, FDA regulations have required such items as storing bottlecaps twenty-four inches from walls, cleaning toilet facilities in a specified manner, filing eighteen sets of reports along with quarterly reports and summaries, maintaining written records regarding the cleaning of laboratory beakers, maintaining housing space for test animals whether or not the drug company involved does its own animal toxicity studies or even *keeps* animals, etc., etc.

The result of all this is not only the evils of drug lag and the removal of competition, but the creation of a super bureaucracy that, like all bureaucracies, not only eventually gets chummy with the very industry it is supposed to be monitoring, but also has the effect of interfering with the first sacred tenet of medicine, the privacy of the physician-patient relationship itself. It has taken expensive federal court cases by doctors and patients seeking access to freedom of choice in medicine to establish what should be a mother's-milk bit of wisdom: Congress never intended the FDA and the Food and Drug Act to interfere with the practice of medicine.

A 1969 congressional study showed that thirty-seven of forty-nine top FDA officials who left the agency took jobs with food and drug companies—that is, members of the two industries the FDA is expected to monitor. Also, the General Accounting Office in 1975 found that 150 FDA officials had violated the government's own "conflict of interest" rules by owning stock in the companies the FDA is supposed to regulate! These facts lead even the least paranoid among us to wonder just how honest the federal regulatory agency can be about food and drug monopolies.

A peek at how the federal agency works was provided in testimony on 19 April 1976 before the Panel of New Drug Regulations of the Department of Health, Education and Welfare by Dr. Richard Crout, then director of the FDA's Bureau of Drugs:

> I want to describe to you the agency as I saw it. No one knew where anything was. There was an enormous documents room—I don't know whether you believe it or not, but this was a place where people said fights went on in a literal sense. There was absenteeism; there was open drunkenness by several employees, which went on for months; there was intimidation internally; and there was a great deal of what I would call feudalism in bureaucracy. I can tell you that, in my first year at the FDA... going to certain kinds of meetings was an extraordinarily peculiar kind of exercise. People—I'm talking about Division directors and their staffs—would engage in a kind of behavior that invited insubordination; people tittered in the corners, throwing spitballs—now I'm describing physicians; people would slouch down in their chairs and not respond to questions; and moan-and-groan, the sleeping gestures. This was a kind of behavior I have not seen in any other institution from a grown man....FDA has a long-term problem with the recruitment of personnel, good, scientific personnel....

And John O. Nestor, a pediatrician with the FDA who spoke out against deficiencies in the agency, told Senate investigators as early as 1963, or just after the Food, Drug and Cosmetic Act was amended, that the FDA "worked too closely with the giant drug companies to be effective."

When FDA is not barring useful drugs, or preventing the use of one "cleared" substance in a situation for which it was not originally licensed, it seems to revel in writing scripts for the Silly Season, based primarily on the American obsession with animal tests. For example, gigantic quantities of saccharine administered to animals in doses equivalent to a human's ingestion of 800 to 1,000 cans of diet soda every day for many years resulted in scattered cases of bladder cancer in the poor animals. This led the FDA to announce a ban on saccharine in 1977—a move which endangered thousands of diabetics and obese people. The Swiss Medical Association promptly noted that "saccharine has helped countless people to avoid obesity and has aided diabetics marvelously for decades....Because it is to be banned on the basis of a scientifically baseless test order and a wrong interpretation of results the FDA has lost credibility on both sides of the ocean."

The FDA has pursued a similar line with its flip-floppery over cyclamates. And the federal government as a whole, aided and abetted by then President Gerald Ford, was left with scientific egg on its face by panicking Americans into swine flu vaccinations, dozens of them proving fatal, as a response to a threat which turned out to be nonexistent.

And when the FDA is not banning helpful remedies and preparations, it seems actually able to rush onto the market products from certain companies—in some cases substances for cancer therapy that may actually *cause* the disease. (For proof, see chapter five.)

Also, should a substance prove too popular, particularly when another product, a patented product, is waiting in the wings, the FDA can move fast and furiously. Ponder, for example, the strange cases of ACE (adrenal cortical extract), available in this country under various brand names for fifty years.

ACE has been found useful as a general metabolic product in the management of hypoglycemia, adrenal cortical insufficiency, stress, shock, burns, and in building resistance to viral diseases. It has, thus, been used for a variety of things across the board, especially by those practitioners who consider themselves metabolic therapists. But in January 1978 the FDA suddenly classified ACE as "a new drug in violation of the Federal Food, Drug and Cosmetic Act."

An incensed *small* drug manufacturer told me, "What this all means, of course, is that ACE is a product whose popularity has grown so much that it is now threatening the major drug companies." He warned that the attempt to substitute for ACE—which is nontoxic and relatively inexpensive—synthetic cortisone (cortisone being only one of the fifty or so hormones found in ACE) is a way to enrich at least three major drug producers, while turning hundreds of thousands of Americans into "cortisone addicts." To take the natural product (originally prepared in China 3,000 years ago) off the market and replace it with one or more synthetic products would, he said, produce "a new generation of captive patients for physicians who don't bother to read the printed inserts."

It is known that cortisone has "hooked" or deranged thousands of users and creates a drug dependency worse than that of amphetamines and many other drugs. More than a generation of ACE users, according to metabolic therapists, has never needed to use the steroid drugs usually given to treat the conditions for which

ACE has long wielded dramatic and positive effects.

But the production of synthetic steriod drugs is already a multimillion dollar industry, and although these drugs carry a variety of harmful side effects, dispensing medics are not apt to read the warnings in the inserts after they have been visited and given a pitch by drug company detail men.

After decades of use in this country, ACE suddenly fell under the FDA axe. The "regulatory letter" 8 January 1978 claimed that the federal agency had "reviewed available data concerning the use of adrenal cortex extract...and concluded that the low level of corticosteroid contained in these drugs represents a substantial risk that these serious conditions will be *undertreated*. [Emphasis mine.] These drugs therefore pose a significant potential hazard to patients."

This is one of the few instances I am aware of in which the FDA used the argument of "undertreatment" to bolster its claims of hazard in the use of a compound. Distributors were given ten days to discontinue the marketing of ACE and, failing this, "FDA is prepared to initiate legal action to enforce the law."

If the FDA *was just then* determining ACE's safety and efficacy, it could mean only one thing: it was under pressure from big drug firms to remove from the market a product that substantially cut into their profits. The ACE matter showed how an important tool in metabolic therapy could once again be blocked by giant government operating in the interest of giant business.

I detail the FDA's shenanigans against laetrile in other chapters. So suffice it to say here that with the onset of the victories accorded the apricot seed derivative and the entire area of metabolic therapy in the mid-1970s, FDA "compliance" officers went into a frenzy of activity to attempt to smash the entire metabolic program of which laetrile is only a part. Vials of material, including emsulsified vitamin A, vitamin B[15], and other substances, were tracked down by the FDA across the country and "notices of recommended prosecution" went to firms and individuals involved in the shipment of a whole series of products when it was assumed such items might be used for the metabolic therapy of cancer.

Turning Physicians Into Criminals

The continued federal harassment of distributors, pharmacists and physicians for their use of or trafficking in substances that are construed as "unproven" has the effect of further criminalizing such individuals. The use of chelating agents such as EDTA (see chapter ten) and of the absorption agent dimethyl sulfoxide (DMSO) occasionally landed such people in hot water. Physicians who dared to use a medicine licensed for one malady to treat another were—and are—hounded by their state medical boards with the same venom accorded those who dared to involve their patients with laetrile.

77

The year 1978 included two important court battles that served notice that the FDA had overreached itself. Chelation therapy pioneer Ray Evers and his patients went to court to secure the use of the chemical EDTA and similar agents in cardiovascular (heart) disease even when they had not been "approved for such use. Ohio pharmacist Steve Michaelis, enraged over the seizure from his store of laetrile, peach kernels, laetrile publications, and even $740 of his son's money by federal agents, won a return of these items at the federal court level.

In Montgomery, Alabama, U.S. District Judge Robert E. Varner denied the FDA a temporary restraining order against Dr. Evers, owner of the RaMar Clinic and a long-time champion of chelation therapy. Judge Varner held that a physician may use medicines for purposes other than those that are indicated in the medicine's package insert. In a nineteen-page opinion issued 28 June he observed, "Congress did not intend the Food and Drug Adminstration to interfere with medical practice and the [Food, Drug and Cosmetic Act] did not purport to regulate the practice of medicine as between the physican and his patient."

Dr. Evers' patients had filed suit for injunctive relief and a declaratory judgment that their constitutional right to privacy and their presumptive constitutional right to receive treatment from a physician of their choice by a system of his choice had been violated by the FDA. The federal government had sought its injunction on the grounds that Dr. Evers promoted and administered calcium disodium versenate in the treatment of hardening of the arteries when the substance is "recommended for heavy metal poisons but not for other things," that patients so treated had been "subjected to an unwarranted risk of grave physical injury or death" as a result of the treatment, and that Evers' use and promotion of the drug, after having utilized interstate commerce in obtaining it, amounted to "mislabeling."

Judge Varner denied all these assertions in what stands as a landmark ruling and pointed out, "When physicians go beyond the directions given in the package insert it does not mean they are acting illegally or unethically and Congress did not intend to empower the FDA to interfere with medical practice by limiting the ability of physicians to prescribe according to their best judgment."

A day later, Judge Robert M. Duncan, U.S. District Court, Eastern Division, Southern District of Ohio, ruled that the seizure of material and money from pharmacist Michaelis on 14 July 1977 was not legal. The seizure had occurred after what Judge Duncan called "an intensive, six-month surveillance of Michaelis and his business operations." The pharmacist was a known distributor of amygdalin and a leader in the Committee for Freedom of Choice in Cancer Therapy. At the time of the raid, the FDA sent a dozen agents to his home and store to seize 1,500 vials and 4,000 tablets of laetrile, as well as ten cases of peach kernels and a stack of laetrile-related publications. They also stole $740 of his son's money, an irate Michaelis charged.

Judge Duncan ruled, in an opinion that sent reverberations through the FDA and may have slowed its 1978 crackdown on amygdalin distribution within the United States: "The validity of the July 14 search and seizure of plaintiff's property...depends upon the validity of the preceding searches of his packages at various common carriers" in Columbus, Cincinnati, and Hebron, Ohio. "Whether the search is characterized as administrative or criminal, it is emcompassed by the Fourth Amendment. The governing principle...is that 'except in certain carefully defined classes of cases, a search of private property without proper consent is unreasonable unless it has been authorized by a valid search warrant....' " He then went on to say that "the manufacture and distribution of food and drugs has not yet been specifically held to be among these exceptionally regulated industries to be included, however, this Court does not believe that the searchers at issue in this case are authorized by statute."

Indeed, should the courts let stand the FDA's interpretation of U.S. Code 21374 (a)—the legal loophole whereby the FDA conducts such raids—then "the statute on its face would authorize the inspection of any place thought by FDA agents to contain the regulated articles without a showing to anyone that the place bears a relation to the industries subject to inspection under the [Food, Drug and Cosmetic] Act, or it is reasonable to believe that it is an establishment where drugs are held," analyzed Judge Duncan.

The judge concluded, "This court does not believe that Congress intended to authorize so broad a search. To construe Congress' intentions as urged by the government would require this Court to invalidate the statute as an unconstitutional authorization of unlimited exploratory searches for drugs 'wherever they might be found' in contravention of the Fourth Amendment. Since the construction the government advocates is neither the only possible nor the most likely interpretation of the statutory language, the Court prefers an alternative that will preserve the constitutionality of the statute."

What Judge Duncan seemed to be saying was, "Push USC 21374 (a) any further and it will be thrown out as unconstitutional."

In both the Evers and Michaelis decisions, the FDA received major setbacks and warnings that it had gone too far as a federal regulatory agency. These court victories for laetrile and EDTA took long steps toward forcing the FDA back into constitutional bounds. But until it is reformed stem-to-stern it will still represent both the policing wing of international vested drug interests and a bumbling, bureaucratic stumbling block to medical innovation in this country, for which thousands of Americans will pay a ghastly price in death and suffering.

The American Medical Association: Guilty as Charged

In the summer of 1978, Nobel Prize-winning economist Milton Friedman, a former presidential advisor, went so far as to directly accuse the FDA and the American Medical Association of hampering the healthy growth of medicine in America. He also called the FDA a "killer" because its restrictions have kept life-saving drugs from reaching ailing Americans. He claimed that "some 100,000 Americans died last year because the heart drugs used in some other countries have not yet been FDA-approved."

In this candid lecture at the Mayo Clinic, Friedman stunned his audience by arguing that physicians should not be licensed and that it has been by governmental intrusion into medicine that the AMA medical monopoly has grown and prospered in the United States, much to the detriment of health care. "The control over that [medical] licensure procedure is what has enabled the American Medical Association to exercise its monopoly power for these many decades," he said, anticipating by a year the Federal Trade Commission ruling against the AMA, and adding that his opinion was based on "considerable evidence, considerable examination of the effects" of the licensing procedures of state boards and the monopolistic practices of the AMA. "You cannot have an open field and an elimination of these monopolistic restrictions unless you eliminate the power of government at that crucial element. If we continue with the licensure of medical practice, then either government or organized medicine is going to have monopoly power in the future."

Eliminating the licensing of physicians and reducing the power of both the AMA and the government would "provide for better medical care, more widely available, at lower cost to the bulk of the people. It is the only effective way of preventing what seems to be a flood-tide toward the complete socialization of medicine," Dr. Friedman warned.

In October 1980 a U.S. Court of Appeals upheld an extensive ruling a year earlier by the Federal Trade Commission that the American Medical Association—educator, arbiter, controller, and spokesman for "orthodox" modern medicine in this country—was guilty of "conspiracy to restrain competition" and that through AMA pressure "new methods of health care have been discouraged, restricted, and in some instances, eliminated."

The FTC documentation and ruling, and the upholding of the ruling on appeal by the AMA, was the most serious propaganda setback in the 132 years of AMA's tangled history. And it came at a time when the AMA, after decades of open-throttle control over the practice of American medicine, was beginning to lose its grip.

The August 1980 issue of *Private Practice* noted that in 1979, AMA membership represented only 39 percent of the nation's practicing physicans, down from more than half in 1970, and that only 18 percent of women physicians and 28 percent of foreign medical graduates belonged. In 1981, according to Ralph Nader's Health Research Group, only 45 percent of all American doctors (down from 60 percent at one time) belonged to the AMA. The Group's Dr. Sidney Wolfe said the AMA was by then only "getting about one-third of the doctors graduating from medical schools to sign up now. I think it's slowly dying, and as far as I'm concerned, the sooner the better."

At the same time, a poll for the American Osteopathic Association (AOA) of 1,008 respondents, conducted by a division of Lou Harris and Associates, showed that 60 percent of those surveyed agreed that people were losing faith in their doctors and 49 percent rated the country's health-care system as fair to poor.

The same poll, which more than offset a positive AMA-sponsored study in 1979, found that substantial numbers of people believe American doctors are indifferent, uncommunicative, charge too much, do not properly explain things, are not really interested in getting to know their patients and overprescribe drugs.

In an era of fragmented, specialized medicine, the AOA-Harris poll showed that most people think there are enough doctors in the country but that 72 percent believe there is a shortage of GPs [general practitioners], physicians people tend to see as less expensive, more flexible, and friendlier than specialists.

In the Appeals Court ruling, the justices said that the evidence before them showed that the AMA "directed and conspired with" the Connecticut State Medical Society and the New Haven County Medical Assoication to restrain advertisement of its individual doctors' services.

The FTC's blistering findings against the AMA included these:

> • The record...is overwhelming in establishing the anti-competitive effects of AMA's ethical restrictions, their economic motivations and their consequent harm to the public interest.
> The ethical restrictions which the medical societies have imposed heavily tip the balancing scales against the needs of the public in favor of the maintenance of the financial security of physicians.
> • The record evidence establishes the existence of conspiracy between the AMA and its constituent and component medical societies.... To find otherwise than that the AMA and state and local medical societies were engaged in a conspiracy to restrain competition would be to ignore an abundance of evidence to the contrary. The record evidence contains a more than sufficient quantum of inde-

pendently admissible evidence to establish the existence of the conspiracy.
  • New methods of health care have been discouraged, restricted and, in some instances, eliminated.
  • The record evidence establishes with clear conviction that AMA has prevented the dissemination of truthful, objective information that could provide substantial benefits to the public.

Like most of the other parts of the American medical miasma, the AMA, spawned out of the efforts of professional medical men to build order out of chaos and to oppose homeopathy is another one of those good ideas gone wrong.

What first AMA President Nathaniel Chapman had pompously styled an assemblage which "presents a spectacle of moral grandeur delightful to contemplate" in 1848 was written off exactly 100 years later by President Harry S. Truman as "just another mean trust."

The AMA grew out of the reality that charlatans, quacks, street-corner medics and proliferating, uncontrolled schools of medicine were victimizing the American public. The attempt to impose standards and rout out quackery, as was the case with the original Food and Drug act, was mostly meritorious and well-intentioned.

But absolute power corrupts absolutely, as the aphorism goes, and with centralized medical licensing and educational support came centralized compliance. Too, the unstoppable marriage of convenience between drug companies and centralized medicine provided an administrative/legislative juggernaut which lined the pockets of the medical profession while vastly expanding the profit potential of the drug empire.

Along the way, unwanted or challenging approaches to drug-based or allopathic medicine had to be ground out. Centralized medicine, which has taken on the cloak of state-mandated medicine, has been able to draft laws in every state which have had the effect of protecting the allopathic medical and drug monopolies while blocking or thwarting anything which stood in their way.

This combination has waged ceaseless war on all other schools of medicine, leading the layman to believe there really *is* only one school of medicine—the AMA kind, which is to say *allopathy,* a word rarely heard. The AMA allopaths have come to a *modus vivendi* with osteopaths, whom they opposed before, but continue to do brutal battle against chiropractic, naturopathy, and homeopathy.

The degree of entrenched bias and conspiracy of the AMA against its primary competitor in the medical marketplace, organized chiropractic, surfaced in the matter of five chiropractors who sued the AMA charging violations of the antitrust laws of the United States.

In 1981 a trial in the long and complicated action brought into the record an incredible series of AMA confidential memoranda which clearly set forth the medical monolith's stated goals as they referred to chiropractic: "first, the containment of chiropractic and, ultimately, the elimination of chiropractic." The memoranda are replete with phrases such as "the chiropractic menace" and descriptions of chiropractors as "cultists."

Later, the New York Attorney General's suit against AMA resulted in a ruling that henceforth doctor members of the AMA could freely associate with chiropractors "without fear of sanctions from the AMA," and that the AMA must recognize the physician's right to refer patients to chiropractors and to accept referrals from chiropractors.

In the meantime, the tyrants of medical education and medical licensing suffered a severe propaganda loss as the public, raised to a fever pitch over the dangers inherent in cigarette smoking, was informed that AMA held $1.4 million in tobacco company stocks. The situation had become ludicrous: AMA doctors grudgingly joining the American Cancer Society and medicine in general in damning the use of cigarettes while the association itself made money off a stock portfolio including R. J. Reynolds and Philip Morris. Finally, in late 1981, AMA divested itself of the stock, a spokesman admitting that "the publicity hurt."

In this decade, AMA, as a pivotal member of the Club, is as panicky in overracting to chiropractic—and continuing to deny Americans medical freedom of choice—as it is in damning laetrile and all it represents (natural management of cancer) as well as chelation and all *it* represents (nonsurgical treatment and prevention of cardiovascular disease).

Winds of Change?

Strong opposition to the FDA's control of new drug development in this country is what led small drug manufacturers, many physicians and a host of congressman to lend support to measures introduced in the 1970s to amend the Food, Drug and Cosmetic Act, particularly bills authored by then Rep. Steve Symms and Sen. Jesse Helms, and later by Rep. Larry McDonald. The essence of this freedom of choice legislation was to remove the "efficacy" clauses from the act. It is the requirement that efficacy be proven that is the roadblock which bars thousands of drugs and medicines from the American market and which greatly expands the FDA's regulatory powers, saddling drug developers with a sea of paperwork and prohibitive expenditures.

As physicians correctly see it, the demand that efficacy be shown transfers to government edict what ought to be the province of the practitioner. *Only* the physician and patient, working together, can really ever know whether a medicine is "working" in a

83

particular case. No amount of animal tests, recommended daily allowances, or stereotyped dose levels can ever settle the issue.

Proponents of the FDA position consistently harp on the thalidomide crisis of the late 1950s as *the* reason for the amendment to the law. Truth to tell, the injestion by pregnant mothers of thalidomide had indeed left a wake of deformed babies across Europe. Yet the reality is that the dimensions of the tragedy were first studied and reported in Europe at a time when American medical orthodoxy was on the way to licensing thalidomide, and only a single researcher within the FDA was heatedly anti-thalidomide. That is to say, the tragedy of thalidomide was reported and known about before the American Establishment had to act on the issue. It was a "victory" for which the FDA could take little credit. But reforming the nation's food and drug regulatory agency to equip it to demand efficacy was hardly the solution to a problem of safety, and few Americans would deny the federal agency the right to be concerned with product safety.

Despite broad support for FDA reform legislation, a single legislator single-handedly blocked efforts to get such bills to the floor for a full vote. By the time it was obvious that the Symms and Helms bills had something approaching majority support, the Carter administration countered with a sham "FDA reform bill," offered to confuse the issue. While the outcome of the national debate on food and drug regulation is far from over, and indeed entered a new dimension under the Reagan administration, the hand of massive vested interests in both the pharmaceutical and processed food concerns is only slightly veiled in efforts to head off authentic reform.

There is, of course, something to be said for a society wishing to protect its consumers against medical and pharmaceutical fraud. Whether we like it or not, the FDA has been designed, in part, to do just that. When the regulatory organization was established shortly after the turn of the century, it was indeed a response to need—the control and monitoring of unrelieved medical and pharmaceutical hucksterism that as often as not promoted poisons and polluted substances to a guileless public. But like so many good intentions, the "cure" of the FDA has become worse than the "disease" it was originally designed to combat. Witness the federal agency's lengthy, and ultimately losing, struggles to control the dose level of vitamins. It took a battle of almost a decade and a half for consumer groups, particularly the National Health Federation, to win the unhampered right to over-the-counter vitamins against a sea of propaganda about the presumed dangers of vitamin A and vitamin D, which, in mammoth and unreasonable doses, like anything else, *can* cause negative reactions. The FDA has since attempted to reassert its authority in this area.

Enter the Killer Diseases

One could reasonably expect the payoff of the rush to overprotect ourselves in the health field would be a healthier, more vibrant people. But this is hardly the case. More and more Americans are being struck down at earlier ages than ever before with degenerative diseases, that is, pathological conditions not so much caused *by* something as by the *lack* of something. It is obvious that the killer infectious and parasitical diseases, still the priority health concerns in the less advanced countries, have been replaced in the West by degenerative disease, primarily cardiovascular disease and cancer. But vast segments of the population have undiagnosed or barely perceptible hypoglycemia and hypertension (early-warning signals of calamities to come), arthritis in several forms, and a variety of degenerative ailments for which there are no known cures. The nation's toll from heart disease and cancer now surpasses 1.5 million victims a year, with hardening of the arteries showing up at ever-lower ages and cancer now representing the major killer of children fourteen and under.

Has the protection of drug-based medicine by the FDA and the government's efforts to overprotect us—quite aside from the scandal of the drug lag—resulted in greater longevity and greater overall health? Many people think not. Even the earlier triumphs over infectious disease by antibiotics were secured, in the main, after the diseases themselves had "peaked out." The advent of insulin, far from forcing diabetes statistics lower, parallels the almost geometric increase in the incidence of that malady. Ivan Illich holds that physicians have been given far too much credit for disease control, and he argues forcefully that institutionalized medicine is now one of the major hazards to the nation's health. Many others agree with him.

Illich notes that *maximum* lifespan has not changed in the U.S.—it still hovers around sixty-five despite every new advance in medical technology—even though *average* lifespan has. This is because more children survive in the Western world, no matter how sickly, deformed, or in need of special care and artificial environments they may be. In fact, it may be said that American babies are *forced* to survive, and in the service of this survival all the most complicated gadgetry a technological society can bring to bear is utilized. The fact that the vast majority of babies survive colors life expectancy statistics.

The "diseases of civilization" now kill as many people as succumbed to pneumonia and other infections generations ago, a reality that, when coupled with accidents, causes a stabilization of life expectancy levels for those in wealthier countries between ages fifteen and forty-four. There may be more "senior citizens" around, but the quality of their lives is hardly something to shout about. Sophisticated equipment forces the aged and infirm to survive, even against their will, down to the last electronically traceable vital sign. It is an open question how many of the stricken elderly, surviving in clinic beds attached to expensive machinery and with tubes dangling from them, can be said to be "living."

In my frequent visits to the Philippines, I have often been struck by high infant mortality in the countryside. It is safe to say that it is a real battle for a tiny Filipino to make it to age five. Not provided the technology the West has to offer, the ill-equipped baby is simply not going to make it. Yet, the dramatic difference is that if the child makes it to age five, something virtually taken for granted in America, he has a far better chance of making it to eighty-five without being visited by one or more of the killer diseases.

My visits to villages in Luzon and Mindanao have turned up case after case of centenarians, octogenarians, and other oldsters enjoying life outside the confines of an old peoples' home—people still spry and usually with good vision and without the drastic effects of heart disease, cancer, and intermediate ailments. "Quality of life" is measured not only in years.

As Illich has noted, "Medicine just cannot do much for the illness [in America] associated with aging. It cannot cure cardiovascular disease, most cancers, arthritis, advanced cirrhosis, not even the common cold. It is fortunate that some of the pain the aged suffer can be lessened. Unfortunately, though, most treatment of the old requiring professional intervention not only tends to heighten their pain but, if successful, also to protract it."

So what has America bought by overprotecting itself in the disease field? The answer would seem to be: a worse problem than the one it started out to solve.

Note: In November 1982 the FDA finally approved chymopapain for the kind of back problems discussed here. On October 19, 1982, the *Federal Register* published forty-five pages of recommended reforms in the FDA, the Reagan Administration's delivery on promises to trim this federal regulatory agency and its activities. While the proposals were Administration-backed recommendations only and some would need legislation to enforce, the constituted the most thorough attempt at overhauling the FDA in twenty years. Legislation to remove "efficacy" from the Food, Drug and Cosmetic Act had still not been approved as this book went to press.

Chapter Four
The American Food Disaster—
Culprit Number One

Challenge At The Check-Out Counter

In October 1979 the National Cancer Institute (NCI) stunned much of the medical community by announcing that Americans could markedly reduce their risk of getting cancer by eating less, by ingesting a balanced, low-fat, high-fiber diet, and by drinking only moderate amounts of alcohol.

The double take by many physicians was because, just a few years before, the nation's cancer orthodoxy, reflected in NCI leadership, ridiculed the very idea that there are definite links between cancer and diet, a line argued by the metabolic/nutritional "quacks" for decades.

In 1980, researchers at Sloan-Kettering in New York demonstrated that dietary manipulation enchanced longevity and the immune system, and prevented cancer in cancer-prone laboratory animals.

A 1979 Canadian study found that more than half of cancer in humans is related to diet and suggested that vitamins C and E may provide some protection against cancer-causing nitroso compounds in processed foods.

In 1977 the Senate Select Committee on Nutrition and Human Needs released a report that covered more than a year of hearings. Called *Dietary Goals for the United States,* the volume urged Americans to cut down on the very things they most love to eat, red meat, soft drinks, candy, baked goods, potato chips, and pretzels. All of this because, chairman George McGovern told a news conference, "too much fat, too much sugar or salt can be and are linked directly to heart disease, cancer, obesity, and stroke among other killer diseases."

However belated, this was the first official American report that directly linked degenerative disease with the nation's eating habits and recommended steps to deal with the problem. Even so, the report, the result of prodigious input from many experts, was not without its problems. The first version reportedly asked Americans to "decrease consumption of meat and increase consumption of poultry and fish." The changed version read: "decrease consumption of animal fat, and choose meat which will reduce saturated fat intake." Pressure from the livestock lobby was suspected in the change of phraseology.

A year later, the Senate committee also had to cope with opposition from the sugar, dairy, canning, egg, and beef-raising interests when it advised Americans to reduce their intake of processed sugar, salt, and eggs and to substitute skim milk for whole milk.

The American Medical Association, not surprisingly, was on hand to claim that there is no proof that diet is related to disease(!) and to warn that changing American eating habits might lead to economic dislocation. Stunned observers wondered whether the AMA was more interested in the state of the food-processing industry than in the nation's health.

The AMA's opinion, though, should not have amazed anyone. As the institutionalized voice of drug-based medicine, the AMA has been a vital force against any move that would tend to get Americans out of the hospitalization-and-visit-your-doctor syndrome. It correctly senses that an identification with the national food problem is a direct attack on the economics of the "health-care delivery system"—the sick business. If the major component in the sick business is degenerative disease, and the major preventive factor in degenerative disease is dietary and food reform, there is at least an implied threat to the sick business and its enormous backup system, the pharmaceutical cartel.

For years, the AMA and food-processing companies have been telling the American people that they are the healthiest and best-fed on earth, that they get all the nutrients they need with a "balanced diet." Even vitamin and mineral supplements are not needed, runs this standard Establishment line, unless there is a specific, recognized, pathological condition or deficiency to be treated.

Hence, neither the food-processing industry nor the medical Establishment was happy with the 1977 Senate report and its annual followups since then. Yet the report was actually timid. For decades preventive medicine had noted links between degenerative disease and food, and the reality is that evidence of that connection has been rising geometrically for the past several years.

The 1978 report stated, again, that cancer, heart disease, diabetes, and hypertension are associated with the American diet, stopping just short of claiming they are *caused* by the diet. That was prudent because at this time, while we can see the links between the food problem and disease, we cannot dismiss other factors as well. The health-food faddists who are committed to the "you are what you eat" school of logic, a perspective 180 degrees removed from the AMA position that food has very little to do with degenerative disease, are probably closer to the truth than they know, but they do overlook the genetic inheritance aspect of human health. Dr. R. O. Brennan of Texas, founder of the International Association of Preventive Medicine, is among those aware of the genetic factor. It is his reasoned view that nutrition and existing genetic predispositions determine disease susceptibility. He has called this fusion of factors *nutrigenetics* (see his *Nutrigenetics,* M. Evans, N.Y., 1975).

Dr. Mark Hegsted, professor of nutrition at Harvard and one of the three nutritionists who helped prepare the 1977 Senate report, told the media, "There undoubtedly will be many people who will say we have not proven our point; we have not demonstrated that the dietary modifications we recommend will yield the dividends expected." In any event, if the report's recommendations were followed by most Americans, the authors agreed, a number of food manufacturers would be forced to cut back on or drastically alter the nature of their products.

The report recommended a decrease in sugar, salt, meat, and other foods high in fat and cholesterol and suggested Americans increase their consumption of fruits, vegetables, and whole grain products, precisely the recommendations made for years by physicians involved in metabolic therapy and preventive medicine. The report noted that Americans took in more than 100 pounds per year per capita of refined sugar (the unofficial figure was closer to 130 pounds per person per year) compared to 76 pounds in 1900. It called for a 40 percent reduction in sugar consumption and added that "the most obvious item for general reduction is soft drinks."

It also called for a 50 to 85 percent reduction in salt consumption (overconsumption of salt has long been linked to hypertension), noting that we can get all the salt we need without actually adding the refined product to our diet, just as all the sugar the body needs is available in natural forms in foods without there being the slightest need for addition of the refined product to the foods we eat.

The report also called for a 10 percent reduction in overall fat intake and the replacement of some unsaturated fat with polyunsaturated and mono-unsaturated fats. This was in response to growing evidence that the human body is not designed to handle— that is, metabolize—the enormous amounts of animal fat that the "affluent" diet contains.

By the beginning of this decade, the U.S. Department of Agriculture had available a monograph (*Benefits of Human Nutrition Research)* which told readers that improved American nutrition could reduce heart attacks and vascular diseases by 25 percent, respiratory and infectious diseases by 20 percent, mental health disabilities by 10 percent, infant deaths by 50 percent, dental disease by 50 percent, prevent or improve diabetes by 50 percent and reduce osteoporosis by 75 percent. But, as California physician Stephen E. Langer, M.D., found in 1981: "To the best of my knowledge, this monograph was only printed in limited quantities (5,000 copies) and very shortly after publication went out of the print. It is inexcusable for anyone to downgrade optimal nutrition in the treatment of illness."

Unhappily for Americans, part of the conservative sweep in 1980 which brought more legislators in favor of medical freedom of choice into office also brought with it an even greater de-emphasis on dietary aspects of disease, particularly where important lobbying groups (dairy, poultry, beef interests, for example) were concerned.

There is nothing more subtle than the scope and nature of the American food disaster, primarily because things don't *look* as bad as they are. The American teenager, for example, has been growing in height and weight since the beginning of the century. The typical American teen looks ruddy-cheeked, well-built, and energetic when compared to the scrawnier specimens of under developed countries. For years, the "Gerber Baby" was rendered on millions of baby food labels as a fat, rosy-cheeked, smiling cherub, conveying the implicit message that a fat baby is a healthy baby—particularly when compared to the weak-looking offspring one might find in an emerging tropical country.

The vast majority of Americans have been weaned on what some call the meat-and-potatoes diet, high in animal protein and starch and garnished with "junk" foods, products actually devoid of most of their actual nutrients and yet "filling" in the sense of leaving the consumer with the feeling of "having eaten." We have been taught that "milk has something for everybody" and consume vast amounts of this tampered-with natural liquid. The three-egg breakfast with coffee and white bread toast is commonplace. The school and office snackbars are part of the American tradition.

Well, we *look* healthier—as long as we are in our teens, our twenties, and, to some degree, our thirties. Beyond that, the picture changes drastically. The first brushes of pot-bellied young executives with heart disease usually occur in the late thirties or early forties, with heart disease problems only reaching the clinical stage when they are advanced. For example, a heart attack is not apt to occur until there has been widespread shutting down of the body's circulatory system.

But with expensive drugs, dilating agents and the like, our technology allows us to keep the heart-attack-prone citizen alive, even if he does not change his eating, drinking, and smoking habits. If he makes it, somehow, through his fifties, he will become a statistical candidate for clinically observable cancer. If he possibly survives through the "early retirement years" without dying from heart disease, then prostatic cancer, which the vast majority of over-65 American men have, will eventually get him.

Women seem to be a heartier race. Statistically, they may avoid more observable heart disease in their early-middle years, and they will probably outlive their mates even while suffering from cardiovascular ills—that is, if they have survived the critical middle-age period in which breast cancer has become the number-one killer of women.

The fact is, Americans consume a "football player's diet" in terms of the nature and amounts of the food they take in. Were we all in our early twenties and playing football every day, a case might be made for the healthy nature of that diet as long as junk foods were not too large a component. But when Americans stop burning off the calories and enter their middle years with sedentary jobs and without changing their eating habits, they simply become prime targets for degenerative disease.

In *How You Can Beat the Killer Diseases,* Dr. Harper and I made the case for the fact that Americans are the most overfed, yet undernourished, people on earth, even though the food situation in the United Kingdom is even worse. Dr. Harper's thesis, now seconded by many metabolic physicians, is that the degenerative diseases are all interlinked, whatever names we give them—arthritis, arteriosclerosis, cancer, heart disease, stroke, schizophrenia, alcoholism, hypertension, diabetes—and that the early-warning system in identifying the problem is the body's inability to metabolize refined carbohydrates, primarily refined sugar. This early-warning stage, *glucose metabolism dysfunction* (GMD), which is rarely diagnosed, will almost certainly become hypoglycemia, or low-blood sugar, an ailment which until recently the AMA even denied existed. Hypoglycemia's links to the degenerative disease states in general is now relatively accepted. That a fourth to a third of cancer patients are also diabetic is accepted, and that both schizophrenia and alcoholism may be controlled by diet is ever more apparent.

In 1978, experiments with spider monkeys by a Louisiana researcher showed clearly that a diet similar to the salt-and-sugar-loaded junk foods of American children could produce high blood pressure in the test animals. The evidence seemed to show, said Dr. Gerald S. Berenson of Louisiana State University, that sugar and salt reinforce each other in developing hypertension, or high blood pressure. What most concerned Berenson was that a continuing program he directs, the Bogalusa Heart Study, has found that children in Bogalusa have diets similar to what he fed the test monkeys.

Other studies have suggested connections between "hyperactivity" in children (an increasingly commonplace problem normally "solved" by doping the youngsters with all manner of tranquilizers and other drugs) and junk food, as well as between junk food, excess sugar, and criminal activity. Barbara Reed, chief probation officer in Cuyahoga Falls, a Cleveland suburb, told an autism seminar in 1978 that the majority of the offenders referred to her committed acts of shoplifting and other petty crimes after their judgment became impaired by eating sugared and/or caffeinated foods. Some 82 percent of her referrals had problems with their diets, and hypoglycemia was a major problem, she said.

Reed told of the case of one woman who thought of herself as the very opposite of a junk food addict but whose eating habits provoked problems anyway. She was arrested for shoplifting and she did not remember committing the misdemeanor. "We found out that she was a health nut and ate all the foods with high natural sugar contents like raisins, bananas, dates, plums. A banana immediately caused her to break out in a cold sweat, have blurred vision and feel exhausted," Miss Reed said. "Putting these people behind bars doesn't help. In fact, their conditions worsen because they drink more coffee and eat more sugared foods. We have got to get back on the basics—a good diet."

The path to overall better health and less degenerative disease through abandonment of the "standard American diet" (SAD—an appropriate acronym) was established in 1978 through the unlikely medium of a study of Navy pilots imprisoned by the Vietcong during the Vietnam War. A study at the Navy's Center for Prisoner of War Studies in San Diego strongly indicated that the natural rice and vegetable diets the American men received at the hands of their captors greatly contributed to their long-term physical health, particularly in terms of cardiovascular disease.

John A. Plag, who headed the study, said he compared seventy-eight former POWs with non-POW pilots who had flown missions over Vietnam during the same period as had the POWs. "Each one of the pilots in the control goup was matched with a returned prisoner of war, according to such variables as rank, marital status, years of schooling, and number of flight hours," he said. The control group agreed to undergo annual medical examinations of the same scope and complexity as those given the POWs.

"Contrary to expectations, the control group, the non-POWs, were less healthy," Plag reported. The most significant finding was a higher rate of cardiovascular disease among the non-POWs.

"When shot down many of the POWs were well above their ideal weight," he pointed out. "On the reduced rations of captivity, which undoubtedly were lower in cholesterol and fat than that of the average American diet, many of the POWs fell to their ideal weight and remained at that level....In contrast, the control group members usually had access to an abundant diet high in animal fat, and to alcohol and tobacco, while at the same time undergoing the stresses of their jobs in which only excellent performance was rewarded by promotions."

In addition, autopsies of young Americans killed in both the Korean and Vietnam episodes consistently turned up evidence that even by age twenty-two Americans have arteriosclerosis, hardening of the arteries, even though there are no outward symptoms of the problem. In contrast, similar investigations performed on bodies of Vietcong dead revealed young men free of arteriosclerosis. Their dietary history was one of living off the land and consuming natural whole grains, fruits, and vegetables.

Indeed, there are now cases of American babies being *born* with the early evidence of arterial plaquing, the accumulation of toxic minerals on a fatty bedrock caused by overingestion of refined carbohydrates. Some aborted fetuses reveal such plaquing underway even before birth because the mothers, while "eating for two," were already sugar addicts and did not realize it.

The dietary dilemma is not only an American problem. In fact, *all* the industrialized, technological nations of the Western world, plus Japan, Australia, and New Zealand, are showing similar statistics, even though they are less noticeable in Japan, which, while technologized, tends to adhere to more traditional eating habits.

Wherever mass, urban, industrialized society is predominant, reliance on processed foods is the norm. The great majority of the citizens of such countries do not grow their own food, eat off the land, or even have a hand in the preparation of most of the foods they ultimately consume. By and large the foods we eat are machine-processed and stripped of their natural nutrients, not because of a venal plot by conscious polluters, but as a direct response to the needs of urban civilization. In the interest of preserving food, and also in the interest of food profits, the majority of what we consume is a chemically treated, preserved, emulsified, canned, frozen, or precooked simulation of the real thing. The very treating of foods with chemicals, though in some cases necessary as a health measure, tends to remove their *natural* ingredients.

Man's food technology has ranged geometrically beyond the body's ability to deal with it, and the only wonder in it all is why *more* people in the "civilized countries" don't die faster and younger from the interconnected degenerative disease maladies.

Man has been on the earth for several million years, and in the majority of that time he has been a hunter and gatherer. For a much smaller period of time, he has been a farmer, and only for a fleeting moment of cosmic time has he been a producer of artificial, preserved foods. Living off the land, avoiding starvation, even undergoing ritual fasts, were part of the normal human experience for thousands upon thousands of years. These activities became the "biological experience" of the human race, one genotyped into its biological inheritance. Fruits and vegetables were consumed in their natural, whole state, and grains were only "refined" by pounding them with stones, their natural goodness left intact.

It was the impact of industrialization in Europe and America that brought about the revolution of food production and handling. With the new technology we learned to move away from reliance on a few staples. Suddenly, the quantity, quality, and distribution of food changed. The revolution in the milling of grains and the processing of sugar changed with it, and as this century began, the advent of ever-more-refined foods was paralleled by the growing pandemicity of the so-called diseases of civilization.

Comparisons may be made not only in food but in *life style* between the civilized West and surviving populations and subpopulations that still consume natural, whole grains and fruits and small amounts of meat. In this regard, the Abkhasians of the Soviet Union, the Hunzakuts of Pakistan, the Vilcabamba Indians of Ecuador, the rural peoples of much of Southeast Asia, and the (pre-food-stamp) Indian tribes of the American West are populations marked either by spectacular longevity or lower levels of degenerative disease, or both.

It is also true that these populations are far less prone to the mental factor in degenerative disease—stress—and that they also do not drink industrially polluted water or breathe industrially polluted air, two other big factors in the degenerative disease crisis. But I mention stress, water, and air as lesser factors here because the vital ingredient in setting the stage for the degenerative disease calamity is not nearly so much stress and polluted air and water as it is polluted food.

While these are still other variables to be considered, there is now evidence pointing to diet as our major problem. This is revealed simply by looking at subpopulations within the United States, subpopulations exposed to the stress of modern civilization—and to its polluted water and air. In the 1970s, for example, separate studies turned up an incredible gap in cancer incidence between Seventh Day Adventists in the Los Angeles basin and all the other identifiable groups in that same polluted area. With stress, water, and air accounted for and being approximately the same for all groups, *only* the dietary factor—the general reliance of Adventists on a vegetarian diet and their abstinence from alcohol and smoking—can account for the considerable difference in cancer rates. And the same is true for Utah's Mormons, who are more natural-food-prone and more abstemious from alchohol and tobacco than are their neighbors, and who have appreciably lower rates of cancer.

In 1976, the National Cancer Institutes's Dr. Gio B. Gori testified before the Senate Select Committee on Nutrition and Human Needs on the connection between diet and degenerative disease, mainly cancer. At the time, his was virtually a voice in the wilderness. Only a few other respected researchers, such as Dr.

Ernst Wynder, had been arguing for the need for food reform and establishing the connections between diet and disease. Even as they did so, champions of allopathic medicine were wont to say that "the first sign of quackery" in medicine is drawing any such parallel.

But Dr. Gori, who was later to run into trouble with the NCI for suggesting that there actually are "safe" cigarettes whose consumption in moderate amounts does not present a major medical problem, was on hand in 1976 to testify:

> Nutrition science is coming of age. For years the experimental difficulties in this field have discouraged scientists, who found other subjects more interesting, and, apparently, more fitting to human health.
>
> Indeed, until a few years ago, the role of nutrition in disease was recognized only for certain deficiency syndromes, such as beri-beri, scurvy and rickets, for which rapid nutritional therapies were found. Until recently, many eyebrows would have been raised by suggesting that an imbalance of normal dietary components could lead to cancer and cardiovascular disease. Today, the accumulation of epidemiologic and laboratory evidence in man and animals makes this notion not only possible but certain....
>
> All this evidence is reinforced because many of these coincidences [dietary patterns and disease] have been found to hold not only for cancer alone, but for a variety of other disease as well, notably cardiovascular diseases. This indicates that some common nutritional balance is at play and that the solution of this problem is likely to have a beneficial impact not for cancer alone, but also for a variety of nutrition dependent disease....
>
> Based on this evidence, potential carcinogens present in the enviroment or as food contaminants do not appear likely to play a significant role in the relationship of nutrition and certain forms of cancer ....Rather, it is plausible that nutritional deficiencies and/or excess influence metabolic processes that, after many years of insult, result in the appearance of certain forms of cancer.

Tragically, the established governmental and medical forces have tended to pay little heed to remarks like those of Dr. Gori, who in the same testimony committed the heresey of mentioning that "some recent experiments have suggested the intriguing possibility of using nutrition as a direct form of cancer therapy."

So the nation went its own merry dietary way, consuming, by 1980, about 125 pounds of fat per capita per year, over 120 pounds of sugar in all its forms, and 295, 12-ounce cans of soda per person per year. All-night doughnut and coffee shops competed with major hamburger chains for the right to pollute the American diet further, and promoters of candy-coated cereals dominated the Saturday morning television fare for children—just as promoters of symptom-maskers (aspirin, antacids, laxatives, etc.) dominated many an evening program for adults. "Poison in the morning, cover the symptoms at night," seemed to be the implied message of a good many commercials paid for by either the food-processing or pharmaceutical industries.

But signs of change were occurring by 1981, and they indicated a major wave in the revolution of medical thought beginning to sweep this country. Natural foods and supplements industry profit was reaching multiples of billions of dollars, the bulk vitamin market was exploding with an annual projected growth rate of 10.2 percent per year, and there were indications that the American sweet tooth was finally loosening, a direct response to unpleasant information brought forward by champions of the "new medicine." Indeed, the U.S. Department of Agriculture reported in December 1981 that Americans had consumed in 1981 the lowest amount of refined sugar in their eating and drinking habits since 1946, though the U.S.D.A. did not define "sugar" in precisely the same way as the orthomolecular people do. Certainly the consumption of its deadliest form, sucrose, is showing a much-needed drop.

At the same time, a Knight-Ridder News Service Survey pointed out that more than 60 million Americans were popping vitamin tablets every day and hence stimulating an industry which had ballooned to $1.2 billion annually. As early as 1977, a Harris poll showed that three out of four Americans were concerned about cholesterol in their diets and that two out of five believed they would be healthier if they ate more wholegrain food, fruits, and fish and consumed less sugar, salt, white bread, and coffee.

Sugar Junkies, Sugar Pushers

A flurry of recent books and articles has indicated that the major addiction in America today is not to opiates, stimulants, tranquilizers and the like but to sugar, that is, refined processed *sucrose*, the major refined carbohydrate in the degenerative disease picture. This is because of the well-developed sweet tooth in the Western world, the discovery of how to refine and process sugar, which was originally a luxury item, and the fact that refined sugar is available in many forms aside from the white, crystallized form that we usually think of when we use the term *sugar*.

Sugar is abundant in a host of foods a mother eats while she is pregnant, it is present in amounts of up to 40 percent in baby food, it is in catsup, salad dressing, TV dinners, virtually all major cereals, and shows up under many different labels—corn syrup, corn sweetener, turbo sugar, for example—in addition to its technical names, sucrose, lactose, maltose and fructose, the latter three being its usual forms in nature. It is in jams, jellies, and gelatins, and, of course, is the major component of all candies. It is to be found in all kinds of canned and treated meats and is a primary ingredient in most pastries.

Even if an individual makes a conscious effort to avoid the actual refined white sugar that is found on every restaurant table he cannot avoid absorbing tremendous amounts of the chemical when he consumes food from the supermarket. It is a relatively cheap preservative, hence its close relationship to the food-processing industry, and the fact that the ingestion of a "naked"-calorie food like sugar *does* cause a quick "pick-me-up" has enabled the sugar lobby to make outrageous claims about the necessity and benefits of their product.

In *Nutrigenetics,* Dr. Brennan correctly described sugar as a "metabolic thief," a food that does not contain the ingredients needed for its own metabolization, as most other foods do. The nutrients needed to break down "pure cane sugar," for example, must be "stolen" from other foods or from the body's tissues. This produces an early malnutrition syndrome that the great majority of American physicians are unable to diagnose, and one that many of them still do not admit even exists. Even raw, unprocessed sugar, Dr. Brennan noted, contains one-half of one percent of the presumed daily requirement of vitamin B^1, 1 percent of vitamin B^2, 2 percent of calcium, and 5 percent of iron.

By the time an American baby is born, he is already apt to be a "sugar junkie," dependent on sugar. And there is nothing in his milieu to retard this, but rather a whole constellation of factors encourages it. Many of the foods he receives at home from even the most conscientious mother will be laden with sugar, and the snacks he consumes between meals and at school will be equally contaminated.

The ultimate outcome of overconsumption of sugar is hypoglycemia, whose symptoms are so myriad—ranging from insomnia, vague pains, a feeling of anguish, persistent drowsiness, and general fatigue to dizziness, outright trembling, conscious craving for sugar, and suicidal impulses—that they normally are misdiagnosed or simply missed by examining physicians. Most hypoglycemics, if left untreated, move on to diabetes. Diabetes, if left untreated, can progress to blindness or even death. In fact, the general statistics are that 80 percent of untreated hypoglycemics eventually become diabetics. By that time, of course, the patient has an excellent likelihood of having developed arteriosclerosis, or some form of arterial deposit problem (atherosclerosis) and/or of having incipient cancer.

Five organ systems are involved in the GMD process—pancreas, liver, adrenals, pituitary, and hypothalamus—whose disturbance may reflect itself in a wide variety of ways. Sugar itself is not the problem, for a degree of natural sugar is necessary to the body, which cannot survive without glucose, or blood sugar, available in the appropriate amounts at the appropriate times. But for sugar companies to equate refined *sucrose*, the product, with *glucose*, the natural substance, as an energy-builder, is immoral.

A proper glucose level is vital for the health of every cell in the body. Each cell must be adequately "fed" and must adequately "breathe." Glucose and oxygen, then, are of utmost importance to cellular health; internal cell functions are dependent on adequate amounts of these factors. The levels of nutrients brought into each cell are of key importance to the longevity and overall health of the cell. Sick cells ultimately mean sick people.

When refined sugar or caffeine is ingested, the level of blood sugar, glucose, is raised and the pancreas is stimulated, which causes the release of insulin, a hormone necessary in the metabolism of carbohydrates. The rising insulin forces down the glucose level by causing its transfer across cellular membranes and triggering the conversion of glucose into the storage form of sugar, glycogen, in the liver. But when the glucose level dips to the "fasting level," or the lowest point at which the body can still function normally, the adrenal gland is stimulated to release adrenalin. This causes the blood sugar level to rise as the liver switches glycogen back to glucose.

The continual "challenge" to the system of stimulating it with excessive amounts of refined, nutritionless carbohydrates in the form of sugar and products made from or containing sugar guarantees a continual whipsaw, or roller coaster, effect on the body, one of continuing ups and downs, highs and lows, which come to be perceptible to the victim. When acutal hypoglycemia occurs, the automatic mechanism for glucose metabolism is thrown out of kilter. The overstimulation of the pancreas by excessive amounts of refined carbohydrates—and/or caffeine—causes the release of an excess amount of insulin. This in turn causes the blood sugar level to plunge below the fasting level, which in turn forces the adrenal gland to work overtime in trying to raise the blood sugar level again. The continual carbohydrate overload exhausts the adrenal system, and by then a variety of symptoms is occurring.

At the same time, the ordinary American is also overloading his diet with such amounts of animal protein and animal fat that the body has difficulty ingesting them. Inability to metabolize such material contributes to obesity, as well as pancreatic exhaustion, a probable preliminary stage for cancer. The obesity-diabetes connection is also well established. In an "ordinary" meal, the average American is apt to be pouring in more refined carbohydrates and absorbing more animal protein than he needs. His body can take an abundant amount of this abuse, depending on many factors, until something "gives." It is only then that diabetes, or heart disease, or cancer, or some intermediate or related condition, is diagnosed.

Sugar's considerable contribution to the development of arteriosclerosis resides in its helping create the bedrock, or matrix, in arteries to which toxic minerals are fastened. The result is the buildup of plaque, and the result of that is hardening of the arteries, which brings about a blockage of circulation and the wide spectrum of disastrous results which ultimately ensue.

The addiction to sugar is gradual and subtle, far subtler than the known process of addiction to opiates. The craving for sweets may be masked by a seeming yen for specific forms of sweets, a certain pastry, a certain cola drink. But in extreme hypoglycemia, all the subtleties are cast aside and the outright need to feast on sugar is apparent. I interviewed one girl who described her years-long ordeal with hypoglycemia as a whipsaw from one emotion to another, a zooming from an exhuberant high to a quasi-suicidal low. She intermittently subsisted on candy bars and junk foods. At one of the lowest of her lows, she awoke trembling and dashed to the kitchen to scoop up a cup of white sugar and eat it raw.

The connection between the sudden appearance of sugar or other refined carbohydrates in a culture and violent changes in the culture's temperament has been documented. It is approximately the same as foisting off on nonalcoholic indigenous populations the liquid refined carbohydrate known as alcohol. The results are dramatic and damaging. But in America and most of the Western world, the addiction to sugar has been slow but sure. It is reinforced by every "pusher" imaginable, as Dr. Harper often notes—the candy counter at the corner store, the snack machine in the office or the school gym, even the harried housewife and mother who starts her family's day with a traditional American breakfast and is apt to begin her own with a few cups of coffee, liberally laced with sugar, and a few cigarettes.

In the meantime, the world consumption of sugar has gone up faster than that of any other food—100 percent between 1938 and 1958—with only minimal signs of letup. Of course, if the price of the white stuff jumps to $50 a pound....

The Feeble "Staff of Life"

One of the most disastrous consequences of the Industrial Revolution was a change in the milling of grains. By going from stone mill to machine what had once preserved 85 percent of the whole grain now kept only 25 percent of it or less. The new wheat milling procedure could turn out more flour faster than ever, but it destroyed most of the grain's wheat germ, oil and protein. By removing the grain's outer sheath it stripped away most of the vitamins and minerals necessary for nutritious bread.

The milling process change was as catastrophic as society's moving away from millet, a natural cereal source of many vitamins and minerals, and substituting wheat. But now, the nutrients even of wheat are mostly removed by the new process. What is left is a white, refined flour out of which refined bread is aged, bleached, and preserved with chemicals that further destroy its nutrients. What we now have is, much as with sugar, a quick-energy producer with no long-lasting effects, save gradually deleterious ones for the whole body.

The body rapidly converts refined white flour into sugar. Hence, food products which contain both refined sugar and refined flour are doubly harmful. The body, after all, does not "see" the separate products as cola drinks and toasted buns; it simply interprets them as what they are—refined carbohydrates practically devoid of real nutrients.

It has been proved that the wheat milling process removes some twenty-two natural nutrients from the raw material, including vitamins A and D, a host of B vitamins, and twelve minerals. The flour industry did nothing about this until 1941, when it replaced some of the essential ingredients that are normally removed. This gave rise to the myth of "enriched" bread. Various bread products now compete in the level of "enrichment" each is said to have. But enrichment simply means that a few of the many nutrients taken out have been replaced—and only in part. More than one nutritionally oriented physican has likened this to a Central Park mugger who divests you of your clothes, watch, and wallet and then returns your shorts. Has he "enriched" you?

The health food troops and nutritional therapists argue that stone-ground, whole-grain bread remains the most nutritious of the bread products available. Now that it has also been accepted that increased fiber in the system seems to help prevent some forms of cancer, a number of bread manufacturers have gotten the message, and both whole wheat and stone-ground varieties of "the staff of life," however altered, are being returned to the marketplace.

What has been true for wheat is also true for rice. The "polishing" of rice removes most of its vital nutrients, leaving the final refined white product virtually devoid of nutrition. The supreme irony in the rice business was reached during the Vietnam War when the United States shipped South Vietnam, a rice-producing country, tons of *refined,* polished rice. The Vietcong in the field, however, were thriving on unrefined, unpolished natural rice, which is loaded with nutrients.

I remember visiting several Huk villages in Central Luzon in the company of the "supremo" of the Philippine Huk movement, Luis

Taruc. I was consistently amazed at the great longevity and general good health of these thin, brown people, many of them septuagenarians and octogenarians who recall struggles against the Americans, the Japanese, and the Filipino central government. I asked them how they had subsisted during the Japanese occupation, and their answer was uniformly the same: "The way we do now"— that is, eating unpolished wild rice, several varieties of wild beans and grains, minimal amounts of meat, and a wide variety of natural whole fruits and vegetables. They were—and are—*tough,* even at seventy-five and weighing in at ninety pounds.

"Civilized" rice may look nice, white, and neat; and it may be puffed, toasted, and sugar-coated. But, even though touted as "nutritious," it is far from that.

The nutritional facts are, of course, that human beings simply don't need to ingest any refined carbohydrates. They get plenty from the enormous lunch table God, Mother Nature, or Force X provided eons ago. They inundate themselves with empty calories through candy bars, cola drinks, polished rice, puffed-up white bread, endless pastries, and alcoholic products at their own risk.

The Trouble With Salt

And they do the same with salt, another addictive product that is either not necessary at all, at least in refined form, or recommendable in much smaller amounts. For the link between hypertension, a precursor of stroke, and salt is being more firmly established every day. It can be said that not only are Americans sugar junkies, but they are also salt-happy.

In fact, great parallels exist between the two. Both refined sugar and salt (or, rather, the sodium that is in salt, for it is sodium that is the culprit) have accompanied the exponential development of the food-processing industry and lurk in many thousands of foods most unexpectedly and in far more forms than the white crystals we are accustomed to seeing in the bowl or shaker.

It has been estimated that since World War II, and owing primarily to the American addiction to presalted junk foods and sodium-laced preserved and frozen foods, American have been taking in up to 2½ teaspoons of salt a day, or more than twenty times what the body actually needs.

And as this sodium consumption has jumped, so too has hypertension. The figure of 35 million hypertensives in this country is based on estimated hard-core cases; an estimate of 60 million hypertensives is more in the ball park if mild cases are included. Nearly half the population of Americans sixty-five years and older is affected. Says one expert, Dr. Lot Page, chief of medicine at the Newton-Wellesley Hospital, "The link between salt and hypertension is as firm as the link between high cholesterol and heart disease," (*Time,* March 1982.)

Just as sugar exists in many forms and in many names and in many varying amounts in many unexpected places, the sodium content of our foods is likewise amazing, and pernicious, according to the U.S. Department of Agriculture.

For example, while 69 mg. of sodium are contained in a half breast of chicken, a fast-food chicken dinner has 2,243 mg. of the chemical! A raw lemon has 1 mg. of sodium, but a teaspoon of salt has 1,938 mg. of it. A tomato characteristically has 14 mg. of sodium, but tomato sauce has 1,498 mg. in a single cup. Corn right off the cob has 1 mg. of sodium—but a cup of canned corn has 384 mg. These exponential rates indicate an explosion of the use of sodium far beyond what the body was designed to handle.

The addiction syndrome in sodium abuse is not as well understood as that of refined sucrose (white sugar), but it is just as real. "Salt junkies" lace practically everything with the white crystals as if their taste buds were so addicted to the single taste of salt they are trying to hide, rather than enhance, the natural tastes of their food.

At an American Medical Association symposium in 1978 in Washington, food scientist Robert M. Kark told fellow savants that "Americans take in high amounts of salt on everything from pretzels and cocktail tidbits to salads and soups," in addition, he might have added, to the sugar and other refined carbohydrates they are getting in most of those same products. Dr. Kark added that one in five Caucasians and one in three blacks in the United States suffers from hypertension.

Dr. Kark and other scientists were concerned with the rates of sodium and potassium in the American diet—too much of the former and not enough of the latter. The Japanese, they pointed out, consume up to four times as much salt as Americans, but Japan's hypertension rate is not that much higher, though stroke is Japan's second leading cause of death. The indications are that Japanese might keep the hypertension rate livable because they get large amounts of potassium from the high percentage of fresh vegetables in their diets.

Utah State University instructor R. Gaurth Hansen pointed out that not enough has been done in researching an average recommended salt diet for Americans. He noted that dozens of fruits and vegetables, including bananas, spinach, winter squash, brussels sprouts, and beet greens, provide significant amounts of potassium, but by and large they are not consumed on a grand scale, particularly, as other researchers have noted, by the lower economic strata, whose children make do almost entirely on a junk-food diet. But up to now there are no established dietary guidelines for the amount of salt in the diet. All we have are belated, if welcome, admonitions from the Senate Select Committee on Nutrition and Human Needs on the need to reduce the amount of salt we consume.

By 1982 legislation was drafted, but so far not passed, to require salt content labeling on all processed and canned foods governed by the Food, Drug and Cosmetic Act. Tennessee Congressman Albert Gore, a backer of such legislation, noted: "Salt is the cheapest flavor enhancer. There is an enormous competitive advantage to loading food with salt and not telling people about it." Added California Congressman Henry Waxman, "We are having difficulty getting the votes to pass this legislation because of industry pressure."

Poisoning The Food Supply

It is one thing for civilized society to switch from dependence on a few trusty staple foods to today's fast-food orgy, and quite another to pollute even that. But that, at least to some extent, is what has happened in the food-processing business. Again, this is not an evil conspiracy, but a response of manufacturers to market demands in an urban, industrialized society requiring more food more easily available and satisfying sugar and salt addictions whose early developments are interesting footnotes to human history. The need to raise, manufacture, distribute, and store an even greater variety of foods in an ever more urban and ever more mobile society has been, well, the bread and butter of the food processing industry.

In 1955 it was estimated that about 419 million pounds of chemical additives—everything from coloring agents to dough conditioners, from flavor-enhancers to thickeners—went into the American food supply. Only part of this was necessary for the actual conserving of the food from farm or factory to the home shelf. The rest was added to make the food look and taste better—that is, to make it more saleable.

Since 1958 the Food and Drug Administration has approved well over 3,000 chemicals and food additives as "generally recognized as safe." The true number of chemicals that go into food will never be known, but some estimate the number to be as high as 10,000—virtually all of them unnatural to man, deviant from his biological experience.

So, in addition to anywhere from 90 to 130 pounds of sugar in various forms per capita per year, Americans are also ingesting an additional five pounds of chemical additives from their unnatural food supply, a growing number of them suspected of being carcinogenic, cancer-producing, at least in terms of laboratory animal experiments.

It happens that most of our food is raised with the help of chemical fertilizers and pesticides, which bring to us an unknown amount of poisonous substances ranging upward and downward from DDT. For years, Dr. Jacqueline Verrett, a veteran researcher with the FDA, argued against the use of the hormone diethylstilbestrol (DES), which is used for the rapid fattening of cattle, and sodium nitrite, used to help give red meat its reddish color (and to prevent botulism, sure enough), because these products may be connected with cancer induction. A number of researchers argued that food processors pressured the FDA to allow such possible cancer inducers to remain on the market even while laboratory tests on them finally put a stop to such items as DES.

The FDA, as we have seen, is quick to move against unwanted substances in the medical and pharmaceutical marketplace—laetrile, ACE, DMSO, EDTA among them—but extremely sluggish in tampering with an industry that is estimated to be in the top or second slot in American business, all aspects of that industry considered. The FDA is able to flipflop decisions and attitudes with the flick of a press release.

For example, take the case of Red Dye No. 2, once the nation's most widely used food coloring, used in everything from cola drinks to strawberry ice cream to lipstick and pill coverings. By 1976 it was going into $10 billion worth of food every year. In December 1975, then FDA Commissioner Alexander Schmidt insisted that there were no studies in the fifteen-year controversy over the substance indicating that No. 2 caused cancer, adding that "the evidence is quite solid that it does not cause birth defects." But by January 1976, the FDA's National Center for Toxicological Research claimed the dye appeared to cause a "significant increase" in malignant tumors when fed in high doses to rats. FDA biochemist Verrett reported that her experiment with chick embryos fed No. 2 resulted in "skeletal defects, stunted growth, some malformed eyes, but the striking effect was that... so few chicks survived long enough to hatch."

The FDA banned the substance in 1976.

Another illustrative example of the FDA's susceptibility to food industry pressure was the long-simmering controversy over the use of cyclamates, the nonsugar sweetening additives that help preserve precious calories for dieters and diabetics. Although cyclamates were successfully and safely marketed for more than a decade, they presented a direct threat to the sugar interests, and in early 1970 the FDA yanked them off the market because of reports that the sweetener caused bladder cancer, birth defects, and other horrible things in laboratory animals.

Much of the information was initiated by the sugar industry, which also spent hundreds of thousands of dollars in propaganda against cyclamates and even nonsugar cola drinks. Abbott Laboratories, the largest producer of cyclamates, provided enough of the substance to its test rats to equal eleven pounds of the chemical per day for two years in a normal human. Only at this and greater levels did negative reactions set in.

Luckily, medical publications in both the United States and Europe took the FDA to task for its precipitous banning of cyclamates on such faulty evidence. The standard joke became, "Cyclamates may be dangerous to your pet rat."

By spring 1976 a government advisory panel had meekly concluded that there was not enough evidence to place a cancer-causing label on cyclamates, but much of the damage had already been done.

Terror At The Tap: Our Polluted Water Supply

The chemical danger in unnatural food holds not only for solid comestibles; it is growing for water as well. Water gets the chemical runoff effect from farmlands treated with pesticides, fertilizers, and thousands of chemicals, and it also receives the chemical fallout from the polluted air blown in from both coasts, which carries with it amounts of manmade pollution on a scale vast enough to boggle the mind of even the most hidebound anti-environmentalist.

It is estimated that each year in the United States 200 million tons of pollutants are belched into the air, including not only such major killers and cripplers as lead (which is poured into the air of the Los Angeles basin at the rate of 30,000 pounds per day) but also nitrogen oxides, carbon monoxide, ozone, sulfur, particulates of tar, heavy metals, and asbestos. This polluted atmospheric fallout finds its way into the nation's food supply both through the grazing grasses on which animals are fed and the tissues of the animals themselves. Some of them find their way into our rivers and streams.

Hence, the water we drink is usually laced with pesticides, chemical salts, detergents, heavy toxic metals, all manner of dangerous chemicals, occasionally radioactive waste, and even human and animal excrement. Up to now, water-supply technology has not kept pace with the continual threat of the poisoning of our water, and for that reason water purifiers and distillers are doing record business.

The water problem has grown so severe that in a September 1980 report to the House Subcommittee on Environment, Energy and Natural Resources, legislators learned that 2,100 sites in the U.S.A.—involving every state and every major city—have "hazardous drinking water" due to pollution and waste. One legislator deemed the situation so serious that he predicted the water problem will become "the most volatile issue of the 80s."

The hottest issue in the polluted water controversy, however, remains the pitched battle over fluoridation—though controversy over chlorination is not far behind—with the weight of Establishment opinion brought to the fore to defend that wholesale poisoning of municipal water supplies in the interest of preventing tooth decay in children.

The reality is that fluoride—a highly poisonous substance—is a byproduct of the steel-manufacturing, aluminum, and related industries. It also seems true that a *small* amount of it, in children is effective in combating tooth decay. But does this excuse the mass fluoridation of water supplies affecting millions of Americans where there is at least scattered evidence that fluoridation can cause a whole host of pathological problems? A growing number of Americans think not, even though their voices are often muted by the multi-million-dollar fluoridation campaigns put on in city after city in support of dumping the known poison into water supplies.

At this writing, there has still been no reliable rebuttal to the claims made by Dean Burk, Ph.D., biochemist, and retired head of the cytochemistry division, National Cancer Institute (and a major figure in the laetrile controversy), and Dr. John Yiamouyiannis. On the basis of statistics gathered from eighteen years of fluoridation in selected cities in America, Drs. Burk and Yiamouyiannis claimed that fluoridated water is linked to a "minimum figure" of 10,000 cancer deaths per year. "But in reality that figure is much higher," Dr. Burk told me. "I calculate there are 35,000 American deaths per year connected with fluoridated water, or about a tenth of all the deaths from cancer in this country." The 10,000 fatalities figure comes from the risks run by the 74 million Americans who are "forced to drink fluoridated water," he added. Dr. Burk argues that the steel and related industries "made unwitting dupes of the dentists and other health organizations."

New fears about chlorination were brought to the fore by a government report in 1977 that chlorinated water—consumed by more than 100 million Americans every day—is a major source of cancer.

"Except for cigarette smoking we haven't identified anything else that accounts for potentially as much cancer as drinking water and chlorination," according to Dr. Robert Harris, associate director of the toxic chemical program for the Environmental Defense Fund, a non-profit consumer group.

One study funded by the federal Environmental Protection Agency found that the death rate from cancer among drinkers of chlorinated water was 44 percent higher than among those who did not drink chlorinated water. A second study indicated an elevated cancer rate in areas where chloroform—which results when chlorine interacts with certain organic material in water—is higher.

That the sum total of chemical pollution in water, air and food may be having composite lethal effects aside from direct disease causation is suggested in growing evidence that as much as 20 percent of the entire male population of the United States may be functionally sterile—that is, less able to have children than preceding generations.

The point was driven home forcefully to Congress in 1980 by researcher Erik Jansson and Dr. Ralph Dougherty, who released the startling information that 23 percent of the male student body at Florida State University was functionally sterile. Other studies have tended to confirm an estimatd 20 percent functional sterility rate for

American males, up from .5 percent in 1938. Reported Jansson: "Most of the dramatic decline [in male potency] is due to the exposure of Americans to hazardous substances. Thirty percent appears to be due to manmade chlorinated chemicals found to contaminate the human sperm cell."

Evidence from the Medical College of Georgia and the University of Arkansas suggest that between 67 and 83 percent of all birth defects in the nation are now caused by men. Too, research suggests that low sperm counts are highly correlated with cancer, Jansson said.

Male functional sterility, and all it implies, is of course only one unexpected outcome of the profound alteration of the human environment by chemicals. The immediate connection is to pandemic rates of degenerative disease.

I am not emphasizing either air or water pollution as much as food pollution, however, because the information is becoming more abundant that the food problem, *per se,* is more severe than either of these. For, as we have seen, differences in dietary habits, as among Seventh Day Adventists and Mormons, apparently can inhibit or slow down the noxious effects of polluted air and water.

The Myth Of The Balanced Diet

As the nation's nutritionally-oriented therapists know, large quantities of refined carbohydrates, as well as our constant exposure to such toxic chemicals as lead, mercury, and cadmium, all this accompanied by deficiencies in needed natural nutrients of all kinds, ultimately affect the health and division of cells. This continual insult to the cells—blocking their natural respiration and ingestion, coating their membranes with toxic substances, interfering in may other ways with their internal machinery—can only have one ultimate result—degenerative disease. And,—as we have seen, the primary culprit in this is what we eat.

But, no matter, the Establishment and the few Establishment-knighted "nutritionists" to whom such matters are referred, go their merry way assuring us that we are the best-fed people on earth and that there is no need even for vitamin and mineral supplements as long as we eat a "balanced diet." There might be some substance in this claim, *if* the components of that balanced diet were themselves balanced, that is, natural. But this is hardly the case. Even if an American of adequate economic means takes in the presumed proper amounts of leafy greens, fruit juices, meat, eggs, and other proteins and carbohydrates, he is getting already deficient food substances the great majority of which have been tampered with in some way.

A century ago, Americans were consuming wheat with a protein count of up to 20 precent, pure meat and "organically" grown fruit and vegetables. The balancing of *this* diet was, indeed, something to crow about. But now our bread, if healthy at all, is 9 to 12 percent protein, our meats are artifically colored and are apt to come from artificially fattened cattle, hogs, and poultry, and rare is the table set with homegrown and naturally prepared fruits and vegetables and whole grains, as against 40 percent in 1900 (see "The Pure, The Impure, and The Paranoid," *Psychology Today,* October 1978, for an excellent account of the change in American dietary habits).

Americans foolhardy enough to believe they will be metabolically sound by taking refuge in the food-label testimonies of compliance with the U.S. Department of Agriculture's "recommended daily allowance" of substances or the "minimum daily requirement" of vitamins have been brainwashed by the propaganda of the FDA and the American Medical Association. First of all, logic dictates that there cannot really *be* either an RDA or an MDR appropriate for all people at all times. Surely the allowable amounts of certain things vary between a Swedish longshoreman and an African pygmy, between a ninety-pound octogenarian retiree and a nineteen-year-old fullback. In fact, these alleged recommended amounts are based on what the National Nutrition Board calls the "reference man and woman," an individual further described as being of "normal" height and weight, living in a temperate zone, and being twenty-two years old.

The legislator who did most to take on the notion of recommended daily allowance and the food industry's influence on the government was Sen. William Proxmire, who warned that "at best the RDAs are only a 'recommended' allowance at antediluvian levels designed to prevent terrible disease. At worst, they are based on conflicts of interest and self-serving views of certain parts of the food industry." He styled the Food and Nutrition Board of the National Research Council "both the creature of the food industry and heavily influenced by the food industry." In testimony to Congress in 1976, Senator Proxmire said, "The RDA standard is established by the Food and Nutrition Board of the National Research Council, which is influenced, dominated and financed in part by the food industry. It represents one of the most scandalous conflicts of interest in the Federal Government."

Can We Trust What The Nutritionists Say?

Most loyal AMA physicians and dedicated readers of the *Journal of the American Medical Association* will readily admit they know little about nutrition and had no more than one or two hours of nutrition science in their medical school courses. When they need information about nutrition, they turn to the few "A-Okay"—stamped nutritionists who are supposed to be worthy of the name, including—sometimes first and foremost—those of the Deparment of Nutrition at the Harvard University School of Public Health. Yet this school has accepted millions of dollars in grants from such food giants as General Foods, Kellogg, Nabisco, the Sugar Association, and the International Sugar Foundation. One of the school's foremost professors of nutrition has been a consultant to the sugar and drug industries as well as a member of the Continental Can Company board of directors. It is an honest exercise to speculate about how fair and objective food science instructors can be when linked one way or another to the food industry.

Congressmen Benjamin S. Rosenthal brought part of the problem to the fore in 1976 when he and a consumer study group claimed that some eminent American nutritionists "have traded their independence for the food industry's favors." He introduced to public gaze a study entitled *Feeding at the Company Trough,* produced by the nonprofit Center for Science in the Public Interest. One of the study's major points was that some of the nutritionists who make public analyses of consumer problems are on the boards of or have other ties with food companies. Dr. Michael Jacobson, co-director of the center, said, "One can only come to the conclusion that industry grants, consulting fees and directorships are muzzling, if not prostituting, nutritional food science professors."

Representative Rosenthal and the Jacobson study found that the Harvard Department of Nutrition had received $2 million in donations from industry between 1971 and 1974, some of them coming from such food companies as Amstar, Beatrice Foods, Coca-Cola, Kellogg, Gerber, and Oscar Mayer. Harvard confirmed that it had received some contributions from the food industry for research, doubted the $2 million figure, and vehemently denied that such contributions had influenced any research.

In 1980, the *Washington Post* reported that two members of a scientific panel which investigated the link between fat and cholesterol and heart attack risks reportedly were paid consultants to industries affected by the report. The newspaper said their relationships with the dairy and other food industries had not been revealed when the National Academy of Sciences' Food and Nutrition Board released a report saying that there is no conclusive evidence linking fat and cholesterol to heart attack risks.

That was not terribly surprising, since at the time two other food industry representatives were sitting on the board, the *Post* noted.

However, the old adage that one does not bite the hand that feeds him is as true today as it was yesterday. The fact is, much of the information coming from "nutrition experts" bankrolled by the food industry can—and should—be taken with the proverbial, and indeed somewhat dangerous, grain of salt.

Chapter Five
The Scandal of Cancergate

Sloan-Kettering: Of Mice, Men and Amygdalin

It was in August 1975 that I was "radicalized" on the subject of "conspiracy" as it related to amygdalin (laetrile) in cancer research. It was then that an event occurred which left me no rational explanation other than that a conspiracy of some sort existed.

A copyboy for the *Berkeley Daily Gazette,* of which I had been editor up until a few months before, rushed to my Oakland apartment some laboratory notes and memoranda that had arrived at the newspaper office from Sloan-Kettering Institute in New York City. He was up enough on the laetrile controversy to realize the documents were indeed important. The cover letter to me, on SKI stationery, bore the message:

> Dear Mr. Culbert:
> Here are some [sic] results of Sloan-Kettering experiments with Laetrile. Due to political pressure these results are being suppressed. Please do your best to bring these important findings to the attention of the people. Krebs' theory is very promising, and Laetrile should be tested to see if it really holds water.

There was no signature. But attached to the cover letter were thirty-two pages of tables, memoranda and notes, which included *six* series of experiments run by Dr. Kanematsu Sugiura, a veteran scientist who had been testing new drugs on laboratory animals for the better part of this century. *All* of these experiments, dated between 3 August 1973 and 8 February 1975 showed positive effects from the injection of refined amygdalin (laetrile) into mice, particularly in blocking the spread (metastasis) of cancer.

I had been waiting for almost two years to see some sort of follow-up to the earlier bombshell that had developed at America's most amply funded and prestigious cancer research complex (Sloan-Kettering Institute and the Memorial Sloan-Kettering Cancer Center jointly received $46.1 million in 1976 from the National Cancer Institute, the federally funded institute's largest single grant for that year). For, in 1973, information leaked from Sloan-Kettering to attorneys representing Dr. Richardson in his "cancer quackery" trial confirmed that tests run by Dr. Sugiura had shown that amygdalin caused "significant inhibition of the information of lung metastases" and "possibly prevents, to an uncertain degree, the formation of new tumors."

SKI had moved swiftly to point out that the ostensibly purloined material was incomplete. Despite this, the "leaked" Sugiura report constituted the first gap in the armor of American cancer orthodoxy, which had been insisting up to that time that no animal experiments had ever proven amygdalin effective. While such statements were consistently rebutted by the NCI's own cytochemistry chief, biochemist Dean Burk, the raw information on which they were based had never been made popularly available.

The 1973 release left SKI (I will use this abbreviation throughout to indicate the entire Sloan-Kettering complex) with considerable egg on its face. It was already in the process of being badly burned by a cancer-research scandal in which research scientist William Summerlin faked test data in response to bureaucratic pressure at the complex to produce good results. This whole, incredible episode was revealed by a former director of public affairs for Memorial Sloan-Kettering, Joseph Hixson (*The Patchwork Mouse*. N.Y.: Anchor Press/ Doubleday, 1976).

But to me, as an investigative reporter who intermittently had been covering laetrile since 1971, the early Sugiura work indicated a breakthrough that seemed a good omen for the apricot seed derivative. I actually imagined, as of fall 1974, that the whole issue was on the way to a happy resolution, since Sloan-Kettering had already confirmed to me, in time for inclusion in my first book, that, while amygdalin had apparently failed in a second series of tests, a third set had been run, had been positive, and on the basis of that, some kind of human trials would result. It looked like now, at last, laetrile was on the way to a fair test at a reliable Establishment institution, that a fresh new insight into the cancer disaster was in the offing.

I was cautioned by hotheads within the laetrile movement not to trust the Establishment, despite its sanguine assessment of the Sugiura results. At that time, I was still a nonadvocacy journalist observing the laetrile story with some degree of objectivity, even though, as my first book points out, I had reached a layman's conclusion that the substance obviously had something going for it and that there was no good reason to suppress it.

However, between fall 1974 and summer 1975, "the fix was in," as I came to learn. Somebody, somewhere, had decided that all preliminary remarks about laetrile efficacy simply had to be countered by new statements in effect denying the "leaked" material and even casting doubt on the reliability of the patient, veteran researcher involved—Dr. Kanematsu Sugiura, an octogenarian scientist and gentleman who, throughout the tempest that was soon to break, rigidly maintained a posture of utter honesty and scientific integrity.

To set the stage for what was happening, allow me to go back in time. The "war on cancer," actually the Conquest of Cancer program, was to be President Nixon's major contribution in the cancer field. There was optimistic talk not only of millions of extra dollars in research but of an all-systems-go, heads-up effort to wrap up the cancer riddle by 1976. The philosophy was not all that naive. After all, the money pump, national pride and coordinated science had landed men on the moon and had brought America triumphantly into leadership of the Space Age.

The Test Laetrile Now Committee, mostly operative in California, had bombarded Nixon with petitions demanding that some kind of testing of the taboo material begin at once. This was the first actual political action involving laetrile and had begun before the Committee for Freedom of Choice in Cancer Therapy—operational by fall 1972—was actively involved. At least a partial result of the Test Laetrile Now petition campaign was that Benno Schmidt, an attorney, vice chariman of the Memorial Sloan-Kettering Cancer Center, and the head of President Nixon's recently appointed Cancer Panel, took the matter up with veteran SKI men Lloyd J. Old and C. Chester Stock, who helped begin the testing program.

On the basis of information that SKI employees themselves later made available to the press, we can reconstruct the chain of events, beginning sometime in the middle of 1972. While a first series of tests, using laetrile on *transplantable* tumor systems, had turned in essentially negative results, by fall of 1972 Dr. Sugiura was able to report on positive findings in CD8F1 mice (a special research strain). This was confirmed during the Richardson trial a year later. Dr. Sugiura had also noted improved health and well-being in the animals. A December 1972 meeting resulted in a decision to go ahead full-bore with the amygdalin testing program at SKI and additional positive results on the CD8F1 mice were obtained in the period February-May. I was kept partly informed of the progress within the research center by the McNaughton Foundation's founder-president, Andrew R. L. McNaughton, who had worked openly and behind the scenes for the vindication of laetrile since the mid-1960s.

What I did not know was that shortly thereafter, an initial

collaborative experiment was underway between Dr. Sugiura and Dr. Daniel Martin of the Catholic Medical Center, who would become one of the most vociferous of the anti-laetrile scientists called upon to denounce the compound. Most intriguingly, Dr. Martin (who bred the CD8F1 mouse colony on which Dr. Sugiura drew for the laetrile tests), reportedly was informed in summer 1973 that the National Cancer Institute, the federal conduit of funds for the Conquest of Cancer program, considered the colony to be of "obscure" value, and his request for funds had been rejected.

Within months, the Suguira memoranda on positive results were leaked. It is appropriate to note that by then a fairly extensive "underground" was in existence at Sloan-Kettering—dissident employees and scientists who held a number of grudges against the complex, some of them politically motivated, and who cultivated outside media and other contacts so that "the other side" of what was going on within might become public knowledge. I was only one recipient of selected information from "within," and to this day I admire the courage and integrity of the individuals who were involved in this, most particularly the man who later, and dramatically, was to "surface" as a major Sloan-Kettering undergrounder.

Between the time of the first Sugiura lead and August 1975 when the full series of reports reached me, Sloan-Kettering spokesmen, now constantly hounded by the media to say something about laetrile, the "quack apricot-pit cancer drug" so roundly denounced by all sections of officialdom for so many years, outdid each other in contradictory statements.

We know both from information subsequently released to the press by the Sloan-Kettering underground and also from documents secured by a Michigan state representative that, as late as spring 1975, Sloan-Kettering had been involved with the following positive aspects of laetrile:

• A Mexican study of the substance on human patients had shown a 46.4 percent *objective* response—that is, tumor shrinkage of 40 percent or more, results so promising to Sloan-Kettering that an American research team was ready to begin an investigative collaboration with the Mexicans. But it was never carried out.

• Research, primarily at Sloan-Kettering, had demonstrated once again the utter nontoxicity of laetrile even at very elevated dose levels. This research considerably undercut the credibility of the Establishment when, particularly from 1978-81, it attempted to make a case for the poisonous characteristics of amygdalin.

• It was generally known to and agreed by the Sloan-Kettering research team that amygdalin administration slowed tumor growth and lung metastases and caused pain relief in laboratory animals.

• Agreement was reached in 1974 that both Sloan-Kettering and NCI should consider human trials for laetrile for pain relief, and would consult with the American Cancer Society to do so.

The above information was not made publicly available until spring 1978, by the office of Michigan State Representative John T. Kelsey, at that time sponsoring a "freedom of choice in cancer therapy" bill in Michigan. It was not public information a year earlier, when Sloan-Kettering held an ostensibly no-holds-barred press conference that ultimately only further tarnished its credibility.

Hence, in the period spring-summer 1975, Sloan-Kettering spokesmen vacillated between insisting that no positive results had ever been seen from the use of laetrile and admitting that at least some "inconclusive" ones had been seen. Sloan-Kettering President Lewis Thomas was quoted in April 1975 as saying that "laetrile has [been] shown after two years of tests to be worthless in fighting cancer." In August 1975, SKI Vice President C. Chester Stock had claimed that "we have found amygdalin negative in all the animal systems we have tested."

Yet, in February 1974 Dr. Sugiura ran still another successful test on CD8F1 mice. By late March 1975, Dr. Elizabeth Stockert had completed a negative experiment with amygdalin but reportedly had changed Dr. Sugiura's experimental protocols. In May, at or about the time the NCI, changing tunes, provided substantial funding to breed CD8F1 mice, Dr. Franz Schmid, who earlier had found suggestions of responses to the Sugiura testing program, completed a second CD8F1 experiment—this one using only *one-fortieth* of the dose recommended by Dr. Sugiura. Dr. Schmid came up with an interesting finding. Though treated animals had more metastases, they lived 50 percent longer.

We now know, thanks to the Sloan-Kettering underground, which summarized for the media results of tests that the complex itself had not seen fit to mention, that between November 1974 and August 1975, Dr. Sugiura performed eight experiments with amygdalin in AKR leukemic strain mice, achieving "certain inhibitory action on the growth of leukemia." He also had reported positive results with the substance on spontaneous mammary tumors in another strain of mice (Swiss albino).

But by August 1975, with Dr. Stock claiming negative results in all experiments, and Benno Schmidt quoted as saying "there's no way, I believe, that they can convince the people at Sloan-Kettering there's any basis for going further," all seemed lost. The established line was the *failure* of laetrile in animal tests, the necessary first step toward human trials.

But then came the full set of memoranda on Dr. Sugiura's tests. I did not know then the scope and degree of the work that had gone on at SKI—I only knew, from "leaked" information, that a lot of positive tests had indeed been performed, and that the statements from top-level spokesmen were misleading at best. As the full impact of what I was looking at hit me, I was swept by a mixture of rage and disbelief. My reaction was very simple: "Here, indeed, is evidence of *some kind of positive effect* from laetrile in animal tests. How *dare* Sloan-Kettering flatly claim it has seen no positive results!" The fact that Americans continued to die of cancer at a faster clip than ever before paralleled the reality that a promising avenue of research was not only *not* being followed up on but was even being lied about. For minutes to hours, I could not believe it. I checked several ways on the authenticity of the data I had received from Sugiura. It was all his, though he had *not* written the politics-tinged note to me. I slammed down these documents before Committee for Freedom of Choice officers Robert W. Bradford and J. Franklin Salaman and said, in so many words, "Count me in." From that moment on, my position as to the need for open exposure of all facets of the laetrile controversy—and distrust of the Establishment—moved from moderate to radical.

Since that time, Dr. Sugiura confirmed his findings both to me and to several other reporters and writers. And he never budged an inch, despite the propaganda that later ballooned as Sloan-Kettering made one disastrous bad turn after another in dealing with its hottest of all potatoes. He died in 1979 without ever having departed one iota from his conviction of amygdalin's usefulness in treating cancer.

"Most of the time when other people repeat my experiments they confirm them—especially in the chemotherapy of cancer," Dr. Sugiura told *Medical World News* as early as October 1975. He was further quoted as saying, "I don't remember ever doing experiments that were not later confirmed. It is still my belief that amygdalin cures [sic] metastases."

He would later tell *American Medical News*, "Laetrile is not a cancer cure. I haven't found the complete destruction of tumors. I think laetrile's place is in prevention of metastases—not a cure—but that's not proved yet." That is, Dr. Sugiura's assessment of laetrile use was far from an enthusiastic endorsement. He was not a laetrile flag-waver, amygdalin ideologue, champion of the trophoblastic or laetrile-cancer prevention theories (see chapter six) or in any way involved with the pro-laetrile lobby. In fact, he was thought of so highly by the New York research complex that SKI's C. Chester Stock himself said of the Japanese-born scientist in 1965, "Few if any names in cancer research are as widely known as Kanematsu Sugiura's.... Possibly the high regard in which his work is held is best characterized by a comment made to me by a visiting investigator in cancer research from Russia. He said, 'When Dr. Sugiura publishes, we know we don't have to repeat the study for we would obtain the same results he has reported.'"

Sloan-Kettering was now, it would seem, in a panic. Dr. Sugiura was standing by his guns and the Committee for Freedom of Choice had published his memoranda, with choice commentary added by laetrile "god-father" Ernst T. Krebs, Jr., in *Anatomy of a Coverup,* which the committee saw fit to print and reprint several times for distribution nationwide and internationally. The publication showed that (a) *some* evidence for laetrile efficacy in animal experiments had been achieved and (b) there was evidence of conspiracy to mute this fact.

From contacts I had with one leak in particular, and, indirectly, from others, I came to realize that the *scientists* involved with the laetrile program on a day-to-day basis were in no way responsible for the public relations battle and the issuance of contradictory statements. These were coming from the complex's officers. Somewhere between the lab and the executive offices determinations were being made to fudge on the issue of amygdalin.

The research center attempted to get off the hook by running joint experiments by Drs. Sugiura and Schmid, and when Dr. Schmid's results bolstered the Sugiura finding that laetrile tended to inhibit metastases, Sloan-Kettering then embarked on setting up arrangements for a "blind" experiment, to be carried out at the Catholic Medical Center, an experiment about which a volume could be written.

In the meantime, fall 1976—a target date Sloan-Kettering had set for the "last word" on laetrile testing—came and went. But instead of a full report coming from the center itself, a group of employees and scientists issued their own report, called *Second Opinion,* a mimeographed newsletter aimed at Sloan-Kettering's 4,600 employees. For the laetrile camp, and particularly the Committee for Freedom of Choice, it was a breath of fresh air. Up to November 1976 the Committee was alone in claiming that a "coverup" was underway at Sloan-Kettering to hide the truth about the laetrile testing program.

In its first number, *Second Opinion* claimed that the most recent laetrile test had turned out to be positive and that word of the results had been suppressed by the front office. It also announced that efforts for a "blind" study at Catholic Medical Center had been "completely botched... whether by accident or design" through the premature killing of about a quarter of the test animals. Dr. Stock had attributed the aborting of this first try at a "blind" study as due to "clumsy injection procedures."

The *Second Opinion* writers were later to claim on the strength of memoranda and lab notes in their possession that the first effort at a "blind" study failed only after Dr. Sugiura let it be known that simply on the basis of observation of the amygdalin-treated mice and the saline-solution-administered control group he could already tell which ones were responding and which ones weren't. He saw objective, anti-cancer effects in the treated group.

The second blind experiment, held at SKI's Walker Laboratory, turned up results that suggested there was no real difference between amygdalin-treated and control animals, even though Dr. Sugiura was overruled when he asked that the amygdalin-treated and control animals be housed in separate cages and that the cages be randomized.

Some others at Sloan-Kettering believe there may have been serious compromising of the "blindness" of the study through the inadvertent injection of control animals with amygdalin, and vice-versa. Sugiura also had noticed an initial stoppage of tumor growth in 40 percent of the control animals, versus 27 percent in the laetrile-treated ones, a suspiciously high precentage of spontaneous stoppages. The results were, at best, indecisive, but nonetheless, they were publicized by Sloan-Kettering as its major effort at attempting to "replicate" Dr. Sugiura's controversial findings, and then failing.

It was not known to the public at this time that the veteran scientist had earlier performed a positive test with prunasin, a variant of amygdalin, and that Dr. Sugiura's efforts to have SKI publish a paper on nine amygdalin experiments, overwhelmingly positive, were rejected. Dr. Martin, however, put out his own anti-laetrile argument for science and the media, denouncing it as a "hoax." He instantly became a "star" anti-laetrile spokesman around the country.

In February 1977, *Second Opinion* brought to public attention unpublished work in the biochemistry of amygdalin and prunasin. A synopsis of this work had indeed appeared in the 1974 SKI annual report. It essentially provided some scientific support for the general theory of action of the vitamin B^{17} compounds as propounded by biochemist Krebs (see chapter six).

By 1977, the flurry of sweeping statements, rebuttals, leaked information, and the presence of a vigorous underground at Sloan-Kettering, matched by the resounding political triumphs of laetrile in state after state, left the New York research facility with the need to provide its "last word" openly and under the full glare of press attention.

I had been warned well in advance that a snow job was in the works, one final, coordinated effort at providing a propaganda blast at laetrile to bury it once and for all, at least as far as SKI was concerned. Right on schedule, the effort took place on 15 June 1977 at a press conference in which Sloan-Kettering released prepublication papers of its work on laetrile to the press but under the sweeping assertion that "laetrile was found to possess neither preventative, nor tumor-regressant, nor antimetastatic, nor curative anti-cancer activity."

But if SKI thought it would orchestrate a conference at which the nation's uninformed media would easily be gulled by scientific phraseology and the well-credentialed presence of anti-laetrile spokesmen, it was in for a surprise. Both media and Committee for Freedom of Choice members showed up at the conference to blitz SKI officials and Dr. Martin with questions about their statements. United Press International reported the event straight, with UPI's Pat McCormick leading off her coverage this way, "Laetrile does not knock out cancer in mice, but in one set of experiments it kept eight of ten breast cancers from spreading to the lung, research at Sloan-Kettering shows."

The prepublication reports, slated to be published by the *Journal of Clinical Oncology* that same year (but not appearing until 1978, and then in an amended version), omitted several sets of data but reported heavily on the failure of amygdalin in *transplantable* tumor systems.

Within twenty-four hours, the Committee for Freedom of Choice called its press conference to rebut this particular area of research, since the study of what a tumor does in one animal when transferred from another has no bearing on either the total metabolic treatment of cancer or the concept of cancer as a systemic, metabolic disease of which tumors are only symptoms. The committee was not naively standing alone in this assertion; growing numbers of researchers question the validity of using animal tumor systems to study those of humans, and even more question the usefulness of transplanted models.

The Sloan-Kettering press release that accompanied the prepublication data was careful to note that in tests of *spontaneous* cancer—that is, malignancy arising *within* the test animals—Dr. Sugiura had indeed earlier found positive results. The institute carefully noted that other researchers had failed to confirm these, save for one test by Dr. Schmid.

But as newsmen shot questions at him, Dr. Sugiura continued to defend his experiments, disagreeing openly with Dr. Martin on the meaning and methods of testing for evidence of metastases in test mice. When Dr. Sugiura was asked what he would recommend if a daughter of his had breast cancer, he replied, "Surgery, conventional drugs, and laetrile." Asked if he would use laetrile if he himself had cancer, the veteran researcher replied, "It couldn't hurt and it might help."

The press conference, then, failed to put the laetrile matter to rest. The prepublication data, however, provided officialdom with some new ammunition to hurl against laetrile—unless *all* of it was taken into consideration. As it happened the data turned out to be flawed by serious omissions.

Waiting to release its own report until just before the time Sloan-Kettering published its "official" version in the *Journal of Clinical Oncology,* the underground group decided to strike in November with a full compilation of the laetrile test data. The forty-eight-page analysis, based entirely on information provided the authors by sources within the research complex, was released to the media at a press conference jointly sponsored with the Committee for Freedom of Choice.

Since I was instrumental in helping set up that conference with New York State Freedom of Choice Committee chairman Peter Lisi, permit me to relay my own pleasant surprise when I saw entering the room my own best leak at SKI, Dr. Ralph Moss, assistant director of public affairs at Memorial Sloan-Kettering Cancer Center, a gentleman whose identity I had carefully shielded from others in the laetrile movement because he was both a major news source and in an extremely delicate position. It was Dr. Moss, in fact, who had written the carefully worded Sloan-Kettering press release covering the June press conference.

Unknown to his superiors, Dr. Moss arrived at our hotel *not* to cover our press conference for Sloan-Kettering's public information department, but to *participate* in it. He was there, he said, to corroborate the findings of the *Second Opinion* report on laetrile, presented by biochemistry doctoral student Alec Pruchnicki. More than that, he turned out to be an author of the report and a collaborator of the underground group. Dr. Moss, whose doctorate is in classics, told the New York media straightforwardly that "there is a coverup" at SKI and that "I doubt they would have ever said anything positive about laetrile if they hadn't been embarrased into it. Our report doesn't say laetrile works—it proves that there is a coverup." Dr. Moss was summarily fired from his job.

This action hardly shut up Dr. Moss. In 1980 he published *The Cancer Syndrome* (Grove Press, New York), which, among many other things, assails the cancer research community's strong links to industry and details the profiteering role in both research and the suppression of "unproven" methods.

Second Opinion's summary of the laetrile test program included these enlightening lines:

> The [official] report... is both incomplete and scientifically invalid. It is incomplete because at least half a dozen experiments with amygdalin performed at the Center between 1972 and 1976 have been omitted.... It is invalid because specious arguments are advanced for the animal model used in most of the experiments.... The nature of scientific controversy over how best to detect metastases, or secondary tumors, in mice is also misrepresented.
>
> There are numerous errors in many of these experiments which allegedly prove amygdalin's ineffectiveness as a palliative or cure of cancer. On the other hand, the positive experiments with amygdalin carried out by veteran researcher Kane-

matsu Sugiura appear to be valid and are not successfully challenged by the report.

The unnamed scientists who contributed to the underground report stressed that Sloan-Kettering's emphasis on the fact that amygdalin failed to work against *primary* breast tumors in CD8F1 mice—in the *host*—completely overlooked the fact that *no* substance had *ever* been found active against primary breast cancer in CD8F1 *host* mice. Sloan-Kettering backed off from this earlier claim in an article by Dr. Richard D. Smith in *The Sciences,* the magazine of the New York Academy of Sciences. The Sloan-Kettering documents distributed to the press in the June 1977 press conference had made the claim that *spontaneous* tumors were susceptible to every drug known to work against human cancer—a claim, Smith pointed out, that was very much in error.

Smith quoted Sloan-Kettering's C. Chester Stock as saying that the erroneous description of the tumor test system involved was provided by his coauthor of the paper on spontaneous tumor tests, Dr. Martin of the Catholic Medical Center. Biochemist-author Richard Passwater has assessed this serious error in the Sloan-Kettering documentation, "That is what you do when you want to fail. It [testing laetrile on the tumor system involved] is like trying to find out if someone is strong by asking him to lift a million pounds." Hence, Sloan-Kettering seems to have gone out of its way to prove laetrile is ineffective against a tumor system that is also resistant to other drugs so tested. By the time the official documents were shown to the New York Academy of Sciences, the erroneous statement had been deleted.

The *Second Opinion* group found a lot more than the breast cancer statement with which to find fault in SKI's "official" report. It found that experiments in which laetrile had been administered together with Bromelain, a protein-digesting enzyme, had been very successful—and had gone unreported by Sloan-Kettering. The significance of these unpublished findings was particularly great in light of findings announced by Loyola University department of Biology chairman Harold Manner and his postgraduate group in late 1977. They reported that a combination of amygdalin, vitamin A and protein-digesting enzymes completely "cured" cancer in 89 percent of cases of spontaneous breast cancer in mice, and achieved positive responses in the remaining 11 percent. *Second Opinion* found that the amygdalin-enzyme dual approach had been "suddenly dropped at the beginning of 1974."

While Sloan-Kettering's official report used language that tended to obscure the reality, a careful examination of the Sugiura-Schmid collaborative tests showed that the results "unequivocally confirmed Sugiura's contention that amygdalin inhibits the spread of metastases in CD8F1 mice." Noted *SO,* "Not only does the official report fail to state clearly that Schmid confirmed Sugiura's findings but, on the contrary, after hedging somewhat it actually states in the concluding section that 'all experiments of three independent observers [Drs. Stockert, Schmid, and Martin]...have failed to confirm Sugiura's results' "—an outright lie.

Though Dr. Sugiura carried out extensive experiments with amygdalin on mice that develop spontaneous leukemia, the studies were accorded only three pages in the prepublication data, and in them "we find that the anti-leukemia features which Sugiura noted in his memoranda have been eliminated from the discussion in the [official] report. Only negative aspects are subjected to comment."

By no means did the *Second Opinion* publication of suppressed data signal the end of the Sloan-Kettering controversy; it simply cast doubt, for all time, on the center's "official" conclusions. In 1978 I received yet another leak from SKI, one signalling the continuing controversy over suppressed reports. A research biochemist, who personally confirmed the authenticity of the suppressed report to me, insisted both that Dr. Sugiura's work *had* been "replicated" at Sloan-Kettering and that promising work had been carried out with prunasin, amygdalin minus one sugar unit. The biochemist was not himself the "leaker," but confirmed that the document—"Cyanogenic Glycosides and Cancer"—was his. Seven pages in length and footnoted with eighteen references, the paper was rejected for publication by higher-ups, he said, because it was not "broad enough."

The laetrile coverup at SKI, as I came to learn so well, was only a part of the entire anti-laetrile hysteria of the Club at work; and the all-out attack on laetrile or amygdalin, which reached its most obscene dimension in the National Cancer Institute (NCI) "clinical trial" of 1980-81, was only a paradigm for the entire scenario of the allopathic, treatment-oriented medical/pharmaceutical monopoly hotly opposing natural substances and the prevention theory in degenerative disease.

During the dispute over laetrile—as in earlier controversies concerning the Hoxsey, Krebiozen, and Glyoxylide cancer treatments—the question of the credibility of vested interest forever arose, and was indeed the toughest nut to crack. *Who* would suppress a cancer "cure" or head off a promising avenue of cancer research? The ultra-wealthy? The government? Don't they have relatives dying from cancer, too? So ran the questions.

Frequently asked to debate this very issue in one minute or less of television time, I tried to avoid using the word *conspiracy* because it has become a flash word, an utterance pregnant with political and psychological overtones. Once an individual talks about "conspiracies" the specter of paranoia and political extremism is raised. It is practically Pavlovian. I usually fended off direct implications of my "extreme paranoia" by pointing out that Julius Caesar would be a great believer in conspiracy theories, and that both the Mafia and the Catholic Church—no offense intended—could be given as good examples of ongoing conspiracies transcending generations and even centuries.

Nonetheless, in answer to the question *"who....?"* I prefer to point to an interlock of vested interests, some of them psychological as well as political, some based as much on ego as economics. There is not, I believe, a central board of directors meeting in New York or Switzerland to suppress a given remedy. But there need not be. I have referred to the Club—and it exists as much in cancer research as in petroleum cartels, as much in medicine as in automobile manufacturing. It is purely human and is as closed a circle, as disciplined a fraternity, as any *other* interlock of vested interests.

In the strictly economic area, anytning that might get in the way of an industry that is now conservatively worth $30 billion a year must be perceived as a threat. Anything that *treats* cancer in a potentially far less expensive way must also be regarded as threatening—not so much to legions of narrow-vision scientists working on isolated aspects of the problem, and certainly not to the great majority of on-line physicians seeing lumps and bumps in their offices, but to the tremendous vested interests of economics, ego, and politics hiding behind them. On top of that, add the fact that the substance, or substances, in question are not susceptible of patents, and you have an additional reason to find unusually strong activity targeted against laetrile. Also, as pointed out earlier, and in strict terms of vested interest, the ultimate issue is not so much laetrile and cancer as it is simple, nontoxic therapies *and* prevention against degenerative disease. For, lurking behind the degenerative-disease-treatment industry, the lion's share of health-care delivery, is the vast world of pharmaceutical interests—a global, intertwining cartel.

From the standpoint of ideology, the dominance of medicine by the allopathic school automatically means that what physicians read, how they are trained, and who does their postgraduate education will have an allopathic tinge. The battle of homeopaths, naturopaths, and chiropractors for a place in the medical sun in this country is not a hidden story, after all. Where research funds will go means in science and medicine—just as in politics and economics—direct or indirect compliance with an implied set of premises. In cancer research, it means relative adherence to the theory that cancer is many diseases, not one; that it *is* tumor disease; that it is almost certainly caused by viruses. Deviations from these *premises* are hardly attitudes for which federal and even large private funds will be allocated. This hardly means that 99 percent of the individuals involved in the funding process are evil. They are simply *human*.

Which brings us to the powerful role of human ego, something I programs for identifying environmental carcinogens as "little more than public relations gimmicks—paper tigers to reassure the concerned public that something is being done when it isn't. This is standard policy in NIH [the National Institutes of Health]. The program on cigarette health hazards is a farce. It consists of noisy scare campaigns which are counter-productive—like most of cancer education."

Dr. Howard Temin, a Nobel Prize-winning cancer virologist at the University of Wisconsin, told the legislators, "We can now say that infectious viruses like those that cause many human diseases do not cause most human cancer. Therefore, we cannot hope to develop a vaccine against a virus to prevent most human cancer... We do not now have the fundamental knowledge to prevent or cure much human cancer."

Dr. Sidney M. Wolfe, a health consultant to the Ralph Nader consumer crusaders, belled the cat as he testified, "Prevention cuts into the profit margin of existing industries, which have thus far been able to escape the costs of the cancer they cause. NCI, under new leadership, must choose to become the leader in the war to prevent cancer rather than the banking operation for the largely unsuccessful war to treat it after it happens." Dr. Wolfe's characterization of the national cancer effort was that it was a "sham battle."

The 1977 testimony was the first major pail of cold water hurled onto the propaganda flames of the war on cancer. It did not stop the American Cancer Society from its annual announcements, usually around fund-raising time, that the "war on cancer is being won." Nor did it stop the tabloid press from reporting in seventy-two-point type on amazing new cancer research turning up promising results in tumor shrinkage of laboratory animals. A reading of the actual texts of most stories usually brought out the reality that such exciting new drugs were very much in the experimental stage, were very costly, were accompanied by side effects, and would not be ready for general human use for years to come. This is not to say that an occasional worthwhile agent, usually an immune-system-stimulating one, is not under study and offers some hopeful prospects.

By 1978, Food and Drug Administration Commissioner Donald Kennedy was correctly styling the war on cancer a "medical Vietnam"—a war the Establishment could seem neither to get out of nor win. Even so, the information was gathering that changes in diet and lifestyle were more and more linked to cancer, a line of research that had been pursued, then dropped, in the 1940s. NCI Director Arthur Upton, asked in 1978 by Senator McGovern's Senate nutrition committee why the NCI was spending only one percent of its budget on the diet-cancer connection when an estimated half of cancer is linked to diet, said, "I wonder about that myself sometimes." This led to Senator McGovern's response that "the suspicion that we are losing the war on cancer because of mistaken priorities has grown strong in my mind as I've listened here today."

Despite the ACS' celebrity yacht cruises, its identification of "cancer's seven warning signals," its clever courting of the mass media, and the backup of favorable press releases from the FDA and NCI, the reality cannot be obscured. Up to now, the war on cancer has, for the most part, been lost. No artful dodging of the facts, manipulations of semantics, or clever juggling of statistics can successfully subvert this horrendous fact.

As a persistent bringer of unpleasant realities, the National Center for Health Statistics announced that in 1976 the overall death rate had declined for the first time in American history (even the number of deaths attributable to heart disease was down). Only three categories of mortality-rate increase were noted between 1973 and 1975: *cancer,* murder, and suicide. The early cancer figures suggested a 4.2 percent increase in fatalities, a real shocker for the Conquest of Cancer program and still a shock when total figures were adjusted downward. The final figures were 2.3 percent overall increase in cancer mortalities and a 0.7 percent increase in "age-adjusted" deaths. This hardly cheered the cancer fighters, either, because the average annual mortality increase between 1968 and 1974 had been 0.2 percent. NCHS Center head Dr. Robert Armstrong noted that cancer was the only leading cause of death for which the mortality rate had steadily increased over the last two decades.

A perusal of the American Cancer Society's annual publication *Cancer Facts and Figures* tells the tale. The "long-term survival" of cancer patients has not increased significantly for a quarter-century. Behind this hidden reality is an outrageous manipulation of statistics and twisting of semantics to gull the American public into believing there has been real progress in the war on cancer.

For example, the 1982 edition of *Cancer Facts and Figures* blissfully repeats what the ACS has been saying for years: "In the 1930's less than one in five was alive at least five years after treatment. In the 1940's it was one in four. Now the ratio is one in three. The gain from one in four to one in three currently represents about 70,000 people this year." This does indeed *sound* like progress. But is it?

It was Daniel Greenberg, editor and publisher of *Science and Government,* who in 1975 challenged the cancer establishment when he reported that the actual survival rates had changed relatively little since 1955. The reason even for *this* change over prior rates, he argued, was very probably due to the postwar introduction of antibiotics and blood transfusions to help reduce the toll from cancer surgery. What this means simply is that more people have survived *operations* for cancer that at an earlier time would have killed them. It says nothing about surviving cancer *per se.*

In *Science* for 4 March 1977 Drs. James E. Enstrom and Donald

F. Austin of the University of California School of Public Health and Tumor Registry reported that "So long as [cancer] incidence and mortality remain unchanged or change proportionately, no genuine change in survival can occur.... Both the age-adjusted total cancer incidence rate and the age-adjusted total cancer mortality rate changed by only a few percent between 1950 and 1970.... The fact that neither has changed significantly since 1950 implies that the total cancer survival rate has also remained essentially constant."

American Cancer Society figures admitted that during 1982 about 835,000 people would be diagnosed as having cancer, a staggering increase eight years after the beginning of the war on cancer program. This figure does not include skin cancer (non-melanoma) or uterine cervical cancer in women. Non-melanoma skin cancer has been "substantially under-reported," the ACS notes, adding that the annual number of new cases is estimated at 400,000. This figure alone brings us to more than 1.2 million new cases of cancer per year, including 430,000 fatalities.

In fact, the flipfloppery of the ACS over its handling of nonmelanoma skin cancer and uterine cervical cancer very likely accounts for the society's perpetual misstatements as to how many lucky Americans are alive today because they opted for orthodox therapy.

In Ruth Rosenbaum's most revealing "Cancer, Inc." (*New Times*, 25 November 1977) it was pointed out that it took ACS vice president of public information Irving Rimer to explain the meaning behind the ACS' titillating claim in its 1975 annual report that "cancer incidence has declined slightly in the last 25 years."

What? Who? How?

"You have to understand," Rosenbaum quoted Rimer, "somewhere around 1972 or '73, we stopped including in our calculations all skin cancers except melanoma, the only one that's fatal, and also *in situ* cervical cancers, because *many experts don't consider these to be cancers at all.* [Emphasis mine.] Since together they account for a large number of cases, that could be why the incidence has gone down."

This may very well be why, as the ACS so merrily puts it in its basic public information publication, *The Hopeful Side of Cancer,* the disease "is one of the most curable of the major diseases in this country." Skin and cervical cancer—not considered by some even fit to be classed as cancer—may in fact account for many of the 1.5 million Americans "alive today who have had cancer." As Rosenbaum adds, "Though their own chief statistician reportedly suggested that the figure be dropped because of its unreliable data base, ACS brazenly upped it to 2 million in 1976." In 1982, ACS reported that "there are over 3 million Americans alive today who have a history of cancer...."

At the end of 1981, the National Cancer Institute (NCI),

primarily through its director, Dr. Vincent DeVita, unleashed a fairly optimistic picture of the cancer disaster through some preliminary data which indicated increases in five-year survival rates—American oncology parlance for "cures"—of at least 45 percent. This would be above and beyond the earlier small gains in five-year survival rates claimed for childhood leukemia and Hodgkin's disease, alleged triumphs in chemotherapy which in themselves account for hardly more than two percent of cancer.

The preliminary data and other NCI figures had some mixed news that was almost as contradictory as it was confusing—Hawaiians were said to have the nation's highest cancer rate, yet Oriental-descent Americans (along with Hispanics and American Indians) had lower rates than everyone else, and the new figures showed one out of every three Americans would get cancer before age 74 (seemingly up from the one out of four across the board reported years before) while one in six (down from one in five) would die from the disease.

Dr. DeVita, a vocal foe of laetrile, said: "For the past decade, we have been more successful in treating cancer patients than we thought."

This was a puzzlement, and criticism of the NCI's data base was not long in coming. Dr. Marvin A. Schneiderman, a leading cancer statistician formerly connected with the NCI, said if there had been a gain in survival rates it might be due to a change in the "mix" of "forms" of cancer, with more people getting "milder" forms and/or being diagnosed and treated earlier, conditions which would have nothing to do with improvements of American oncology's Big Three in the anti-cancer arsenal: surgery, chemotherapy and radiation.

And the *New York Times* quoted John Young, head of the NCI demographic analysis section, as saying he and his colleagues were normally reluctant to release survival figures for all cancers because such a figure is "not that meaningful a measure" of a disease which orthodoxy considers to be many diseases.

The "bottom lines," despite any reading of statistics, preliminary or otherwise, are that more people are getting cancer and dying from it than ever before.

Also, it is easy to forget that the official "cure" statements are based on *five-year survivals*—and are not necessarily cures at all. A recurrence of cancer a decade or more later, which is commonplace, may *not* affect earlier assessments of so-called cures. The fact is, as most cancer specialists admit when pressed to the wall, by any precise definition of the word *cure,* orthodoxy has no cure at all. But it *is* true that in some "forms"—that is, manifestations of symptoms—of the disease there have been longer rates of symptom suppression. Of course, a symptom suppression over seventy years would, by any fair definition, be construable as a cure so long as the underlying disease in no observable or traceable way negatively affected the host.

By 1980, the ACS propaganda line, following on the heels of its perennial "one out of every three people who learn this year they have cancer will survive five years or more after treatment"—a fact which has not meaningfully changed since the mid-1950s—was that "but of course 50 percent *could* be saved" if they had prompter diagnoses and treatment.

There is a fair amount of gobbledygook in all this, of course. Aside from using "saved" for "cured"—and meaning five years free of symptoms—ACS implies that the cancer industry has a "proven" remedy for cancer. It doesn't.

The projections of a better job of symptom-suppression in young bodies able to withstand chemotherapy were accompanied, going into 1981, with ACS's parrotings of Breakthrough Number Umpteen-Plus, the use of interferon in cancer.

Interferon, a natural protein produced by the body and shown to be a natural defense against viral infections, may have anti-cancer properties, according to some reports. The action in the U.S. cancer industry at this time, however, has little to do with natural, intrinsic interferon. By spring of 1980 pharmaceutical companies, picking up the scent of both anti-cancer possibilities and profits, had poured $150 million into interferon research and production facilities, with NCI announcing it would buy up to $9 million worth of the material for future studies and the ACS pledging $5.8 million to test the substance.

Exogenous interferon—produced outside the body—carried a price tag, as of 1980, at between $10 *billion* and $20 *billion* per pound!

The earlier reports of interferon effectiveness dimmed after studies revealed by Sloan-Kettering and the American Society of Clinical Oncology found interferon either of little direct anti-cancer benefit or productive of only temporary effects, though immune stimulation seems definitely to have occurred. Interferon's real role in cancer, many believe, may be in those "forms" of the disease associated with viruses, but not in those which are, for example, hormone-dependent.

Nonetheless, the commitment to providing a *natural* substance, and the ACS' improved rhetoric about immunotherapy, further opened the door of Club thinking into natural and immune-system-stimulating ideas. In a statement which the Society would have rejected a decade before as rank heresy, ACS said in its 1981 report, "Immunotherapy holds hope of harnessing the body's own disease-fighting systems to combat cancer with essentially no overt toxicity. In laboratory animals, substances such as BCG (a tuberculosis vaccine) can stimulate immune mechanisms. These substances are being used in humans alone or with other forms of treatment."

Egad—shades of Coley, Doyen, Deakin, Gerson, and Pauling, to name only a few!

The rhetoric is good. It bespeaks both the failure of orthodoxy and an at least hesitant willingness—one might say desperation—to look elsewhere. Indeed, there is a virtual rush in orthodox cancer research to look at immunotherapy, to find new ways to stimulate the body's natural defenses, all of which gives immunotherapy the fascinating possibility of being a bridge between holistic, or metabolic/nutritional, medicine and allopathic nostrums. Too, the examination of the genetic component in cancer, and the possibility of genetic manipulation through advanced technology that is just now beginning to make itself felt, indicate possibilities of cancer breakthroughs as medicine as usual yields, out of sheer failure, to desperately needed new ideas.

In the meantime, have rates really improved for some "forms" of cancer—at least in terms of longer suppression of symptoms? Sure. But that's the lesser of the facts involved.

As the National Cancer Institute's Dr. Dean Burk consistently pointed out in the 1970s, rates for some "forms" of cancer are actually worse now than they were years ago. Greenberg found this in assessing the cancer debacle in 1975—plus a whole smokescreen of misleading numbers, anonymity, and enforced silence. Researchers spoke openly to him about their real feelings only when guaranteed anonymity, something I found in talks with scientists from several research centers. The most telling quotation of all came from a researcher at NCI, who told Greenberg, "Look, when you've got 10,000 radiologists and millions of dollars' worth of equipment, you give radiation treatments, even if study after study shows that a lot of it does more harm than good. What else are they going to do? They're doing what they've been trained to do. Like surgeons. They're trained to cut, so they cut."

The Failure, Threat—And Cost—Of Orthodox Therapy

The Cancer Society and its allies usually took exception to the Committee for Freedom of Choice's references to data extrapolated by Dr. Burk from former NCI director Frank Rauscher, Jr., that under orthodox methods—that is, surgery, radiation, chemotherapy, which some of us baptized "cut, burn and poison," much to the consternation of the ACS, *et al.* there was a global likelihood of a five-year survival for only 7.5 percent of metastatic cancer cases. Turning this around, it meant that there was a 92.5 percent likelihood of a cancer patient *not* surviving for five years with disseminated cancer. But no good counterfigures were offered, for the modest life extension achievements in childhood leukemia and Hodgkin's were more than offset by big increases in lung, breast, and several other forms of cancer. (Too, the chemotherapy used to treat cancer also is suspected of developing secondary cancer, as is the case with Hodgkin's, in which five percent of patients develop leukemia ten years later, as *Newsweek* concluded in a 1981 survey which was guardedly optimistic about chemotherapy.)

In spring 1977, a man with a quarter-century of experience in analyzing cancer statistics even took apart Establishment claims of great successes in childhood leukemia and Hodgkin's. He was physiologist Hardin B. Jones, assistant director of the Donner Laboratory of the University of California-Berkeley and a personal friend of mine. Dr. Jones, who died in 1978 at sixty-three, was a key witness for the defense in the government's "international laetrile smuggling ring" trial in San Diego, even though the jury was not allowed to hear his testimony, so vital to explain the reason for the clandestine entry of Mexican laetrile into the country. He was on hand to tell U.S. District Court Judge William B. Enright that not only had cancer mortality rates not materially changed in the Western world since the early part of this century, but that the apparent improvement in chemotherapies for childhood leukemia "wouldn't be affecting more than one hundredth of one percent of all the cancers that are occurring in the country."

While orthodoxy was claiming a cure rate of up to 80 percent in Hodgkin's disease, the California researcher, who had reported on cancer statistics for the American Cancer Society years before, said the statistics might be misleading because "it is also possible that cases of Hodgkin's disease are simply dying of other causes having to do with treatment rather than the obvious extension of the disease." In the meantime, "the evidence for curability is distinctly in doubt" for all other forms of cancer.

"If we take mortality from cancer and compare individuals of the same sex and the same age throughout the calendar time in this century, we are hard pressed to see any difference in the mortality rates from approximately 1911," Dr. Jones testified. This was the earliest cancer tabulation in England. The U.S. rates have held steady since they began to be tabulated in the early 1920s, he argued.

Judge Enright did something of a double take when Dr. Jones testified once again that a woman with breast cancer would statistically do four times better—that is, live four times longer—if she remained *untreated!*

Before the California Board of Medical Examiners in 1975, Dr. Jones had testified, "Most clinicians claim up to a 50 percent cure rate for various malignancies. If this were sure we would see a shift downward by up to 50 percent in mortality. However, we do not see this; mortality figures show an overall trend of increase which is unaffected by any attempts to treat the disease. Statistically, patients are as well or better off untreated as those who have treatment, in the sense that the death rate remains the same, or slightly better, for those who are not treated at all."

A key reason for misleading cancer treatment figures, Dr. Jones said, is this, "I discovered that there have been errors in cancer reporting for many years because of the necessity of gathering cases into statistical groupings during which they are not reported. Those who publish results wait until treatment is over before publishing, and so there is a gap in the statistics brought about by their failure to report anything from the time treatment begins until it ceases, which is usually several years." Since patients who die during surgery are excluded from survival results, for example, "in the treated group, deaths which occur before completion of treatment are rejected from the data...With this effect stripped out, the common malignancies show a remarkably similar rate of demise, whether treated or untreated."

In 1969, Dr. Jones assessed the overall statistical problem for the American Cancer Society this way (and he told me in 1977 he was standing by all points of his prior analysis):

> (1) Evidence for benefit from cancer therapy has depended on systematic biometric errors.
> (2) Neither the timing nor the extent of treatment of the true malignancies has appreciably altered the average course of the disease. *The possibility exists that treatment makes the average situation worse.* [Emphasis mine.]
> (3) It is important to consider as a preferred mode of cancer therapy a mild degree of treatment designed to reduce the troublesome symptoms of the primary disease without adding to the health problems of the patient.
> (4) While the evidence of the falsity of claims about cancer therapy is overriding, some infrequent benefits may have been achieved but obscured by the major trend. In the absence of convincing evidence to this effect after 50 years of cancer therapy, however, these postulated benefits must be very rare indeed to have been incapable of proof.
> (5) The combined effect of the mistaken evaluation of the nature of cancer and the failure to recognize that treatment has not produced "cure" has had grave consequences.

The "Cancer Patient Survival" report of the National Cancer Institute in the 1970s noted that the total five-year cancer survival rate in the United States had increased only two percent since 1950. Taking another look at even that misleading statistic, Dr. Lucien Israel, France's leading cancer specialist, who was called in to treat Betty Ford, told writer Philip Nobile in 1978 that:

> This so-called five-year cure pertains mainly to surgery. The limit of five years was chosen because

the after-five number of recurrences drops off between five and 15 years.

But here the statistics are deceptive: The number of recurrences drops five years only because the total number of survivors has dropped significantly by then and continues to do so. The rate of tumor growth remains the same. The fact that nothing is detectable after five years does not imply nothing will be detectable at seven years. . . .

He added that "basically, surgery is a powerless cure. For example, about 20 percent of cancer patients [who] die after having had surgery succumb to local recurrence—that is, the tumor reappears in the same place. But 80 percent die from distant metastases, which existed in germ even before the operation. . . . Surgeons guess wrong 90 percent of the time on the presence of remaining microscopic cancer cells." This is, in fact, the fallacy of the "we got it all" school of cancer therapy, which usually starts with local surgery that mostly *fails* to "get it all," and then, painfully and expensively, progresses to chemotherapy and radiation.

It is one statistical reality that orthodox therapy has failed to dent either the incidence of or fatalities from cancer, at least by any appreciable margin. That would be a grim enough assessment of "business as usual" in the $30-billion-a-year cancer industry. But we must now face the reality that orthodox therapy may even be *worsening* the problem—and, in the case of breast cancer in women, as we will shortly see, decidedly *is* aggravating the situation.

It is known that surgery, the original and exclusive "treatment of choice" in cancer, can actually *spread* cancer. It can stimulate metastases that otherwise may be inhibited by the primary tumor itself, according to the work of Dr. Michael Feldman and others at Israel's Weizmann Institute in 1978. The rush to the knife, then, is *not* a tried-and-true approach to cancer. Primary tumors *themselves*, unless they pose an immediate, life-threatening situation, are not in and of themselves killers. Cancer primarily kills by the spread of cancer cell clusters—metastasis—to vital tissues and organs. Hence the extreme relevance of the Sugiura findings at Sloan-Kettering; amygdalin did little to inhibit *primary* tumors, but was obviously active in blocking metastases.

Also, as Krebs, Jr., *et al.* have noted, the majority of cells in a tumor mass in many cases is normal. A huge tumor may be composed of a large majority of normal tissue, and the ability of cancer drugs and radiation to blast out or poison the tumor is actually an index of the capacity of these modalities to theaten the entire defenses of the host. Indeed, chemotherapy—which is essentially the use of highly toxic chemicals to mimic the action of radiation—is really a race between so poisoning the whole body that the host himself dies or killing enough cancer cells first. The toxic chemicals in and of themselves may be fatal at even low doses, and most are not attempted other than under the strictest clinical conditions. Radiation is a sophisticated burning of tissues and is a modern update of an ancient attempt to treat cancer with fire.

The extreme danger in radiation and chemotherapy, aside from the possibility of helping spread the disease and/or causing secondary tumors later, lies in their blitzkrieg assault on the body's immunological defense against *all* disease. Assaulting cancer with radiation and chemotherapy other than in the most desperate of cases may be likened to the dropping of hydrogen bombs on a hostile state and killing two million people in an effort to knock out the country's 50,000-man navy.

In case after case, a patient may actually respond to "cancer treatment" in the sense that his *symptoms* show a response to the poisons and/or radiation blasts pumped into him, and yet his immune system is so sabotaged that he may die of a simple infection. Needless to say, the use of mutilating surgery, other than where utterly essential, and the administration of toxic chemicals with their brutalizing and life-depleting side effects, constitute a violation of the first injunction of the Hippocratic Oath, "First, do no harm." Indeed, cancer has become a disease in which, by orthodox reasoning, the patient is supposed to feel much worse before he can become better.

Happily, the newer school of immunotherapy has more than a foot in the door of orthodox credibility, and from it have flowed several ways of harnessing the body's immune system to fight back against cancer. Ironically enough, orthodoxy is accepting some of the theory and practice of immunotherapy while still turning a cold shoulder to the use of megavitamins and enzymes, immune stimulators par excellence.

None of this is to say that there have been no responses and recoveries under orthodox therapy. People are walking around today totally free of the symptoms of cancer and free of the debilitating effects of their therapy. They are to be praised and applauded, but their survival has far more to do with the basic health of their immune systems and genetic inheritance than it does with the marvels of modern chemistry.

Overall, as we have seen, there is little statistically to recommend orthodox therapy as practiced and understood up to now, but there *have* been apparent gains, some of which must be viewed with caution. In their *Science* article, Drs. Enstrom and Austin pointed out that the tiny gains in three-year survival rates in acute, chronic and, chronic lymphocytic leukemia between 1955 and 1969—from 3 percent to 7 percent, from 39 percent to 41 percent, and from 51 to 53 percent respectively—are themselves misleading, "Although significant increases in leukemia survival are often cited as evidence of great progress in cancer control...the survival rate for leukemia with all forms has remained constant (20 percent). This is due to the increasing proportions of the highly fatal forms of leukemia," they wrote.

Dr. Matthew Block of the University of Colorado Medical Center noted in *Medical World News* in 1974 that "in the case of chronic lymphatic leukemia as we see it in adults, if the survival time is not better than it was 30 years ago, then we must conclude that there is something we are doing to these people that is making their survival shorter. The use of transfusions as well as other aspects of better ancillary care should have increased longevity in this disease and if it is not any better we must then conclude that...indeed longevity has been decreased by treatment."

The National Cancer Institute disclosed at the Sixty-Sixth Annual Meeting of the American Association for Cancer Research in 1976 that several drugs that the screening process of the Food and Drug Administration had allowed to be used to treat cancer may be responsible for the development of secondary tumors. These include such standard orthodox modalities as vincristine, nitrogen mustard, chlorambucil, procarbazine, and phenylalanine mustard (L-PAM), all of which cause toxic side effects, and the hormone prednisone.

Far more sinister, however, have been the delayed reactions to the invasion, decades ago, of X-rays into therapy of all kinds. Only now are we beginning to pay the bills for the overexposure of our people to radiation, which once was considered sound medical practice for everything from acne and ringworm of the scalp to enlarged adenoids and tonsils. Cancer researchers in 1977 began attributing the increase in both malignant and benign tumors of the thyroid to X-rays, some of them administered forty years before.

Also, the delayed effects of both radiation and chemotherapy in children are suspected of causing new tumors as many as fifteen to twenty years later. The University of Southern California Cancer Center's Dr. G. Denman Hammond announced these delayed effects in 1978, but added that such secondary effects—less severe than the earlier cancers—had not been a problem before "because the patients didn't live long enough to have those problems." One such problem is an inhibition of spine growth.

In 1977, four NCI doctors reported that certain alkylating drugs used in women treated for cancer of the ovaries have apparently caused thirteen cases of leukemia each year in every thousand women so treated, and that leukemia might appear in 5 to 10 percent of patients who survive for ten years.

But pity the researcher who does too much in bringing such unhappy realities to the fore. The aforementioned Dr. Irwin Bross of Roswell Park wrote off the NCI's refusal to renew his $1.5 million research grant as "medical politics" after he and Dr. Nachimuthu Natarajan reported that low-dose radiation of either parent could cause leukemia in children. The two pointed out that leukemia could be caused in a child if its mother was X-rayed while she was pregnant or if either parent was X-rayed before the child was conceived. They based their assessment on a study of the medical records of and interviews with 300 families in New York, Maryland, and Minnesota, and also noted that the likelihood of such low-dose radiation causing leukemic children, while serious, is probably less than one in 100. Dr. Bross pinned much of the blame on physicians who order unnecessary X-rays for their patients and recommended that health care insurance companies sign a statement that the therapy is necessary.

But the sanctity of X-ray therapy is not to be trifled with. The yanking of his funds did not unduly ruffle Dr. Bross, who said the action was in response to "self-interest groups protecting themselves."

He added, "This is a hard game I'm in.... The public is putting the money up for all these research projects, but the public never has a say on how the money should be spent. The medical research grants are given out by medical people. One of the biggest mistakes the public makes is to let technologists make all the decisions on technology."

Dr. Bross put the entire matter of orthodox cancer therapy into a rhetorical question on 10 August 1978 in testimony before the Committee on Health of the New York State Assembly—a body which twice voted in favor of freedom on choice in the matter of laetrile, only to see both bills vetoed by the governor:

> Primary prevention of cancer is a threat because it offers an alternative to the therapeutic control of cancer. Since it offers a choice it raises a question: Which approach is most effective? This, in turn, raises a question that oncologists don't want raised: How effective is orthodox cancer therapy? For instance, most of the $30 billion is spent on cancer patients with generalized disease. However, none of the orthodox treatments, singly or in combination, can cure a patient with generalized disease. So the awkward question arises: Is it worth $30 billion a year just to prolong the agony for a few months?

And just how much does it cost to prolong the agony for a few months, weeks or days? Plenty—and therein, of course, lies a great deal of the rub. A 1978 *Consumer Reports* study estimated the average cost of cancer to be about $20,000 per patient for *direct* medical services. The cost of health has ballooned faster than inflation, however, and the more reasonable figure was closer to $30,000 going into this decade. With hospital rooms running $400-$500 a day and up, and an average hospital visit for cancer patients of

15 days, cancer price tags often pass $50,000.

But the *indirect* costs of cancer are far worse. The American Cancer Society noted in its *1980 Cancer Facts and Figures* that taking into account reduced or lost earning power due to illness and death from cancer, "estimates range from $13.7 billion to $22.7 billion, making cancer and other neoplasms the most costly group of diseases after circulatory disorders." A 1969 Department of Health, Education and Welfare study set the *direct* cost of treating cancer at $5.3 billion in 1975. Inflation will have greatly expanded that figure today. The direct and indirect costs of cancer obviously constitute a total industry far in excess of $30 billion a year. And the price is going up by leaps and bounds every year.

From the testimony of Dr. Bross, the analyses of the late Dr. Jones, the revelations by such probing journalists as Greenberg, the long-held positions of Dr. Burk, and ever-more developing information from cancer researchers who are not afraid to speak their minds, the reality becomes ever clearer that the war on cancer has meant the throwing of good money after bad. Even when the funds are legitimately targeted for legitimate research, the results are questionable enough. But, as in any bureaucratic effort, vested interest occasionally rears its head. The General Accounting Office found in 1977 that a major research facility had apparently used test animals, research material, and equipment, all provided by federal cancer funds, to do work for its corporate clients—which produce chemicals that the research firm was supposedly monitoring for cancer-causing effects! Involved was $22.5 million worth of U.S. funds and a $12 million contract awarded to the same institute first in 1973 and again in 1977 without competitive bids. One of the institute's directors was the chairman of a National Cancer Advisory Board subcommittee that monitored a division of the NCI which awarded the contracts.

But Cancergate is more, much more, than an occasional conflict of interest. It is suppressed information, the suffocation of promising research, the stifling of unwanted and "unproved" remedies, the ruining of careers of those who do not toe the line. Its history started long before the laetrile rumpus. It can only be our prayer that it ends there.

Mammography: Keeping Abreast Of A Scandal

In 1978, and following a delay of six months and much haggling, a report was brought to light that conservatively estimated that forty-eight American women—and probably many more—had needlessly lost their breasts as the result of misdiagnoses in a government-sponsored, American Cancer Society-promoted "breast cancer screening project."

Lurking behind the admission is the reality that probably many more women, stampeded into the campaign to have their breasts screened by an X-ray program—mammography—might develop cancer later from the years-delayed effects of radiation. The twin realities are all the more infuriating in the light of such studies as those by the late Dr. Hardin Jones that, statistically, even women *with* diagnosed breast cancer will live four times longer if they remain *untreated*.

The 1978 disclosures, pushed to the forefront by a group of pathologists headed by Dr. Robert A. McDivitt of the University of Utah College of Medicine, constituted the most recent chapter in the breast screening program, the possible cancer-*causing* risks of which had been warned about from its inception in 1973 by John Bailar III, editor of the *Journal of the National Cancer Institute*. Those who wanted to bring the matter to public attention simply felt, as Daniel Greenberg reported it in the *Washington Post,* that "purposeless mutilation had been inflicted on many women" and that "no matter how embarrassing the blunders might be for the image of medicine, the matter should be brought into the open to preclude repetitions."

The other side, surgeons and clinicians who sought to maintain Club discipline, argued that the practitioners involved were only trying to do their best. The fight between the two groups had kept the statistics from public view and, assessed Greenberg, "the fact that we know anything at all about this sorry business is no small event in the sociology of medicine." Editor Bailar, a physician and biostatistician, had strongly suggested that the actual incidence of needless breast surgery is probably a lot higher than forty-eight cases that the pathologists were able to identify from the confusing records of the Breast Cancer Detection Demonstration Project.

The project was launched in 1973 when the American Cancer Society induced the government's National Cancer Institute, as the money pump of funds for the war on cancer, to put up $45 million in an extensive and expensive campaign to alert American women to the dangers of breast cancer and the marvels of early diagnosis. The ultimate tab for taxpayers is expected to range between $55 and $58 million.

The latest collision between the keepers of Club silence and the dedicated medical men who believe dirty linen should be aired in public, no matter how embarrassing it may be, had been preceded in 1977 by open criticism of the program, which by then already involved 280,000 women 35 years old and over showing up at twenty-seven medical centers around the country.

One 1977 assessment was that at least 13 percent of women who underwent mammary surgery for small tumors located as part of the X-ray screening program had lost their breasts needlessly. At about the same time, a government-sponsored committee called for further restrictions on the use of X-rays to detect breast cancer, citing the risk from X-rays in developing breast cancer ten to fifteen years later.

The findings on misdiagnosis and needless breast surgery and removal were arrived at after analyses of tissue samples taken after surgery on women in whom tiny breast abnormalities had been found at various of the twenty-seven centers. Some 13 percent of tissue samples identified as cancerous at the time of surgery were actually benign, and 4 or 5 percent of others may have been "questionable," though these figures were cast into doubt by program defenders.

Even so, 15 September 1977 the National Institutes of Health called for restrictions on the program, asking that women thirty-five to thirty-nine have mammograms *only* if they already had breast cancer, that X-rays be permitted for women forty to forty-nine only if there was a history of breast cancer in their immediate families, and that X-ray screening for women under fifty be abandoned because of a lack of evidence that mammograms reduce the breast cancer death rate in younger women who have no cancer symptoms.

The *Journal of the American Medical Association* reported that year on early results of the program that in 106 breast cancer surgery patients under forty-five, 84 percent of the tumors had been detected by the patients themselves and only 2 percent had been discovered by X-rays. In an astonishing 63 percent of cases, X-rays had failed to detect the disease.

Medical writers Greenberg and Judith Randal had earlier revealed in the *Washington Post* that the 1963 New York Health Insurance Plan (HIP) study on which the mammography drive was based contained information that, had it been heeded, might have restricted the mammography campaign from the beginning.

"While ACS sought to sway public and medical opinion against the interim [mammography] guidelines...three committees of experts appointed by NCI in October 1975 were quietly engaged in studies that eventually hit the X-ray screening program like a bomb crashing into a munitions dump," they wrote.

From these studies came such information as the fact that of the 132 tumors detected during the HIP project, 45 percent had been *missed* by X-ray examination, and mammography was written off as an ineffectual way to detect breast cancers at the early stage. It was also revealed that 47 percent of the aggressive tumors detected by mammography were so large that they could have been discovered by simple physical examination.

An early analysis of the HIP findings was that the hazards of X-raying women under fifty were not outweighed by the benefits—a point strongly made by Bailar—and a statement at a 1974 meeting by an expert that mammography is of "virtually no value in women under 50" went unheeded.

Also, the Ralph Nader Health Research Group obtained data on fifty-seven X-ray machines used in the national breast screening program and found seventeen of them producing X-ray levels that were "ominously high."

Dr. Irwin J. Bross, who, as we have seen, is no novice at ruffling the feathers of officialdom, reported that "extensive information about the hazards of ionizing radiation used in the mammography of symptom-free women under fifty was available in the early planning stage of the program," and in the words of an ACS statistician, "no one at ACS appears to have looked carefully at these hazards and realized their seriousness."

With such early warning signals, why the effort to push forward with such a program? Simply the "public relations yield" for the Cancer Society, Greenberg and Randal suggest. "The 280,000 women in the screening program would serve as a word-of-mouth force that would spread news of breast screening, and ACS' role in it, to many times that number."

Mammography is held to be so highly sensitive that it can detect the tiniest of tissue changes, ones that normally go unnoticed. This new capability turned up hundreds of tiny lesions, frequently labelled "cancerous" by pathologists who had not had prior experience with them. Breasts were lopped off upon such determinations and recorded as swift victories against cancer based on early detection. Only after the McDivitt group did postoperative tissue reviews was it disclosed that surgery had been performed on many misdiagnosed cases.

By 1978, X-ray dosage in the federal mammography program had been cut to a third of the originally approved level. In the meantime, mammography or no, the surgical removal of breasts—which, at $20,000 a whack, threatens to make breast removal as booming a business in cancer as coronary bypass surgery is in heart disease—is still the "treatment of choice" in breast cancer. As such it is a mutilating leftover from the last century, when the "radical mastectomy" was pioneered. In this operation, which in recent years American women have been undergoing at a rate of 1,000 a week, the entire breast, its underlying muscles, and nearby lymph nodes, are removed. This frequently happens even when women go in for what they think will be only a biopsy—an operation to remove a small piece of tissue for examination.

This "radical" surgery, which often leaves the patient with a great deal of pain, is something of an anachronism, for the removal of lymph nodes eliminates one possible nearby attack on cancer itself, and it now is known that operations *on* cancer can actually *spread* it. And, all too frequently, this first radical mutilation is only the beginning of a long, downward spiral in which, whether further mutilations occur or not, therapy will shift over to radiation and toxic, system-poisoning drugs.

Radical mastectomies still occur in spite of the report in 1976 by Dr. Bernard Fisher of the results of an NCI study of 1,700 patients at thirty-four medical centers. It showed that there was no difference in survival or recurrence of cancer between the radical and simple mastectomies (breast removal) with or without radiation, in cases of Stage I (localized) and Stage II (area) malignancies. They are still performed despite the conclusions reached in 1978 by Dr. Alfred Meyer and colleagues at the Rockford (Illinois) School of Medicine. Their assessment of 1,686 patients found that there were no significant differences in five-and ten-year survivals for "simple, modified radical or radical mastectomy."

In 1972, Dr. M. Vera Peters, studying 162 breast cancer cases at Princess Margaret Rose Hospital in Toronto and comparing radical mastectomies with "lumpectomies"—removal of the tumor alone—found the five-year survival rate to be about the same for each group, but slightly better for the lumpectomy cases: 72 percent to 70 percent.

But the rush to bring a patient under the knife only underscores the ingrained thinking of Western medicine—treat the symptoms of a disease—and the greatest skill in the treating of a symptom is the surgical excision of it. Through this primeval reasoning, surgeons remain the best-paid of the "health-care-delivery team."

The American Cancer Society maintains a list of "unproven" cancer remedies, one now headed, of course, by laetrile (vitamin B^{17}). But its list is based on the implied premise that there are *proven* remedies. Any disciplined scrutiny of the facts shows this not to be the case. Five-year suppressions of symptoms are not cures, and, billions of dollars later, the war on cancer is no closer to solving the mystery of what cancer is or how to treat it than when the program was designed in 1971.

Chapter Six
The ACS, the NCI and the
War on "Unprovens"

As a "charity," the multi-million-dollar American Cancer Society has to be one of the most profitable on record. And, in terms of fund-raising, one of the most successful. To think *cancer* is not only to think *death* but to think of "American Cancer Society," which at one time seemed as down-home as the flag and mom's apple pie.

But no longer. As the war on cancer seems increasingly lost and scandals such as the mammography program are aired, as the tax bite for cancer research mounts while the incidence of cancer and fatalities from it increase, the society's message of "fight cancer with a checkup and a check" and its announcements of light at the end of the tunnel, near-victory in the protracted war, etc., etc., take on a hollow tone reminiscent of Washington's Vietnam War "progress" pronouncements.

If any single agency was responsible for pushing the war on cancer along, it was ACS. If any group has any more influence on deciding how and where cancer research funds will be spent, it will be news to ACS. Since the mid 1940s—though the society was founded in 1913—the ACS has dominated what the public thinks and knows about the dreaded number-two killer disease of the West. The ACS fund-raising ball, celebrity cruise and annual "information" bash for newsmen are now all parts of Americana, originally as sacred as baseball and Fourth of July parades. But the botching of the anticancer effort has brought the society in for some rough criticism from people who in an earlier time would have been its backers.

Former FDA Commissioner Donald Kennedy, of all people, charged that ACS has dodged positions on environmental and industrial "causes" of cancer. Other researchers have noted that the ACS, while death on prevention theories of cancer, has hardly uttered a peep about industrial carcinogens, while taking the full share of credit for alerting the nation to the perils of cigarette smoking.

A congressional aide said in 1978 that the society "works like a money pump. They don't represent the experts and they promote the government's interest in expertise by lobbying Congress and the public. In effect, their hand reaches right into the appropriations pocket."

Knight-Ridder News Service recalled in 1978 that the ACS declined to take a position during regulatory hearings on suspected pesticide cancer-causers as well as the food additive Red Dye No. 2, the fire retardant Tris and forms of synthetic estrogen. One federal regulator has said this passivity makes the society one that should be called "the infantile society for national paralysis."

For years ACS fund-raisers told the American public that the organization could not finance promising research "due to insufficient funds," and they were not called on this until 1976. At that time, the National Information Bureau (NIB), which monitors charities, said the society could hardly make the "insufficient funds" claim when it already had $31 million in uncommitted funds. After auditing the ACS in 1976 and 1977, the NIB concluded that "questions arise with respect to the ACS' accumulation of assets beyond the amount required for its next year's budget." A careful observation of ACS funding between 1970 and 1973 showed that, while the society had increased its income by $24 million, the percentage allocated to cancer research actually declined. Indeed, this amount slipped to 27.1 percent in 1975.

Even in the 1978-79 budget ($149 million), the ACS allocated only 32.4 percent to research, with the vast amount of the remainder going to "public education," "professional education," "fund-raising," office overhead, and general management. More than $18 million was spent in 1978-79 on fund raising alone. Only a third of ACS's total budget in 1981 was designated for research.

Investigative reporter Peter Barry Chowka detailed (in "The Cancer Charity Ripoff," *East-West Journal,* July 1978) that in fiscal 1976 the society spent $114 million, but its assets totalled $181 million, and that between 1970 and 1973 the organization's net annual profit doubled. "With so many millions of dollars invested and deposited in checking and savings accounts, ACS is a prime banking customer," he wrote. "At least eighteen members of the ACS Board of Directors and House of Delegates are executive officers or directors of banks. As of 31 August 1976, 42 percent of ACS' cash and investments, totalling $75 million, were maintained in banks with which these eighteen men were affiliated."

Taking its own peek at an earlier ACS budget, the *National Enquirer* revealed in 1977 that the 1975 fiscal budget could be construed as showing that fifty-seven cents of every dollar went to officers, staff, and administrative expenses, and that the amount allotted to research was less than it paid its 2,900 employees. Also, only $5.7 million of the total $122 million income went to direct aid to cancer patients, and millions went into the ACS treasury to build up the society's unspent assets to $155 million.

In summer 1977, as part of the ongoing review of the war on cancer national effort, the House Committee on Government Operations, while investigating the National Cancer Institute, found that the NCI and the ACS in effect had interlocking directorates, although neither has taken any pains to hide this. The most obvious example of the comfortable relationship between the NCI as a spender of taxpayer monies in the cancer war and the major lobby for conducting that war in the first place was the hiring of former NCI Director Frank Rauscher as an ACS senior vice president—at a doubling of his annual salary to $75,000.

Chowka's piercing review of the ACS' board of directors pointed out that no crocodile tears should be shed over the fact that the board is not paid directly—being directors of a "charity"—but, not to worry, because much of it consists of physicians and scientists whose work is mostly supported by NCI and ACS grants. By ACS' own happy admission, 70 percent of its 1976 research budget went to "individuals or institutions" with which board members were affiliated.

Medical writers Daniel Greenberg and Judith Randal have pointed to the ACS as a primary reason why priorities in the war on cancer have focused on treatment rather than prevention, and argued that "the origins of this misemphasis lie in a little-known and complex relationship between the [NCI]—the 'Pentagon' of the War on Cancer—and the private but powerful American Cancer Society, which, among other things, serves as NCI's ministry of information for educating the public about cancer."

They wrote off the treatment emphasis in cancer as akin to "dealing with aviation disasters mainly by seeking to reconstruct wrecks rather than prevent them." The strategy continues, even though the NCI, as we have seen, has shown more and more interest in preventive aspects and nontoxic approaches. It *should,* of course, because NCI scientists have publicly stated that environmental sources account for as much as 90 percent of all cancers; others have linked at least 50 percent of cancer to diet.

Greenberg and Randal pointed out that the ACS' compliation of its own research spending in fiscal 1975 showed that it provided scientists with more than $2.1 million for new research projects that year, but only $92,000 went into environmental studies and $145,000 for research on chemical carcinogens, despite the burgeoning information linking cancer to such chemicals. No new awards in the environmental category were made in 1976, when more than $13.2 million for new research projects was available. In the 1976-77 report, Society cancer grants reflected additional interest in studying the immune system, which can only be considered a positive step, but most of the research the society is still talking about in this decade is still based on the viral theory of cancer and on chemotherapy and radiation.

Indeed, the ACS entry into immunotherapy on ever greater scales seems to reflect the tacit admission that cut-burn-and-poison approaches have, by and large, failed to stem the cancer tide. As this was written, the Society was far from any admission of the ability of nutritional and metabolic therapy to stimulate the immune system, for such an admission would grossly undercut the Society's long-held views on "nutritional quackery." The Society, in fact, seemed bent on improving its image by being the leader in assaults on the tobacco industry, a way to get around the criticism that for so long it had reflected so little interest in industrial causes of cancer. Even so, the ACS's assumption that a widespread decline in cigarette smoking would vastly reduce lung cancer (and, hence, thereby finally secure the slight downturn in cancer incidence statistics orthodoxy is so desperately seeking in this country) is built on the faulty premise that smoking is *the* cause of the disease. In some highly concentrated urban areas, such as Tokyo, it is obvious that there are far more cigarettes smoked per capita than in many areas of the United States—but the incidence of Japanese lung cancer remains far under that of the United States. It is a rush to judgment to make the assumption that a vast decline in smoking, however obnoxious and insalubrious a habit it is, will *ipso facto* result in such a decline in lung cancer, the major killer and leader in incidence in American cancer, that will turn in the decline in cancer statistics American orthodoxy needs to bolster medicine as usual.

While the NCI is, in funding terms, much bigger than ACS, it is under heavy ACS influence, a classic case of the tail wagging the dog, Greenberg and Randal analyzed—pointing particularly to the mammography scandal as a case in point. Against the advice of many of its own staff and advisors, the NCI was persuaded by the ACS to pay for more than four-fifths of the breast screening program. John C. Bailar, III, editor-in-chief of the NCI's journal, had warned that the program "contains the seeds of a major disaster," and Dr. Bross warned, "This exposure to diagnostic X-ray will probably result in the worst iatrogenic epidemic of breast cancer in history."

That the much bigger NCI can be so dominated by the smaller ACS is in large measure due to their respective personnel makeups; the ACS is dominated by experts in advertising, public relations, and business. Indeed, the pizzazz with which ACS operates can largely be attributed to the virtual takeover of an otherwise lackluster charity by the team of Albert Lasker, "the father of modern advertising," and his socially well connected wife, Mary, and Elmer Bobst, regarded by some as "the father of the modern drug industry," a self-made man of the Horatio Alger stripe.

To some extent, one can only admire the public relations capacities and business expertise such personalities brought to bear. Before the Lasker era, cancer was virtually as taboo a subject for discussion and explication as was feminine hygiene. Indeed, Lasker did for cancer and the society what he had earlier done for Kotex as the designer of its advertising campaign—he brought previously taboo subjects "out of the closet."

The ACS propagandists can be blamed for a lot of things, including overterrorizing the public with fright programs, but on balance it seems to me far better that the bejabbers be scared out of people over the existence of an awful disease than that its facts be kept hidden. To its credit, the ACS made cancer a household word. But, as in so many overzealous and evangelical movements, the society has become more adept at asking questions than providing right answers, and, like organizations before it, more involved in *looking* for the cure than finding it. Big bureaucracies, be they public or private, are simply loath to phase out of existence. The American Cancer Society, to a large extent a good idea gone wrong, is no exception.

Pat McGrady, who for a quarter-century was the ACS science editor, gave this overview of the society and medicine in general to Peter Barry Chowka:

> Medicine has become venal, second only to the law. The ACS slogan, control cancer with a checkup and a check...it's phony, because we are *not* controlling cancer. That slogan is the extent of ACS' scientific, medical, and clinical savvy. Nobody in the science and medical departments there is capable of doing real science. They are wonderful pros who know how to raise money. They don't know how to prevent cancer or cure patients; instead, they close the door on innovative ideas. ACS money goes to scientists who put on the best show to get grants or who have friends on the grant-giving panels.

Over at the NCI, it's business as usual.

In 1980, the Congressional watchdog General Accounting Office (GAO) accused the institute of using unsound management in awarding contracts and said the NCI's Cancer Control Program had no clear objectives. The CCP is a $70-million-a-year project authorized by Congress in 1971, which is not directly involved in finding cures for cancer but in disseminating information about cancer treatment and prevention.

After reviewing five contracts awarded in recent years, the GAO reported, "NCI did not effectively manage four of five contracts we examined." The chairman of the Cancer Control Merit Review

Committee told the GAO that problems similar to those found in the five reviews contracts probably existed in about 50 percent of all the cancer-control contracts.

In releasing the GAO report, Rep. David Obey of Wisconsin said it left "little doubt that those involved in decision-making in cancer control both in Congress and in the executive branch have not had a clear idea of what they specifically expected to achieve with this $70-million-a-year expenditure."

By 1981 it was more evident that things were not going at all well in the federal effort to wipe out cancer—and that scandals in cancer research both public and private were on the increase.

The NCI, shepherd of the Conquest of Cancer Program, was under the sharpest probe it had ever suffered through, with the gravest charges hurled its way not so much by the congressmen but by the *Washington Post,* hardly a redoubt of anti-Establishmentarianism. The *Post* ran a four-part series following a one-year investigation of the cancer drug-related deaths of 620 patients. The story (which caused a one-day congressional hearing to be called) revealed that hundreds of Americans had been killed by experimental cancer drugs, many of which are still in use even after having been proven worthless.

Ironically, a major anti-laetrile spokesman from the Food and Drug Administration (FDA), Dr. Robert Young, helped deliver telling blows against the NCI, an intriguing display of infighting within the Club and a message not lost on Congress: "Patients who undergo experimental cancer therapy under NCI auspices are often not fully informed of what they are getting into," said Dr. Young. He told the Washington reporters of a Boston hospital that had tested an NCI drug on children and "their kidneys were lost within days. This was no big deal because (NCI) new drugs were routinely given out with no safeguards for people who receive them." In another case, the widow of a leukemia patient learned only two years after the fact, and from reporters, that her husband had died not of the disease but from an accidental overdose of the experimental drug given to treat it.

Dr. Young, perhaps well seasoned by his laetrile debates and the analogies to the Vietnam War the cancer controversy inevitably elicits, said of the use of experimental chemotherapeutic drugs in cancer therapy: "You've got the generals, the NCI, and you have this attitude among the generals, 'We've got to burn the village to save it.' " Before the congressmen, Dr. DeVita reported that the *Post* figures were grossly in error and that "only" 43 of 1,453 patients who had received experimental drugs over the prior eighteen months had died from drug-related causes.

In the meantime, Senators Orrin Hatch and Paula Hawkins began probing the mismanagement at NCI, with Hatch scoring "the cozy relationship with contractors and tolerance of mismanagement and fraud" within the federal bureaucracy in charge of cancer research. He also told the public that, despite declaration of the war on cancer a decade before," we are still demonstrably no closer to a cancer cure than we were 10 years ago." The congressmen flayed DeVita for NCI's issuing a $910,000 grant to a Boston University researcher who had been forced to resign amid charges he had falsified research.

Indeed, that particular case was only one of several cases of major cheating in cancer research around the country. A similar scandal rocked Cornell University at about the same time. Other major cheating cases occurred at the Yale School of Medicine and the Massachusetts General Hospital, an affiliate of Harvard University. Sloan-Kettering, the stage for the laetrile cover-up controversy, had already been pummeled by bad publicity over a famous and fraudulent research project involving painted mice.

The scope of cancer research cheating, let alone the mismanagement of funds within the NCI, an allocator of $2 billion per year (as of 1982) of taxpayer largesse in cancer research, and the sorry state of cancer treatment progress in this country, are ample reasons why the American public is increasingly losing faith in the ability of medicine—and government—to get some kind of meaningful grip on cancer.

Research "Outside The Pale":
The Case of Cecil Pitard, M. D.

The Food, Drug and Cosmetic Act makes it virtually impossible for any meaningful cancer breakthroughs to originate outside the bounds of drug research which is controlled and directed by the major pharmaceutical companies, but this reality does not stop some innovative medics from doing things on their own, particularly if their own lives are at stake.

Hence the strange case of Cecil Pitard, M.D., a soft-spoken otorhinolaryngologist and bacterial disease specialist in Knoxville, Tennesse, whose personal life-and-death cancer discovery should be shouted from the rooftops rather than kept, as it has been up to now, in relative secrecy.

In May 1980 Dr. Pitard was diagnosed at the Mayo Clinic, he told me, with terminal stage IV lymphocytic lymphoma, a kind of lymphatic cancer originally diagnosed from a node in the groin. By the time he was at Mayo, his cancer involved significant tumefaction, and he was told he was beyond operation and that—frankly— chemotherapy would do no good.

This is one of many cases I have come across in which doctors, nurses, or other medical personnel, felt to be "members of the family," so to speak, are able to elicit from their medical comrades the private admission that chemotherapy just won't do any good. This kind of frank appraisal is rarely given to non-medical victims of the cancer industry, who do not have the benefit of such open dialogue due to their lack of medical degrees and training.

Dr. Pitard recalls that he was informed that this kind of cancer had a prognosis ranging from just a few weeks to "a long time." But there was no doubt he was "terminal."

Not one to give up easily, Dr. Pitard decided he would find out all he could about this "form" of cancer and learn if there was anything that could be done at all, despite American orthodoxy's insistence that he was beyond hope. The Knoxville ear-nose-and-throat man observed the rapid spread of his lymphoma until he had abdominal, bone, chest and jaw area involvement. He began consulting medical libraries every night and making calls around the country to other doctors and researchers. "I have that advantage—I can just pick up the telephone and ask doctors important questions," he recalled.

Hence, Dr. Pitard was happily surprised while making these calls to pick up leads on cancer research that had been either substantially under-reported, overlooked, or simply not pushed in the U.S.A., areas of research absolutely unknown to the American people because they involved either unpatentable substances or special substances patented for uses other than cancer—stunning evidence of the chilling effect on independent scientific research by orthodoxy and the scope of the Food, Drug and Cosmetic Act.

The two lines of research that turned out to be most meaningful to him centered, ironically, on the anti-flu bacterial antigen, staphage lysate, "which I actually already had in my own refrigerator," and the relatively common chemical sodium butyrate, a fatty acid found in milk and butter—an "unlicensed new drug," as it were.

He was amazed to learn that a fairly substantial, if scattered, literature existed linking sodium butyrate (butyric acid) to anti-tumor effects in animals. Some 250 articles on the substance exist in the literature. This nontoxic, inexpensive chemical (costing at the time about $17.65 per quarter-pound, he said) was, in effect, just sitting out there, ready to be experimentally used on humans.

Dr. Pitard was excited about the immune system-stimulating possibilities of staphage lysate vaccine, which he described as a "germ's germ" known to devastate staphylococci without producing any side effects, and the tumor-destroying potential of sodium butyrate. Fighting for his life, he began treatment with both.

He told me that tumor diminution was noticeable within two days and that by the end of a full year *all* tumors had vanished. He was still free of cancer in 1982 and continuing the therapy. He was not prepared at the time to announce total victory, yet his own probing mind had obviously come across something of great significance for lymphomas, tricky cancers which indeed may pass through long periods of quiescence.

At present, of course, neither he nor any other American physician has the "right" to announce the treatment of human cancer with these substances within the U.S.A. despite some interpretations of law allowing doctors to use a medicine for something other than that which is described in the "package insert." Hence, relevant followup began, as usual, outside the U.S.A. At this time, the butyrate complex-staphage lysate combination is being experimentally used by American Biologics-Mexico, which is turning in promising results. AB-Mexico and Bradford Research Institute scientists also found a fairly extensive literature on sodium butyrate and saw in its existence one more rage-producing situation in the American cancer debacle: lack of follow-through on a promising avenue of treatment because of lack of a profit motive and the continuing roadblock of the Food, Drug and Cosmetic Act.

My suspicion is that literally hundreds of useful substances are out there in the literature, waiting to be picked up at the appropriate time by mavericks and others fighting life-and-death battles. The extreme tragedy, the awful immorality of it all, is that the American people are not made aware of such substances because research into them is blocked or chilled by the Club.

Decades Of Deceit: The Cancer Establishment's War On "Unproven Remedies"

I have argued that there is a Club of vested interests, both economic and ego-centered, whose concentrated clout can be expressed through politics. The only way to counteract it has been to engage in political action—as has been the case, with striking results, with laetrile. But had *other* anticancer remedies also become political issues, I have no doubt that the nation would now have a free marketplace of available nontoxic cancer remedies. Indeed, laetrile is only the latest in a series of "unproved remedies" that has felt the full brunt of the Club's wrath. The history of the persecution of cancer remedies developed outside the pale of the Club is long and agonizing, and we will only observe the high points here.

There are *reasons* that the treatments of choice in cancer are surgery, radiation and chemotherapy. Unhappily, science is the least important of all these reasons. Economics is the bigger part—vested interests in *things* and substances. When that economic interest becomes political, we find that even channels of information become clogged. The ordinary American is simply not supposed to know that immune-system-stimulating agents, vitamins and nutritional therapies, and even anticancer vaccines of a kind have been tested and found useful. They don't know until a scandal is big enough to get press attention.

The unproved remedies-list of the American Cancer Society is concerned primarily with plant-derived vitamin and bacterial substances, all showing some promise—plus some authentically shady remedies as well. By no means do I insist here that every unproven remedy has something going for it and that orthodoxy is utterly bereft of results and truth.

As we examine in chapter eight, part of the development of laetrile was vested in the trophoblastic theory of cancer enunciated at the turn of the century by Scotch embryologist John Beard. Out of his work came the use of the enzymes trypsin and chymotrypsin in cancer therapy. While the enzymes have achieved notable success in anticancer effects, their promotion early in this century collided with the high pontiffs of surgery—at that time, the only treatment of choice in cancer. The enzyme treatment, while fostered and developed in Germany, pretty much got the bum's rush in America. Orthodox medicine in this country had essentially killed this approach by 1910.

But even before Beard's enzyme approach, a noted New York City surgeon, William Bradley Coley, discouraged at the low-success rate from subjecting large tumor masses to the knife, took the first steps in what would now be regarded as using immune system stimulators to combat cancer.

He took his cue from the discovery by Germany's Friedrich Fehleisen in 1833 of the streptococcus of the disease erysipelas. Fehleisen had observed that for over a century there had been reports of cancer patients being cured when they had a severe attack of erysipelas. Dr. Coley found that by giving erysipelas to a fellow physician, W. T. Bull, a hopeless cancer patient, his tumors disappeared. He then achieved ten more complete remissions out of streptococcus, to which he added a bacillus. He began using the vaccine on terminal cancer patients, and London surgeon C. Mansell Moulin reported similar results with the substance, to become known as "Coley's fluid" and "Coley's toxins." In 1906 Coley was able to report that 124 out of 312 inoperable cancer patients were alive and well after five years—by today's misleading definition, "cured" of cancer.

But when the American Medical Association investigated the Coley treatment, this close-minded body decided that there was no evidence of its efficacy, that it might be dangerous—and worse of all, it might persuade people to abandon "proven remedies"—that is, surgery. This line of reasoning is exactly that pursued seven decades later by the opponents of vitamin B^{17} (laetrile or amygdalin) and the other metabolic/nutritional therapies. Nonetheless, several physicians continued to use the substance until hundreds of persons had positively responded to the therapy.

The work of Coley has been carried on by Helen Coley Nauts and her New York-based Cancer Research Institute. Due to pressure from scientists still working with Coley-like preparations, including those—much to its credit—at Sloan-Kettering, the Coley fluid was quietly removed from the list of the American Cancer Society's unproven remedies, but there is still no open espousal of it. To keep it on the "quack list," though, would be terribly embarrassing to the ACS, since it indicates the first in a wave of substances that may turn out to be common treatment modalities in the future.

Dr. Ralph Moss, the courageous Sloan-Kettering public information official who was fired for helping expose the coverup of positive laetrile test results at SKI, wrote (in *Second Opinion,* September 1978) that hundreds of case records at Memorial Hospital, many scientific articles by Coley, and numerous monographs had assembled a thousand positive cases of proven responses to the Coley substance. He quoted Sloan-Kettering vice president Lloyd Old, a key figure in the laetrile testing program, as saying that the Coley approach "later fell into virtual disuse, no doubt in part because of high hopes raised in introduction of radiotherapy, and afterwards chemotherapy." Moss also noted how James Ewing, "Coley's nemesis and arch rival," turned Memorial Hospital into a "medical branch of the radium trust."

It is interesting that results of a "double blind" test on Coley toxins at New York University-Bellevue turned up the assessment by the research coordinators that "it is the impression of the authors that Coley's Toxin had definite oncolytic [tumor-destroying] properties and is useful in the treatment of certain types of malignant disease." Even these modest assessments resulted in a demand that the chief author leave the hospital involved.

At about the same time, highly interesting work—now being revived under other names and essentially based on immune system stimulation—was being done by individuals working against the surgical grain of their times. Oddly enough, it was one of France's greatest surgeons, Eugene Louis Doyen, who set the revolution in motion by making cultures of a cancer tissue he had removed in surgery. He killed the culture with heat, made a vaccine from the dead bacteria (*micrococcus neoformans)* and its toxins, and used the substance on 238 patients. Of these, forty-two seemed cured, and another forty-two responded favorably. Follow-up work in England and Belgium indicated that Doyen was decidedly on to something.

But orthodox medicine in the West had now discovered the greatest of the new gimmicks, the X-ray machine—and the high costs that went with it—and these promising early approaches at cancer-vaccine development were relegated to the trashcan of history.

At the same time the "microbe of Doyen" was being developed in Europe, Tom Deaken, an obscure American laboratory technician, was working along similar lines. For two decades he worked on his theory and ultimately made a serum from the blood of horses he had inoculated with a bacterium he had cultured. When a Montana surgeon tried the anticancer serum on two patients and they both became well, he gave up his practice and spent most of his time and wealth fighting for the Deaken serum. Interestingly enough, as Wayne Martin notes in his excellent *Medical Heroes and Heretics* (Devin-Adair, Old Greenwich, Conn., 1977), Deaken was actually travelling the same road the Durovics would later follow when Krebiozen—after laetrile, the most notorious of the "unproven remedies" advanced in the U.S.—was developed.

But J. M. Scott, the altruistic surgeon in question—although he interested a number of physicians in the Deaken serum and "miraculous regressions" were achieved in hopeless cancer patients—found out that no major medical journal in the United States would publish his successful case histories. It was not until 1926, and in an Irish medical journal, that this promising approach was published in a responsible medical publication. But Western orthodoxy was now fascinated with radiation therapy and still relied on nineteenth century surgical techniques. The money was in both of these areas. The Deaken serum died in the U.S. as the Doyen vaccine died in Europe.

Robert Houston (in "How the War on Cancer Is Being Lost," *Our Town,* September 3, 1978) made the point that, "although the ACS and FDA foster the notion that unorthodox therapies are developed by unqualified charlatans, examination of the unproven remedies list reveals quite the opposite." The chief proponents of the substances and therapies on the ACS-FDA list of "unprovens" in 70 percent of cases are medical doctors and in 20 percent of cases are professors of medicine. Ten percent of the therapies were pioneered by Ph.D. biologists and biochemists. Eighty percent of the unprovens come from qualified individuals, some of them bordering on genius—not the least among them Max Gerson, M.D., founder of the nutritional approach in cancer therapy, and hailed by Dr. Albert Schweitzer as a medical genius; Morvyth McQueens-Williams, M.D., Ph.D., developer of KC, a botanical agent, and who Dr. Lewis Terman at Stanford University found to be the most brilliant of the prodigies he followed in the classic survey of IQs of gifted children; Andrew Ivy, M.D., who pioneered Krebiozen in this country; and the Ernst T. Krebses, father and son, who codeveloped vitamins B^{17} (laetrile) and B^{15} (pangamic acid). In an earlier era, Coley, Deaken, Doyen, and their collaborators were all qualified in one or more scientific fields.

Another fully qualified researcher later branded a "quack" was William F. Koch, M.D., professor of physiology at Detroit Medical College (Wayne State) and the University of Michigan. As Nat Morris has recorded so well (*The Cancer Blackout,* Regent House, Los Angeles), Dr. Koch believed cancer to be caused by toxins that remain in the blood system and that a function of sugar oxidation is the destruction of toxins that result from metabolic processes. He was, in fact, presaging free-radical pathology treatment. The answer to cancer, he reasoned, should lie in providing more active catalysts to stimulate the body's own capacity to oxidize toxins—a theory that led to the development of Glyoxylide, a preparation that he argued converted toxins into antitoxins. While Koch's chemistry has been criticized, no scientific arguments have been advanced to refute it.

Dr. Koch combined Glyoxylide with a special dietary regimen and enemas as part of a total treatment program. Its threat to established science was that his preparation and diet could handle cancer and remove it from the hands of surgeons and radiologists. The therapy was also—as Morris described it—the "ultimate dream of cancer research: a one-shot treatment that allegedly made tumors vanish—and other diseases as well." Dr. Koch also ruffled Establishment feathers by correctly arguing that biopsy and surgery *spread* cancer.

Despite evidence that the Koch program was securing victories over cancer symptoms, some of them dramatic in nature, a Wayne County Medical Society hearing denied both cancer diagnoses and the evidence of cancer "cures" in Koch patients. The AMA was already lobbying by 1921-23 against the Koch approach, despite support for it from a number of widely respected physicians and growing evidence of its positive effects.

The story of the persecution of physicians who used Glyoxylide in this country is a lengthy one and spans several decades. Only hearings by the Cancer Commission in Ontario, Canada, between 1939 and 1949, provided objective forums surveying Glyoxylide cases, and they turned up one positive reponse after another. Canada became an area of support for Koch despite his virtual banning as a heretic in the United States, with Dr. Forbes Godfrey, an eminent Toronto surgeon, and for twenty-six years minister of health and education, praising the Koch remedy as superior to radium.

Dr. Koch worked in 1940 and 1941 in Mexico and Brazil on leprosy, tuberculosis, and mental conditions and claimed a rapid cure of dementia with a single Glyoxylide injection. Morris writes, "This reputedly so incensed a representative of a big pharmaceutical firm that was then reaping huge profits from useless drugs injected repeatedly into mental patients he was reputed to have shaken his fist in Doctor Koch's face and warned him that he would not be interfering much longer in Brazil."

When Dr. Koch was arrested in Florida in 1942 on a charge of false labeling, a federal official demanded to know why a high bail of $10,000 was set. The district attorney said he had been ordered from Detroit to ask for the higher sum to help keep Dr. Koch from returning to Brazil and finishing his research there.

Dr. Koch was the subject of two bitter Food and Drug Administration trials in 1942 and 1946 in which the federal agency argued—as it still argues today—that the Koch agents were indistinguishable from distilled water. A permanent injunction against the Koch Laboratory was issued in 1950, and Koch, in essence, gave up his fight. Several other physicians who continued to use the substance either lost their licenses or were subjected to other forms of official harassment. Needless to say, there are still patients walking around today who believe they owe their lives to Dr. Koch and Glyoxylide—and to its modern day analogues.

In the 1930s and in the World War II era the primacy of surgery and radiation was being challenged by a growing interest in nutrition as a means of dealing with cancer, a line of research dropped and only recently resurrected. And it was largely abandoned at the time because of the wholesale move into cancer research by chemotherapy. Indeed, the early disputes between radiologists and chemotherapists, some of which continue to this day, were no less lively than those between the defenders of orthodoxy and unorthodoxy in cancer therapy are now. Dean Burk told me that in the 1940s the National Cancer Institute, whose cytochemistry division he headed, "breathed" nutrition, but that all such interest sagged as the postwar introduction of chemotherapy and an increased hunt for human cancer-causing viruses (not a single one of which had been discovered by 1982) took over standard thinking about cancer.

The NCI was losing interest in nutrition just as real evidence about the connection was being established by Max Gerson, M.D., a German physician who came to this country and ran a clinic in New York for twenty years. In his native country, Gerson had found that a vegetarian diet with raw fruits and vegetables and no salt could cure both migraine headaches and lupus erythematosis. He was hailed for his theory by Dr. Albert Schweitzer after using the same diet to cure Schweitzer's wife of lung tuberculosis. But his main contribution, which continues today, is his dietary and detoxification approach in cancer. His nontoxic, diet-only modality, of course, got him into trouble, but there is little to refute in the legacy of cases he put in published form in 1958.

The modified Gerson program, still used, calls for the vegetarian diet, a detoxification program usually emphasizing coffee enemas, and liver extracts. Dr. Gerson was the first unorthodox practitioner ever to get the ear of a congressional committee. His patients, and their evidence of total cancer control through diet and detoxification, appear in the record of Florida Senator Claude Pepper's 1946 Senate subcommittee on cancer research.

Senator Pepper had before the Senate a bill that called for a $100 million federally controlled cancer research program, a baby war on cancer, as it were. But despite the impressive evidence for the Gerson approach, the wonderful world of orthodoxy was able to suffocate the meaning and scope of the Pepper hearings completely. For his efforts, Dr. Gerson was suspended by the New York County Medical Society. The American Cancer Society stated that no food had any effect on any form of cancer, and the American Medical Association relegated the Gerson treatment to its "frauds and fables" list.

Charlotte Gerson Straus, Dr. Gerson's daughter, has continued the work of her late father, though, as in the case of laetrile for years, she finally had to go to Mexico to do so. I have interviewed several cancer patients who have been alive and well on the Gerson therapy when everything else failed. Most of the Gerson diet, and, to some extent, the detoxification program, are widely used by metabolic/nutritional therapists, frequently in conjunction with other treatments. As late as the 1970s, spokesmen for the ACS were still styling the arguments for nutrition in cancer treatment as "the first sign of quackery."

Another therapy based on natural substances and which was involved in forty years of controversy with American medical orthodoxy are the Hoxsey herbal preparations, whose origin dates back to 1840 but whose primary promoter in this century was Harry Hoxsey. His fabled battle with the American Medical Association and its magazine editor, Morris Fishbein, makes fascinating reading, and I would recommend the perusal of Hoxsey's *You Don't Have to Die* for anyone who wants the full, incredible story.

Suffice it to say that Hoxsey inherited the formulas for the preparations originally made by John Hoxsey in the nineteenth century. The latter, Harry Hoxsey has related time and again, observed the seeming spontaneous cure of cancer in a horse. By observing the animal's eating habits, he found a clump of shrubs and flowering plants which seemed to be its favorite "dining area." He identified red clover, buckthorn, and prickly ash as among the vegetable matter the horse was eating. There were other plants he could not identify. Among all of these or combinations of them must be the substance which ultimately had allowed the horse's tumor to literally drop off, Hoxsey reasoned.

As Harry Hoxsey recorded it, "He picked samples of all the plants growing there, took them to the barn, ground them up with a mortar and began a series of experiments. He mashed the flowers and berries, ground the stalks, boiled the roots. Patiently, month after month, he tried them separately in various combinations on sick horses in the neighborhood. He studied the ingredients of old home remedies, adding and subtracting them experimentally.... Finally he hit upon three formulas that proved effective in many cases of cancer." Ostensibly, these were a liquid medicine administered orally. He became known as a healer of horses and passed on the formula only to his son who passed it on to Harry Hoxsey, the latter claimed.

Nat Morris summarizes Hoxsey thus, "In the life-and-death struggle Hoxsey has waged with AMA, he has been fined, jailed and prosecuted more times than any other man in the history of cancer. He has fought back tooth and nail; matching his cunning and ruthless opponents with equal cunning, craft and resourcefulness .... In the fight, Hoxsey has not been too meticulous in his choice of allies, several of whom were pretty unsavory characters."

Through it all, Hoxsey proudly said of himself, "For 35...years I have been kicked, hounded, persecuted and prosecuted because I've treated cancer with medicine and without the use of surgery, X-ray or radium."

And so he did. It is certainly not my province to defend the controversial Hoxsey preparations, but I can report that they are still being used, that hundreds of people today claim benefit from them, and some of the patients date back to the earliest Hoxsey clinics. He operated in Illinois, Pennsylvania, and Texas during his long and expensive battle with the AMA, and realized little satisfaction from it all other than besting the AMA's Fishbein in a libel suit.

Harry Hoxsey attributed the beginning of his survival-oriented battle with the AMA to the fact that, in the early days when his treatment was looked upon favorably by several physicians, one of them, Dr. Malcolm Harris, tried to force Hoxsey to turn over his formulas to himself and his colleagues in Chicago. As Hoxsey, a naturopath, recalled it, the Harris plan called for him not only to turn over the formulas but to relinquish all claims in favor of the Harris group, to deliver existing supplies of the material and to instruct the Harris group on their manufacture and to close his clinic and stop treating patients forever. When Hoxsey understandably refused, Harris threatened to run "that quack doctor...out of Illinois." And the battle was on.

Attorney Benedict F. Fitzgerald, Jr., who more than any other man outside the area of unorthodox therapies helped get insinuations of the cancer conspiracy into the record during an investigation of the Krebiozen and Hoxsey controversies, wrote the following to Sen. William E. Langer:

> From the evidence I have gathered, it appears that as early as 1924 the Hoxsey method of treating cancer was considered so effective by a former president of a medical association that he personally presented its sponsor with a written proposal which, among other things, provided for the relinquishment of valuable property rights in the Hoxsey method and medicines and formulas to this same official. The evidence indicates that when the proposition was spurned, Hoxsey was advised to sign and accept the proposal or face ruination. Such tactics, if true, constitute blackmail of the rankest order and this evidence should be examined closely to ascertain its credibility.

The Fitzgerald letter also noted that "the record in the Federal Court discloses that this agency of the Federal Government [the National Cancer Institute] took sides and sought in every way to hinder, suppress and restrict this institution in their treatment of cancer."

In 1953, Fitzgerald, general counsel for the senate investigation into cancer treatments, authorized by New Hampshire Sen. Charles Tobey, summarized the Hoxsey-AMA fight this way:

> A running fight has been going on between officials, especially Dr. Morris Fishbein of the American Medical Association through the Journal of that organization, and the Hoxsey Cancer Clinic. Dr. Fishbein contended that the medicines employed by the Hoxsey Cancer Clinic had no therapeutic value; that it was run by a quack and a charlatan. (This clinic is manned by a staff of over thirty employees, including nurses and physicians.) Reprints and circulation of several million copies so prepared resulted in litigation. The Government thereafter intervened and sought an injunction to prevent the transmission in interstate commerce of certain medicines. It is interesting to note that in the Trial Court, before Judge Atwell, who had an opportunity to hear the witnesses in two different trials, it was held that the so-called Hoxsey method of treating cancer was in some respect superior to that of X-ray, radium and surgery and did have therapeutic value.
>
> The Circuit Court of Appeals of the 5th Circuit decided otherwise. This decision was handed down during the trial of a libel suit in the District Court of Dallas, Texas, by Hoxsey against Morris Fishbein, who admitted that he had never practiced medicine one day in his life, in a verdict for Hoxsey and against Morris Fishbein. The defense admitted that Hoxsey could cure external cancer but contended that his medicines for internal cancer had no therapeutic value.
>
> The jury, after listening to leading Pathologists, Radiologists, Physicians, Surgeons and scores of witnesses, a great number of whom had never been treated by any Physician or Surgeon except the treatment received at the Hoxsey Cancer Clinic, concluded that Dr. Fishbein was wrong; that his published statements were false, and that the Hoxsey method of treating cancer did have therapeutic value.

Fitzgerald also noted that a great number of doctors the government called as witnesses admitted that X-ray therapy could actually *cause* cancer, and Fitzgerald read into the record several statements to this effect.

But his major investigation concerned the use of Krebiozen, which controversy was breaking just as several California physicians began the use of Ernst T. Krebs, Jr.'s, refined amygdalin (laetrile), hence setting in motion what would ultimately become the major battle to break Cancergate. (It should be pointed out that there is no connection between Krebs—whose name, interestingly enough, is German for "cancer"—and *krebiozen,* which is Greek for "growth regulator.")

Krebiozen is another of the substances which today would be regarded as immune-system stimulators. When Yugoslav physician Steven Durovic theorized that the immunological defense system of a horse or cow could be used to fight cancer in humans, he was a good quarter-century ahead of his time, but already following in the footsteps, at least to some extent, of Coley, Doyen, and Deaken.

The Krebiozen story has it that Durovic inoculated cattle and horses with a bacillus that caused actinomycosis ("lumpy jaw"), during which a tumor is formed. Durovic's view apparently was that by being challenged with the inoculation, the animal produced in its blood an anticancer substance. It was from the dried blood of such animals that he produced the yellow powder that he called "Krebiozen."

It was in 1949 that Durovic travelled to the United States and met Dr. Andrew C. Ivy, a vice president of the University of Illinois, professor of physiology, M.D., and Ph.D., and considered so reliable in ethics as well as his own field that he had been sent to the Nuremberg war crimes trials thrice to interpret the code of medical ethics.

Dr. Ivy, possessed of an open mind, tried out Krebiozen on several terminal cancer patients. When they showed positive results, he decided to go ahead with its use. It was reported that two major drug companies each offered Durovic a million dollars for rights to manufacture and distribute Krebiozen and that Durovic turned them down. Assuming this is true, it explains part of the great hostility and venom with which the Club later pursued Dr. Ivy, a man widely respected and well credentialed and whose very use of the substance lent it a fair measure of credibility. It would also be a scenario repeated through the annals of the Establishment's dealings with outside-the-pale compounds—be they Krebiozen, the Hoxsey preparations, laetrile, or—as we assess in another chapter—Dr. Peter DeMarco's Procaine PVP. Rejections of takeover offers from major drug firms always spell trouble for inventors.

Although the AMA had already published a report on Krebiozen and had written it off as being of "no benefit"—despite gathering reports of analgesic effects and improved well-being from its use—Ivy published his own assessment in 1956. In 1962 he left the

University of Illinois and moved into facilities at Roosevelt University in Chicago to continue his work, ultimately coming up with his version of the substance, Carcalon.

But by the time he was well along with his unorthodox approach, the Food, Drug and Cosmetic Act had been amended, an act which has pushed American medicine back by a century and set the stage for the Gestapo-style actions which were to be used against all popular—if "unproven"—remedies that had not been proven "effective" through hosts of animal studies. The federal grand jury's 1964 return of indictments against Ivy and Durovic was one of the first major uses of the new legislation, and it meant a multi-million-dollar prosecution against Ivy and his colleagues and a 289-day trial. Falsified testimony and the deft manipulation of the media were part of the Club's battle against Ivy, but in truth the Krebiozen side was found wanting in several areas. Despite all the hoopla that surrounded the case, to this day the Club likes to forget that Dr. Ivy was cleared of all the counts against him.

The Durovic behavior in the Krebiozen matter is at least suspicious, and there were enough holes in the promotion, claims, and use of the substance to lead the Club to believe it had an open target in Krebiozen. Among the most telling blows against the product was the possible profiteering motive of Durovic, who allegedly made millions off Krebiozen sales. (The issue of profiteering—to obscure the reality of efficacy—would be raised once again in the pitched battle over laetrile, which was not to break for another decade.) But by the time of the Krebiozen furor, there were some 20,000 testimonials to its efficacy—case histories the Club would call "anecdotes," as they did to explain away the seeming effects of laetrile and metabolic/nutritional therapy later.

Recall that the first effort at taking a close look at cancer research in this country had been attempted by Senator Pepper in 1946 at the time of the Gerson disclosures. That was also the first time that the cancer establishment sallied forth to lobby against anything as unwanted as a congressional look into its activities. Led by the AMA—of course—the cancer research lobby had influenced enough legislators to defeat the $100 million appropriations bill for federally monitored cancer research, with 170 representatives abstaining.

But now Senator Tobey was on the scent, and he was trying to launch a full-scale investigation into the American cancer industry. And why not? His son had been saved from cancer through unorthodoxy—in this case the Lincoln "bacteriophage" method. It was Tobey who, as chairman of the Senate Interstate and Foreign Commerce committee, retained Benedict F. Fitzgerald, Jr., of the Justice Department as special counsel. In his report to the Senate Interstate Commerce Committee on the "Need for the Investigation of Cancer Research Organizations" carried in the *Congressional*

Record for 28 August 1953, Fitzgerald made some telling disclosures:

> There is reason to believe that the AMA has been hasty, capricious, arbitrary, and outright dishonest, and of course if the doctrine "respondeat superior" is to be observed, the alleged machinations of Dr. J. J. Moore (for the past 10 years the treasurer of the AMA) could involve the AMA and others in a conspiracy of alarming proportions....
> Being vitally interested and having tried to listen and observe closely, it is my profound conviction that this substance Krebiozen is one of the most promising materials yet isolated for the management of cancer. It is biologically active. I have gone over the records of 530 cases, most of them conducted at a distance from Chicago, by unbiased cancer experts and clinics....I have concluded that in the value of present cancer research, this substance and the theory behind it deserves the most full and complete scientific study. Its value in the management of the cancer patient has been demonstrated in a sufficient number of cases to demand further work.
> Behind and over all this is the weirdest conglomeration of corrupt motives, intrigues, selfishness, jealousy, obstruction and conspiracy that I have ever seen.

There! He had dared to utter the ineffable word, *conspiracy*. And remember, this was *1953*. But Fitzgerald had a lot more to say:

> If radium, X-ray or surgery or either of them is the complete answer, then the greatest hoax of the age is being perpetrated upon the people by the continued appeal for funds for further research. If neither X-ray, radium or surgery is the complete answer to this dreaded disease, and I submit that it is not, then what is the plain duty of society? Should we stand still? Should we sit idly by and count the number of physicians, surgeons and cancerologists who are not only divided but who, because of fear or favor, are forced to line up with the so-called accepted view of the American Medical Association, or should this Committee make a full-scale investigation of the organized effort to hinder, suppress and restrict the free flow of drugs which allegedly have proven successful in cases where clinical

records, case history, pathological reports and X-ray photographic proof, together with the alleged cured patients, are available?

Accordingly, we should determine whether existing agencies, both public and private, are engaged in and have pursued a policy of harassment, ridicule, slander and libelous attacks on others sincerely engaged in stamping out this curse of mankind. Have medical associations, through their officers, agents, servants and employees engaged in this practice? *My investigation to date should convince this Committee that a conspiracy does exist to stop the free flow and use of drugs in interstate commerce which allegedly [have] solid therapeutic value.* [Emphasis mine.] Public and private funds have been thrown around like confetti at a country fair to close up and destroy clinics, hospitals, and scientific research laboratories which do not conform to the viewpoint of medical associations. How long will the American people take this?

Apparently, at least a quarter-century more.

But Tobey had died that summer of a heart attack. His successor, Sen. John Bricker, far more favorable to the AMA, told the rambunctious counsel to tone down. But he didn't. The investigation was quashed—and the counsel was fired.

By the mid-1960s, however, independent investigators were putting together pieces of the Club's war on Hoxsey, Koch, and Ivy, and its spurning of Gerson and developers of other unwanted therapies. Morris A. Beall, who wrote on the medical-pharmaceutical-governmental interlock extensively, detailed in his books "the largest drug manufacturing combine in the world" which still uses all its might "to bring pressure to continue and increase the sale of drugs." Laetrile apostles would discover the same combine a few years later.

In *Super Drug Story*, Beall accused the FDA of winking at violations by the "drug trust" but being "very assiduous in putting out of business any and all vendors of therapeutic devices which increase the healthy incidence of the public and thus decrease the profit incidence of the Drug Trust." The FDA, Beall said, "is used primarily for the perversion of justice by 'cracking down' on all who endanger the profits of the Drug Trust." He wrote off the AMA as being little more than a "powerful subsidiary of the Drug Trust."

Through Beall's pages, Dr. Emanuel M. Josephson argued that "associations have been formed to 'control cancer.' They have been more successful in controlling the cancer business. If they incidentally increase the financial returns of their doctors' investments in radium—it must be said that the price of radium increased 1,000 percent when they began to use it on cancer victims—that was hardly unexpected or undesired."

When I first read the Beall-Josephson critiques a decade after they were published, I throught they were too heavy-handed. It was difficult to imagine very many people actively involved in an effort to block something worthwhile against cancer. But I was naive. There *are* such people—and the almost frantic efforts of the Club to stamp out laetrile and everything it represents prove it a dozen times over.

Far more than laetrile has continued to be suppressed and oppressed in the modern era, but it was laetrile that "went political" and made waves which are now pounding at the sea walls of the troglodytical medical establishment.

There are many other examples of researchers and scientists, working alone with their own theories and substances, proving that they have something that "works" against cancer. Their histories are similar. They are at first ignored, then studied, then offered a buy-out, then forgotten. If they persist in their belief and endeavors they are harassed to the point of bankruptcy.

There is a long and troubled, if fascinating, story to the development of anti-cancer(and other) compounds from the head-shrinking Jivaro Indians of the Amazon Basin. The substances discovered and researched by Dr. Wilburn Ferguson in Ecuador over forty years ago developed an incredible performance record in treating a wide spectrum of cancer in South America. Yet the research, while officially supported at one time in Ecuador and subjected to solid laboratory and clincial research, was never allowed a foothold in the United States.

Of all the promising foreign-derived *natural* substances developed, surely the Jivaro extracts had the most going for them, involving at one time the backing of the Ecuadorian president, interest by a U.S. senator, and field visits by an official of the National Institutes of Health. The evidence for their use was overwhelming.

But the battle for official sanction, for tax-exempt research foundations to carry on work brought to Dr. Ferguson a long, frustrating series of twists and turns, a story that itself would take a book to tell.

Suffice it to say at one point, in the 1950s, in Dr. Ferguson's own words:

> One of my friends suggested that if I visited one of the most eminent cancer authorities in the world and frankly discussed the entire project with him, his influence might be able to change the apparent block [i.e., the reneging by Sloan-Kettering and the cancer society to front funds for further research].

163

He secured an appointment and I visited the eminent specialist in his office, on Park Avenue. I had just started my research account when he stopped me and said, "We know all about your research, perhaps even more than you yourself know about it. We know you are closer to finding a truly effective therapeutic for cancer than anyone else in the world today." He paused for several moments, trying to put his thoughts into the words he wanted to use, then concluded, "Suppose you find an effective cure for cancer next year, or within five years; what the hell happens to my business?" I was absolutely speechless.

Part of the Ferguson research work, which went on intermittently in the U.S.A. and in Mexico, blazing a lonely and pioneering trail, resulted in the setting up of the Blewett Cancer Research Foundation in Texas to further research and test one Jivaro head-shrinking-derived anti-cancer compound and a sister compound.

I was shown information that laboratory tests at three United States universities and two major research centers had shown the substance, which Blewett had called BF 70, effective. Lawton Butler, Jr., executive director of the small and struggling foundation, said that in six years of organized research in the seventies, 73 percent of 85 patients had shown positive responses to the plant-derived compound. Morever, one of the earlier users of the original Ferguson discovery lived an additional fifteen years.

Blewett attempted to cooperate with the cancer industry powers-that-be in securing support and recognition for the discovery. As early as 1975, the NCI had found that the experimental product had "shown significant activity" in the B-16 melanoma test system. Yet in efforts to collaborate with NCI in developing experimental data preliminary to human trials, Blewett ran into an incredible series of events in which NCI kept changing the protocols for experiments ("It was as if every time we started to get close to something they thought, 'If we change the protocol we can put them out of business," Butler said), NCI twice lost the compounds, and NCI totally ignored confirmed anti-cancer activity in one cell study.

In 1977, an incensed attorney Ben A. Wallis complained to the Intragovernmental Relations and Human Resources Committee of Congress:

> Blewett compounds shipped to NCI were repeatedly lost or contaminated, [because of] either incredible NCI mismanagement or deliberate foul-ups. Blewett's attempts to secure funding, testing,

or other cooperation from outside laboratories were thwarted consistently by NCI in a ruthless course of conduct that appears designed to destroy Blewett.

NCI is in a position of total control over all cancer research in this country. Little or no funding is available to anyone who falls from favor with NCI, and great pressure is brought to bear on all others in the field to bow to the wishes of NCI. It is virtually impossible to be allowed to test compounds which NCI has not approved, and the facts indicate a course of obstructionism, rather than furtherance of research by NCI.

Wallis further accused the NCI of attempting to "corner the market" on the plant sources of the compounds on the one hand while on the other claiming they were worthless, despite the evidence of outside laboratory tests to the contrary.

New York health commentator Gary Null in 1979 reported on the plight of Polish physician Stanislaw Burzynski, who emigrated to the U.S.A. after five unsuccessful attempts to leave his native land. He had published ten papers on the positive results of a natural substance which he extracts from urine and calls *antineoplaston*.

The Burzynski group, working in Houston, Texas, reportedly isolated four different antineoplaston peptides which they claimed restrained up to 99 percent of the growth of three different types of cancer cells while causing no inhibitory effects on surrounding normal tissue. Null reported that of forty-one patients treated with antineoplaston therapy:

> a positive response to the treatment and definite clinical improvement were found in 86 percent of the cases with advanced cancer and leukemia. There was total remission...in 19 percent of the cases, including advanced cases of acute lymphocytic leukemia, cancer of the bladder, and cancer of the mouth and tongue....[There have been] very good results with malignant brain tumors....

Dr. Burzynski's research reportedly was confirmed by independent institutions both in this country and in Europe, yet, reported Null, this chain of events occurred:

• After applying "four or five times" to the National Cancer Institute for research funds, he received two grants and a supplemental one and was told the project looked "interesting." Then NCI ran out of funds for him. Funding dried up completely after he presented highly positive results on terminal cancer patients before an annual meeting of the Federation of American Societies for

Experimental Biology. "His work was channeled into other areas of research, and his superior discouraged his pursuit of cancer therapy," Null wrote.
• When he submitted an abstract of his research in 1978 to a meeting of the American Association for Cancer Research, it was rejected—and he could never get a straight answer why.
• His research proposal was rejected by the ACS.
• He was investigated by the Harris County (Houston) Medical Society for "unethical" research.

We report elsewhere on the situation, odyssey, and promising endeavors of Lawrence Burton, Ph.D., literally forced out of the United States to continue his "immuno-augmentative" research in the Bahamas.

The Laetrile Fight: A Showcase Of Dirty Tricks

In this book, I am attempting to develop, among others, the thesis that what laetrile (vitamin B^{17}) represents is far more a reason for its frenetic suppression than its presumptive action against cancer. It could expect Krebiozen- and Hoxsey-style attacks simply by being a threat to the $30-billion-a-year cancer industry. But as the first assault team on the beach of the metabolic/nutritional revolution, laetrile must be stopped *at all costs*. And I *do* mean at all costs.

That is the only way to explain the development of every iota of energy at the Club's command in trying to squelch laetrile, malign its developers and promoters, insult the recipients of its positive effects, and ridicule its proponents. It is the only way to explain the multi-million-dollar campaign, waged by the FDA and the ACS with both public and private monies, to hammer away at every aspect of amygdalin and to use some of the dirtiest of dirty tricks to put it under.

It is the only plausible explanation of the government's use of two dozen agents and undercover cars and a police helicopter to entrap Robert W. Bradford, founder of the Committee for Freedom of Choice in Cancer Therapy—and "convicted conspirator to smuggle" laetrile. (The bust netted thousands of dollars' worth of the material—not millions of dollars in illicit harmful drugs.)

It is the only logical reason why the U.S. government, by admission in its own testimony, actually hired and paid Mexican smugglers to smuggle in amygdalin with which to entrap Bradford and several other individuals engaged in amygdalin distribution, and why the government would smuggle in, then actually package and ship such merchandise to set up vitamin distributors in Minnesota, an act so outrageous that it drew national publicity.

Only panic and shock can explain the persistent and continuing violations by the FDA of U.S. federal orders on the legal importation of amygdalin, achieved in December 1977, and in spreading "Laetrile Warning" posters at taxpayers' expense across the country in every federal hospital, pharmacy, and many post offices throughout 1978. The backlog of FDA violations of the law while balancing the need to "interpret" court orders against the continuing pressure to crack down on laetrile is by now sufficient to fill a separate volume. That FDA agents would tell distributors that, under terms of new court decisions, *yes,* foreign laetrile could be brought in—and then seize the supply—can only be viewed as vicious duplicity.

Until laetrile's rapid-fire political successes in 1976-80, the Club had been able to deal with the substance as it had dealt with Krebiozen, Glyoxylide, the Hoxsey preparations, etc., for years—smear, isolation and neutralization, and the use of the courts and the media as heavy hammers to bludgeon unwanted new ideas. The politicization of laetrile, as we have seen, changed all that.

The NCI "clinical trial" of 1980-81, the coverup at Sloan-Kettering, the arrests and prosecution of amygdalin-using physicians, the entrapment of distributors—whose rather picayune business is hardly a footnote in comparison to the profit dimensions of both "legitimate" pharmaceuticals and addictive drugs—are all parts of a pattern, one of sheer, unmitigated panic.

The FDA was ordered by the U.S. District Court of Western Oklahoma in 1977 to develop a record as to *why* it had been suppressing laetrile for fourteen years without even an "informal" document available to explain its stand. When the FDA called a two-day hearing to establish its fourteen-years-late position, it put on what amounted to a show at taxpayer expense. It flew in eleven witnesses to testify against laetrile, paying them $3,477 in expenses and $2,775 in "fees." Proponents had to make it to Kansas City on their own, their expenses coming out of their own pockets, and received no fees. Cross-examination of speakers was not allowed and no testimony was sworn. As a journalist who has covered many hearings, this was the worst kangaroo court I had ever experienced. It exposed the Club at its worst. Luckily, the thousands of pages of testimony taken failed to offset the case after case of demonstrated or implied laetrile efficacy and it did not dissuade U.S. District Court Judge Luther Bohanon from his earlier decision that the FDA had failed to prove its charges against laetrile. The ghosts of Krebiozen and "quack" cancer cures past could almost be heard laughing in the background.

When I first began researching laetrile in the period 1970-71, I was skeptical. I wanted to know on what basis the government was resting its case as to the inefficacy of laetrile when I was seeing patient after patient slipping away to Tijuana for treatments that each and every one claimed were of benefit. I was referred to a single document—the 1953 Cancer Commission of the California Medical Association report on laetrile. Reading its synopsis was interesting—ploughing through the whole report was even moreso. For, until the Club belatedly began running a few animal tests on amygdalin in the 1970s, this single report from a state government unit was the *only* peg on which the powers that be could hang their case against laetrile. It stated, quite simply, that forty-four terminal cancer patients had received injections of laetrile and that all had died. But it also said a lot more.

First, all the patients received injections that by today's standards would be regarded as hardly minimal, 100 mg being about the average. Of course, no effort was made to provide a total metabolic program, and orthodoxy was only looking at tumors and other manifestations of patients all literally at death's door. That is to say, even the sample of patients selected was unjust (as was the case, 28 years later, with the NCI "clinical trial"). But, most interestingly, the report noted that the administering doctors agreed that their patients had reflected an increase in appetite and well-being and a decrease in pain. The report's authors snidely added the phrase, "as though these observations constituted evidence of definitive therapeutic effect." The fact is, *all* the test's doctors concurred in the "subjective" response reported—and, in the matter of dying cancer patients, wasting away in great pain, even these results, however fleeting and subjective, deserved follow-up. There was none. Yet this *single* report was the one and only "official" study ever done in the U.S. on humans until the belated NCI trials started in late 1980.

But the evidence *for* laetrile, however minimal and sparse, was coming in from the Philippines, Japan, Italy, and Belgium. It was also mounting in the small caseloads of the few physicians who, during the 1960s, used the substance in the United States. Due largely to efforts by the McNaughton Foundation to keep interest in vitamin B^{17} alive, and the continuing embarrassment to U.S. orthodoxy by the then single clinic in Tijuana, to which ever greater numbers of desperate Americans were fleeing for their "forbidden" treatment, laetrile did not die. The series of actione used against Krebiozen, Glyoxylide, Hoxsey, and other "unproven remedies," while mostly successful in discrediting laetrile *within* the United States, failed to do so around the world.

With laetrile beginning to become a political issue, the decision was reached that at least some kind of testing needed to be done. Not only did such a program begin quietly at Sloan-Kettering, with ultimately disastrous results for the Club when SKI's own employees consistently proved the evidence of a coverup of positive results, but one was also under way under the aegis of the National Cancer Institute as well. For one thing, the NCI's Dr. Burk had found the *in vitro* evidence of laetrile's cancer killing effects and was already informing the congressmen that laetrile was not getting a fair shake. Various sets of tests, for example, could be interpreted different ways by different researchers, depending on what they were looking for.

In 1974, the National Cancer Institute announced results of animal tests on the Lewis lung carcinoma system in mice, in collaboration with Southern Research Institute. The results, supposedly "definitive," were supposed to prove that laetrile did not work—yet Dr. Burk instantly observed that in three of the experiments in the NCI-SRI collaboration "any average grammar school student could, any SRI-NCI scientist should, and any sufficiently experienced statistician would, be able to see at a glance widespread evidence of amygdalin MF efficacy, in terms of both absolute and percent positively increased median life span."

In 1976, Dr. Bernard Kenton, of the City of Hope Medical Center in California, wrote off these same "definitive" tests as "a textbook example of how to lie with statistics." He further analyzed, "Most shocking, from the standpoint of scientific ethics, is the fact that, *without exception,* every one of their [statistics] errors was in the direction of lowering the efficacy of the treatment. It is critical to appreciate that there is essentially zero probability that such systematic misrepresentation is inadvertent. There is no doubt to give anyone the benefit of!"

Despite animal tests with results mixed enough that different experts could read them in entirely different ways, the established line remained that laetrile was without *any* efficacy—none whatsoever, neither a "shred of evidence" nor a "valid sign of efficacy" having ever "once been observed." Just why the Club had to be so sweeping in its assertions, Dean Burk wrote one congressman, was that "once any of the FDA-NCI-AMA-ACS hierarchy so much as concedes that laetrile anti-tumor efficacy was indeed even once observed in NCI experimentation, a permanent crack in the bureaucratic armor has taken place that can widen indefinitely by further appropriate experimentation." There was no NCI "underground" to report on the real meaning of NCI-directed tests, as there was at Sloan-Kettering, so the permanent crack was not to develop until the release of the Sugiura experiments at SKI.

Going into the 1970s, the official position on laetrile was simply that it was worthless. No one yet claimed that it was in itself harmful. The argument, raised as well against Glyoxylide, Krebiozen, and the Hoxsey preparations, was that its only danger lay in leading patients away from "proven" remedies so that they wasted time, money, and energy on quackery before turning themselves over to the tender ministrations of cut-burn-and poison. Not much later, the metabolic/nutritional physicians were to argue that the real waste of time, money, and energy was by opting for standard treatments first.

In the meantime, laetrile proponents were placed in a Catch-22 situation when asked to defend their "unproven remedy"—be it laetrile alone or in combination with metabolic/nutritional therapy. The existent but limited foreign data available were dismissed out of hand simply because they *were* foreign. The American animal data was said to be evidence that the material did not work—and all the accounts of human response inside the U.S. were said to be "spontaneous remissions." Laetrile-proponent physicians were continually asked, "What is your evidence?" But should they try to step forward *with* evidence, they were subject to arrest and peer-group harassment. And, since animal tests had not been conducted in sufficient numbers so that laetrile could become "legal" under the amended Food, Drug and Cosmetic Act, and because few proponents actually believed an investment in time and money on a non-patentable item, even if successful, could ever result in recouping the financial loss implicit in the tests, an effort to secure a license for human tests occurred only once. That was in 1970, when the McNaughton Foundation was first issued, then suddenly denied, permission to go ahead with human tests.

For a time, the Club attacked laetrile along the traditional lines—inappropriate animal studies, "ancedotal" human evidence, the lack of an earned degree for Krebs, Jr., the colorful and controversial career of Andrew McNaughton, the suspicion of a profit motive in amygdalin distribution, the political credentials of its new proponents. But with the successful politicization of laetrile, and as one statehouse after another fell to the apricot-seed extract, it was clear that a new tack must be pursued. And the new one was that laetrile, by golly, is no longer worthless though harmless—it is now worthless *and* harmful. This new strategy was to take the Club down perilous propaganda paths it had not trod before, and to leave it with more egg on its face than ever.

It is probably fair to say, too, that a shift in emphasis to the "dangers" of laetrile was also in response to the destruction of the placebo argument because of gathering evidence from veterinarians that laetrile and/or its natural sources, such as apricot kernels and bitter almonds, were achieving anticancer effects in domesticated cats and dogs. This particular evidence, which *did* get fair play in veterinary journals, demolished the idea that cancer patients just thought they might feel better because a physician told them they would—unless the cats and dogs so studied either read minds or understood English.

California authorities had already zeroed in on the sale of apricot kernels, the main source of American laetrile (and California produces some 85 percent of the nation's apricots) under argument that the the kernels themselves could cause toxic effects. This is true, of course, since—as I note in chapter eight—there is a safely bound cyanide radical in amygdalin that is a putative anticancer agent thereof. Overingestion of too much of the natural material in the *oral* product *can* produce a toxic reaction, but then so can too much water, air, salt, or sugar. The 1972-76 apricot kernel scares, mostly in California, in which there were scattered cases of toxic reactions from doing such things as drinking a slurry of ground-up apricot kernels in water left standing overnight, were quickly accompanied by efforts to claim that two "laetrile foods," Aprikern and Bee Seventeen, neither promoted as medicine, might also be toxic.

At least three million capsules of Aprikern and 100,000 packages of the milkshake-like Bee Seventeen had been sold before the FDA released an amazing report claiming that five capsules of Aprikern "could be fatal" to a child, twenty to an adult. No evidence whatsoever of this was advanced, and no recorded cases of poisoning from the ingestion of either product were reported. In analyzing the FDA's analyses, Dr. Burk was amazed to find that the University of Arizona tests which were used to support the FDA action had involved the hydrolyzing—that is, breaking down—of the product to release cyanide under conditions that in no way correspond to human eating habits, and then administering it to rats at a level equivalent to a human's consuming a third of a pound of the product per kilogram of body weight. Prehydrolyzed material consumed at any such level would, as hydrolyzed material given at astronomical levels and in a manner at variance with human ingestion habits, became the hallmark of "official tests" to prove the danger of vitamin B^{17}-containing products.

Nonetheless, on the basis of these incredible tests the products were removed from the shelves in several states. Also, state and federal action began against the distribution of amydgalin-containing "bitter food tablets," and attemps to seize packaged apricot and peach kernels, natural sources of B^{17}, were made. The campaign reached ludicrous proportions with raids and confiscations that, in Florida, netted 470 pounds of kernels—and, fantastically, forty *tons* in a Tennessee warehouse. In the latter case, vitamin distributor Douglas Heinsohn, also a Committee for Freedom of Choice organizer, took the FDA to court over the confiscation and finally won.

The scenario of federal agents lying in wait to seize packages of apricot kernels proved too much for the nation's media cartoonists, and they unleashed a volley of graphic ridicule of this latest tactic. I learned early in my probe of the apricot kernel capers that not a single case of apricot kernel fatality had ever been reported in the Americas, and that the material on which such scare information was based came from anecdotal reports in Turkey. It was obvious to many normally skeptical journalists by 1976-77 that the government was "reaching" when it announced open war on apricot kernels. Those who were aware of the high vitamin B^{17} content in a wide range of foods waited breathlessly for FDA action bulletins on confiscation of alfalfa sprouts, lima beans, chokecherries, macadamia nuts, cashews, and buckwheat pancakes (all rich in B^{17}) to say nothing of the banning of all fruits that contained bitter-tasting black seeds (the most potent sources of B^{17}).

Behind the laughter, though, lurked the Club's urgent need to get the toxicity goods on amygdalin (laetrile) at all costs. Contrived statistics on mice and rats failed to impress state legislatures and physicians, and there simply were not any human fatalities on hand from laetrile overdoses—at least not yet. Finally, there appeared a case that *suggested* possible laetrile toxicity. While there are still unknown aspects of this highly ballyhooed case, it is now apparent from statements by both her mother and father that ten-month-old Elizabeth Hankin did *not* die by overdosing on laetrile tablets from the supply her father was taking for his own fight with terminal cancer.

But because the little girl was admitted to a hospital with symptoms suggesting some kind of toxicity, and because it was reported she had somehow had access to her father's medication while the family was preparing to move from one house to another, the story clicked over the wire services that the child had died from consuming laetrile tablets. Both Mr. and Mrs. Dale Hankin told me, repeatedly, and also said so for official hearings, that Elizabeth did *not* consume the tablets. First of all, a 500-mg laetrile tablet would have been difficult for the baby to ingest, and its bitterness would probably have been a warning to stop eating anyway.

Even more suspicious, at the hospital in question, Elizabeth survived for almost *four days* and was off the critical list before she took a turn for the worse and died. If in fact she died of cyanide poisoning, she set a record, for free cyanide kills in a matter of minutes, not hours and days. Indeed, in the cult mass murder-suicide in Jonestown, Guyana, which claimed more than 900 lives in November 1978 from ingestion or injection of cyanide, all the victims were dead within five minutes. Three physicians writing in the Nyack, New York, *Journal* of 27 September 1977, advanced these observations, "One of us, who appeared as an expert at a recent trial involving laetrile, had the privilege of examining the child's medical records and was therefore able to make observations that were not released to the press. This information, in conjunction with well-known medical facts involving cyanide poisoning, has led us to the conclusion that the child did not die of laetrile or cyanide poisoning." Another theory advanced was the alarming possibility that by being treated for cyanide poisoning when there was no free cyanide present, Elizabeth might have suffered a fatal trauma.

Despite depositions by the parents and their continual statements denying the story, the FDA and Club spokesmen gave wide circulation to the Hankin case, which they presented as established fact in hearing after hearing. Later, they were able to report on the death of a teenage girl who reportedly broke open four vials of laetrile and *drank* the contents—12 grams, or far over the 1.5-2 gram maximum recommended oral dose. She had apparently not been told by her doctor to do this, and more details of her case were sketchy at best. Yet this irrational act was widely promoted as evidence that "laetrile can kill."

Incredibly, as the FDA did everything in its power to subvert the court-approved legal entry of foreign amygdalin into the country, the fact that both understrength tablets and vials would turn up in the black market, and that some of these were contaminated, was also used as an argument against laetrile. Since I was usually knighted to do battle with this particular set of data, I responded to anyone who would listen that, *of course,* as long as laetrile remained illegal by governmental action, it would be a blackmarket product susceptible to all the problems involved in black-marketeering. I argued strenuously for the legal manufacture and use of the laetrile in *this* country, under FDA-approved standards of purity and sterility, as the only guarantee of absoultely reliable material. But this argument was lost on the FDA, which continued to seize laetrile shipments and raided and closed the only facility in the United States that at the time was openly manufacturing laetrile tablets.

The Club's data on laetrile toxicity reached geometric new proportions in 1977-78 with "new evidence" designed to strike fear into the heart of the stoutest laetrile defender. First, there was the circulation by the FDA of a study that claimed that amygdalin had caused thirty-seven poisonings and seventeen deaths, as reported in world literature. These figures were reeled off by multi-degreed savants as they appeared in state after state to attack laetrile. But what did the raw data *actually* say?

Incredibly, the information covers more than a century of scattered reports and deals with natural plant sources of vitamin B^{17} (and many other things). The thirty-seven poisonings and seventeen deaths are those attributed to the overconsumption, for example, of cassava. The *only* death attributed to laetrile itself was, again, the Hankin case. Also, the data from which the information was drawn came from many different countries and they were reported under all kinds of conditions. Laetrile proponents shot back that a century of such "anecdotes" meant nothing at all scientifically about laetrile—but even if there were one or even two fatalities from laetrile poisoning over such a span, just what relevance did any such figure have when given the thousands of toxic reactions to and hundreds of fatalities *yearly* from such a common product as aspirin?

But logic was not a strong point in the toxicity assault on laetrile. In another report, this one from a major research laboratory in Ohio, oral toxicity from laetrile was said to have produced fatal poisonings in monkeys and dogs. But what were the doses? Up to 1.3 grams per kilogram of body weight for the monkeys, up to 6.4 grams per kilogram of body weight for the dogs. The monkeys, thus, were getting from five to sixty times the normal *oral* dose of a 150-pound man. The dogs were getting, at the upward range, *300 times* what a human would receive!

The all-time champion "toxicity study," however, which grabbed the headlines and was used as a double-whammy attack not only on laetrile but on the mostly vegetarian diet that usually accompanies its intensive care use, in the "crisis treatment" stage, occurred in the infamous "Laetrile Toxicity Studies in Dogs" research at the University of California at Davis. It is vital to understand that the report itself, which appeared in the 6 March 1978 *Journal of the American Medical Association,* contains all the relevant information as long as one reads *all* of it. However, most newsmen apparently saw *only* its introductory synopsis or simply a press release based on the article's overall contents, and the information from these sources was widely circulated even before the *JAMA* reached professional hands.

The press articles reporting on the research by Eric S. Schmidt, *et al.* were accompanied by such scare headlines as "Laetrile Poison with Some Foods," "Laetrile Can Kill," and the like. It represents the most extreme reach of the Club to somehow "get the goods" on laetrile, and is still used by opponents as proof positive that not only is the compound itself dangerous, but it is doubly so when consumed along with many fruits and vegetables.

The synoptic summary of the research, on which the press liberties were either taken or based, said, and the emphasis added throughout is mine:

> Dogs were *fed* laetrile and fresh, sweet almonds under *various conditions.* The doses of laetrile were similar to those prescribed for patients with cancer and ranged on a basis of gram to square meter from an equivalent of the *oral dose* to five times this dose. Six of the ten [though the report described seventeen] dogs died of cyanide poisoning. One dog recovered, and three dogs, at the time of sacrifice [officialese for "killing"], demonstrated various levels of neurologic impairment.... These studies demonstrate that *oral* laetrile is highly toxic when *taken* with some common table foods. We predict that there will be an increased incidence of cyanide poisoning in man as laetrile becomes more readily available.

Pretty stong stuff, right? Any newsman would think so, since the verbs *fed* and *taken* immediately conjure up visions of animals eating or chewing laetrile along with "some common table foods"— and then dropping dead. Virtually nobody in the media bothered to read what the "various conditions" referred to were, or even to report that Schmidt *et al.* clearly stated their announced bias by noting that "our studies were designed to confirm our prediction that oral laetrile, when ingested with certain uncooked foods containing beta-glucosidase, would result in HCN [cyanide] toxicity." A study "designed to confirm" a prediction is hardly a bulwark of scientific integrity.

Quite alarmed over the press releases, and aware that thousands of Americans were indeed ingesting oral laetrile with "common table foods" every day—without a single known fatality being reported—I went over the *JAMA* article line by line. Had I not already been "radicalized" by the Sloan-Kettering coverup to the point where I actually expected orthodoxy to lie, cheat, and distort, this report alone would have done the job. First of all, as the fine-print "materials, methods and test subjects" section clearly reflects, only one test dog was "fed" sweet almonds alone. He "chewed and swallowed" twenty sweet almonds (these nuts having one of the highest concentrations in the plant kingdom of the enzyme that breaks down, or hydrolyzes, amygdalin). Absolutely nothing happened to this animal. Another dog was fed *fifty* sweet almonds— which itself is a little difficult to imagine—and also given two grams of liquid laetrile, though *how* is not made plain, but probably through the amazing route described below. This second dog was said to have had "trouble standing." So much for the two dogs that in any way, shape, or form were "fed" anything for this openly biased test.

The media chose to overlook the author's admission that the test dogs were *starved* in advance of the tests. They were hungry and were given either sweet almonds in the natural state (that is, two of them were), or in their *unnatural* state. Several of the test animals were given a drug in order to suppress vomiting, which is nature's first stomach reaction to poison, and others were given a drug to "ensure a light plane of anesthesia," as the scientists put it. That is to say, the test dogs were, in the main, *starved and doped* in advance of the incredible experiment that ensued.

The *JAMA* article insists that cyanide poisoning effects resulted in fifteen dogs. And, by golly, they did. But just how? They were not "fed" laetrile and sweet almonds *at all,* other than by the broadest possible semantical perversion of the verb "to feed." But they *were* "force-fed"—and not laetrile and sweet almonds. What they got— *inserted into them by gastric tube*—was a concoction that consisted of laetrile and a mash of sweet almonds ground up and mixed in a plastic blood bag at a temperature sufficient to allow the beta-glucosidase from the almonds to hydrolyze the amygdalin, thus causing the release of cyanide. That is, a prehydrolyzed mixture with free cyanide was rammed into the test dogs. *Of course they were poisoned!* But in this section of the report, we read that the animals received an "administration" of the substance. Here, "feed" is substituted by "administer." This outrageous test, then, had nothing whatsoever to do with the kinds of substances consumed by humans—or dogs, for that matter—let alone ways in which humans (and dogs) eat. It was simply an incredible experiment designed to prove something known to science for decades—that beta-glucosidase hydrolyzes amygdalin.

The Club then paraded this fiendishly misleading experiment, to alert cancer sufferers to the presumptive danger inherent in consuming plants that are high in beta-glucosidase together with oral amygdalin, and then raising the spectre of thousands of cyanide deaths to come—even though none had been reported from any such combination.

Again, bear in mind, only *oral* amygdalin was under direct attack with the cyanide scare. Other than problems inherent with occasionally contaminated vials and other manufacturing problems —*all* of which had to do with the government's driving laetrile underground and thus blocking American production—the Club could find nothing toxic in a cyanide way about injected amygdalin. Used as indicated, injectable amygdalin, manufactured under responsible norms of pharmaceutical preparation, is so utterly *nontoxic* that it has been administered at in excess of 70 grams by intravenous "drip." An LD^{50}, or dose at which 50 percent of experimental animals die, of 8,000 milligrams per kilogram of body weight was established in 1980 for one brand of stabilized, purified, natural amygdalin in aqueous solution. (A level of 5,000 mg/kg is regarded as non-toxic.) Some levels as high as 20,000 mg/kg have been reported. The injectable preparation, then, as the Club very well knows, makes it normally *safer than every other injectable cancer drug* on the market, and safer than many other drugs. As the Bradford research group found, there are specific pathological conditions in which the injectable form *may* present problems, but this is true of virtually any medicine.

Faced with the essential non-toxicity of the injectable form, the Club needed to emphasize the dangers of the *oral* form—which admittedly are present, and at much lower levels than for the injectable one, but which still make the oral product one far safer than most of the thirty or so highly toxic anti-cancer compounds "approved" for human use in this country.

However, any cyanide radical-bearing compound *does* have a toxic danger at some point. Metabolic therapists advised for years that no more than 1.5-2 grams of oral amygdalin should be taken daily during treatment, and research done in 1979-80 by the Bradford group indicated the absolute need to monitor oral amygdalin ingestion with blood serum thiocyanate levels and avoid overingestion of plant foods bearing beta-glucosidase while consuming the oral product. This, however, was serious science—not a study in which cyanide was used to poison starved, doped dogs.

As an incensed Dean Burk wrote to the editors of *JAMA:* "The moral of all this is that if Schmidt *et al.* are really interested in the essential facts rather than their displayed fancies, they will make haste to study *Homo sapiens* instead of *Canis mongrelli,* and to avoid preincubated amydgalin-enzyme mixtures as they would avoid putting air into veins—what's the point?"

Dr. Burk, as an award-winning and highly honored biochemist, is one of several scientists around the world who have demonstrated the essential nontoxicity of amygdalin. It has also been shown in research conducted by Krebs, the McNaughton Foundation, the Bradford Foundation, Dr. Harold Manner's research team at Loyola of Chicago, and by Dr. Bruce Halstead, a veteran cancer researcher and biotoxicologist. In this exhaustive analysis of the history and use of amygdalin, Dr. Halstead wrote in a monograph:

> The safety factor in the use of Amygdalin (Laetrile) can best be appreciated by comparing its toxicity to that of some of the more commonly used medications. It will be noted that Amygdalin (Laetrile) has a much greater safety range than any of the drugs listed that are already approved by the FDA. Aspirin is the cause of upwards of 100,000 intoxications and about 300 fatalities each year in the United States. It will be noted that the usual FDA approved "anticancer drugs" are not only extremely toxic drugs, but are also paradoxically carcinogenic.

In 1978, with the Club ever more desperate to come up with more negative information on laetrile, a Georgetown University physician was quoted as saying that two unnamed laetrile-using cancer patients had developed "adverse reactions" to the material and for that reason "the controversial substance may be dangerous." One news commentator even took liberties with that and reported that "two cancer patients died as a result" of taking laetrile.

One of the two "adverse reaction" patients, very much alive, turned out to be Carol M. Dunn, a journalist. She was so irate that she had been listed as an "adverse reaction" case that she wrote her own rebuttal, noting that her "adverse reaction" had been a rash and a temperature of 102 degrees. The fact, she said, was that her *real* "adverse reactions" had been to the chemotherapy drug chlorozotocin, one injection of which had "damaged my bone marrow to such an extent I was unable to produce platelets, which are an important part of the white blood cell. In fact, three days after receiving six units of platelets, the platelet count was down lower than previously. After extensive vitamin therapy, including Laetrile (B^{17}), I am now just beginning to hold my own."

She noted that she had had far more serious reactions to aspirin and penicillin than to laetrile, and that orthodoxy is silent as to how many cancer patients die annually from chemotherapy and radiation.

In early 1979 the media gave wide attention to the putative death-by-cyanide-poisoning-from-laetrile of a California woman. If the case proved anything, it was that injectable laetrile should not be given by enema—as it reportedly was—just as air should not be shot into a vein.

Evidence that the conspiracy against laetrile is world-wide became obvious in October 1978, when laetrile proponents travelled to Buenos Aires for the quadrennial meeting of the World Cancer Congress, the twelfth such "Olympics of Cancer" jamboree, one attracting 8,000 experts from more than seventy-five countries. The conference is sponsored by the Switzerland-based World Anti-Cancer Union, which is obviously influenced by American medicine at every turn.

We were enthusiastically awaiting the presentation before this prestigious world body of the evidence gathered by Mexico's Dr. Ernesto Contreras of the Del Mar Medical Center in Tijuana. His fifteen years' experience had resulted in a closely monitored and tabulated group of 4,800 case histories, divided into two sets of five-year survival studies. They showed the overwhelming evidence that laetrile is active against some "forms" of cancer by itself, that its total program had achieved 65.17 percent positive responses over a five-year period, and that it is also useful in combination with orthodox drugs. Here, we thought, would be a world forum to announce such vital information.

Funny things had already happened. Dr. Contreras, who was invited to speak, had first been told he could address the world body and that his data would be published. Then he was informed that he could speak but that his data would not be published. You can imagine his considerable chagrin when, arriving in Buenos Aires, he was told that he would not even be allowed to speak—the orders allegedly "came from Switzerland."

At the same time, the Philippines' Dr. Manuel Navarro, despite his quarter-century of experience with laetrile, was also denied a place on the program. He was to present a paper on cancer diagnosis, not on laetrile itself, and was to have seven minutes before his peers. But when his name showed up on a leaflet announcing the press conference at which we presented the Contreras evidence to a group of Argentine and Brazilian physicians and media, he was denied the right to go on the program for even seven minutes.

So the plot thickened. And continues to thicken.

But the prospects for the vindication of laetrile within a framework of metabolic/nutritional therapy have never looked better. And the slow vindication of many of the "unproven remedies" is underway even now.

Under the intellectual pressure of German research (after all, who can pooh-pooh German science?), the American cancer establishment is grudgingly looking into vitamin A uses against cancer and is tiptoeing into the area of enzymes, as well. It continues to look at vitamin C in cancer, after years of refusal to do so, and at least one Club project is interested in vitamin E and cancer.

In the meantime, laetrile (vitamin B^{17}) use goes on, with Americans being both treated at home by gutsy, principled physicians not afraid to risk the wrath of peer criticism, and in clinics around the world. Virginia Livingston (see the next chapter) is continuing her fascinating work in new areas of "unproven" remedies. Desperate Americans suffering from a wide spectrum of maladies are finding responses from a wide array of "unproven" methods if they can afford to leave the U.S.A.

Even so, the dinosaurs take a long time to die. As these lines are written, marijuana has been approved for use in several states *to reduce the side effects of cancer chemotherapy*. And research programs have been suggested to see if heroin is more effective than morphine in easing the pain of cancer patients. Defenders of heroin have pointed out, wryly it would seem, that "smack" is a fine analgesic—and of course there is little chance of addiction since the patients will die anyway.

O tempora, o mores.

Chapter Seven
Modern Medicine's Magnificent Mavericks

Of Heresy And History

The battlefield of progress is strewn with the corpses of heretics without whose last full measure the battle could not have been won. Virtually every major breakthrough in science and medicine has been made by people and groups who, when they were actually accomplishing the feat, were branded as heretics and quacks. This seems to be a universal part of the human condition and is constantly repeated today, as ubiquitous evidence attests.

This does not mean, of course, that every scientist or physician who dares rattle the cage of the Club or operate outside the pale of orthodoxy is breaking honest new ground. The rigidity of orthodoxy and the intransigence of bureaucracy are in part reactions to, not causes of, irresponsibility and charlatanry. But the reality that the medical-scientific pioneers are, in their day, frequently held to be heretics must be borne in mind when reading the latest pronouncements of the American Medical Association or any of its state affiliates, or while perusing the American Cancer Society's "unproven remedies" list.

Copernicus and Galileo, in their day, felt the might of orthodox thinking for making assumptions that flew in the face of conventional wisdom. The point has been belabored elsewhere that the "best medicine" of earlier centuries killed as many people as it saved—and that such architects of contemporary history as George Washington were killed by conventional medical wisdom.

How easy it is to forget that today's heroes were yesterday's heretics. We are routinely treated to the reality of the Salk vaccine against poliomyelitis as a triumph of Western medicine, while being allowed to forget how Jonas Salk fought a long, hard struggle for vindication and was in the main opposed by the Establishment medicine of his time. While the ACS today parrots the virtues of the "Pap smear" for early detection of cervical cancer, the fact is that Papanicoleau's procedure was ignored for years before achieving acceptance.

Sir Alexander Fleming noted more than once that penicillin was consigned to the shelf, for well over a decade before its use as a major antibiotic was accepted. Louis Pasteur's long, often bitter, battle to establish the germ theory of disease, now such a vital cog in the allopathic thought process, is one of the most illustrative examples of scientific heresy slowly gaining credibility. Orthodoxy in its day reviled the theory and its proponent with the same venom and spite as are now accorded the promoters of metabolic/nutritional therapy, vitamins E and C in disease, vitamins B^{15} and B^{17} in cancer and other degenerative diseases, and chelation therapy in cardiovascular ailments.

The story of establishing the vitamin-deficiency nature of pellagra, rickets, scurvy, and beriberi is a recitation of challenges to orthodox thinking by researchers, spanning continents and time, who dared to speak the unspeakable, think the unthinkable, and then do the undoable. How easy it is, in this day of reliance on antiseptic measures in operations, to forget that Ignaz Semmelweiss was driven to a lunatic asylum by opposition to his insistence that physicians wash their hands between deliveries of babies. At a time when orthodoxy now promotes insulin as utterly necessary in the management of diabetes, it is easy to forget that Fredrick Banting battled long and hard against impossible odds to secure the rightful place of insulin in the treatment, and that, luckily, insulin was developed and in general use before a law such as the Food, Drug and Cosmetic Act as amended was around to stop it.

Humanity owes as much to Christian Eijkman, who found the vitamin nature of the killer disease beriberi, to Armand Trousseau, who did about the same for rickets, and to Joseph Goldberger and Thomas Spies, who did the same for pellagra, as it does to Banting, Fleming, and Salk. It is my view that it will ultimately owe as much to such unsung champions as Krebs and Krebs, Warburg, Burk, and Bradford and the chelation pioneers as it does to Pasteur and Lister. Some of the pioneers of medicine past, and those of medicine present, never lived, or will live, to see their theories and breakthroughs vindicated. But many will. For the American medical revolution is now breaking all around us, led—as stated earlier—by the unlikely apricot kernel.

Elsewhere we will examine the battles for the recognition of vitamins C, E, and B^{15} and B^{17} in degenerative disease, as well as the story of chelation therapy, for these are all vital entities in and of themselves in the developing scenario of medical revolt and innovation. But stressing their importance is to give the idea that they and they alone constitute the only elements in the clash of ideas and inventions. There are many other facets to be considered, far from the least of which are the following.

Otto Warburg And Dean Burk

It is ironic that Otto Warburg should be on American cancer orthodoxy's heretics list, for, unlike many proponents and champions of "unproven remedies," none was more credentialed for the field than Warburg, nor was the scientist who espoused his thinking in this country, Dean Burk—whose name appears time and again in these pages. Warburg, for many years director of the Max Planck Institute for Cell Physiology in Berlin, was a two-time Nobel Prize winner, one (1931) for his discovery of the oxygen-transferring enzyme system of cell respiration, and again (1944) for discovering the active groups of hydrogen-transferring systems. But, as two-time Nobel laureate Linus Pauling has found in fighting for the recognition of vitamin C's role in combating cancer, the American cancer Establishment is not necessarily impressed by such lofty credentials.

It was Warburg who, years ago, solved part of the cancer riddle, only to have his words fall on deaf ears in America and, to a large extent, Western medicine. Among his other notable achievements, this respected German savant found that all normal cells are oxygen-using (aerobic) and that cancer cells are not (anaerobic), and that when normal, oxygen-using cells are partially but not completely deprived of oxygen they will revert to a fermentation process (conversion of glucose to lactic acid) for energy—that is, they will become cancerous.

He demonstrated that more than thirty complex chemical reactions are involved in the use of oxygen for the derivation of energy within cells, and that many food factors are involved in the process, very much including iron salts and the B vitamins, B^1, B^2, B^{12}, nicotinamide, and pantothenic acid, which he termed the "active respiratory groups." He postulated that by adding the "active respiratory groups" to the diet before and after cancer surgery, the spread of cancer—metastasis—may be prevented. As Kanematsu Sugiura was to demonstrate later with vitamin B^{17} (amygdalin or laetrile), Warburg pointed out that these substances would have little or no effect on a primary tumor. It is, of course, the spread of cancer-cell colonies to vital organs and tissues—not, usually, a primary tumor—whereby cancer kills.

Following up on his work, Warburg in 1966 proposed a four-point program that he argued would reduce cancer in humans by *80 percent:* making sure enough B vitamins and iron are in the diet, maintaining a high concentration of hemoglobin in the blood, keeping bloodstream velocity high enough for venous blood to contain sufficient oxygen, and staying out of contact with known carcinogens (cancer causing agents). Once again, the *prevention* of cancer had been elaborated. And simply. But not even a double Nobel laureate was to be listened to in this country when making such a proposal.

In 1967, a constituent of Sen. Edward Kennedy wrote the latter a letter criticizing the medical Establishment for ignoring the Warburg approach. In return, she received a letter from National Cancer Institute Director Kenneth M. Endicott in which she was told that "as far as the universal use of vitamins and minerals to enhance the activity of the respiratory groups is concerned, Warburg's concepts have been the focus of controversy in the scientific community for thirty years. And, at the National Cancer Institute, we are more concerned with the danger of producing hypervitaminosis in some members of our population."

It was this kind of remark that was enough to trigger Dr. Dean Burk into action. Burk, a founder of the NCI, and after thirty-five years at his retirement in 1974, the head of the institute's cytochemistry division, edited and translated the English version of Warburg's "The Prime Cause and Prevention of Cancer" lecture before Nobel laureates in 1966. He was also a long-time friend and student of the German scientist. At the time, Burk replied that "hyper-vitaminosis" (toxicity from an excess of vitamins) had been found only in remote cases and only with vitamins A and D—and that even an average teenage student would know that the danger of overdosing on the B vitamins is practically nil.

Burk, a biochemist who spent forty-five years of his professional life investigating cancer, not only was the primary apostle of Warburg in this country and within the NCI, but eventually he became the single research voice within the Club arguing for a fair hearing for laetrile. He was the first credentialed scientist of stature within this country to accord laetrile its status as a vitamin—B^{17}—after its designation as such by its codiscoverer, biochemist Ernst T. Krebs, Jr.

Burk also argued long and hard against the use of toxic drugs in cancer chemotherapy and *for* the research of nontoxic food factors—vitamins, such as Warburg's "active respiratory groups," amygdalin and vitamin C—in cancer therapy. His continual arguments, protestations, letters to congressmen, and the like failed to move the NCI, at least while he was there, but they provided ample ammunition for proponents of nontoxic therapy who were operating outside the blessing of orthodoxy. As we have seen, it was also Burk who lent his professional credibility to the fight against fluoridation of the nation's water supply and continued hammering home the semantic —and juridically vital—difference between vitamins and drugs in the matter of laetrile. He also wrote in defense of the use of classifications of vitamins B^{13} and B^{15}.

To all of those in the battle against cancer orthodoxy, Burk is best remembered as the single man within the Establishment to point out consistently and forthrightly that orthodoxy played fast and loose with cancer treatment response statistics. He argued time and again that traditional methods of cancer therapy have achieved only a five-year survival rate of less than 10 percent. It was Dr. Burk who was on hand to inform a congressman of the "extensive falsification, duplicity, deviousness, red herrings and literal lies... promulgated by the FDA with respect to laetrile."

At the time this is written, Burk continues to be enthusiastic about another "unproven remedy" that has established at least a partial record of credibility in cancer therapy—hydrazine sulfate. He is thus forwarding the work of Dr. Joseph Gold of the Syracuse Cancer Research Institute in New York, who was led to the hydrazine sulfate theory by the work of Otto Warburg.

Dr. Gold theorized that the answer to interrupting the degenerative metabolic process, whereby cancer cells use up enormous energy by the recycling of their wastes and converting normal body mass into tumor substrate, lies in the inhibition of gluconeogenesis, the synthesizing of glucose in the liver and the kidney cortex. This interruption can be accomplished by blocking a key enzymatic reaction in the gluconeogenesis process, and hydrazine sulfate, used as a rocket fuel in World War II by Nazi Germany, does this best, Dr. Gold decided.

He reported in 1973 on "favorable responses in a wide array of different kinds of cancer in human patients without serious side effects. While information is far from conclusive on hydrazine sulfate, it has been used by several thousand American cancer patients, usually in conjunction with other therapies, and favorably received and scientifically advanced in the U.S.S.R.

In the meantime, Western medicine had paid scant attention to Warburg's "active respiratory groups" and his oh-so-simple approach to the prevention of cancer. It has failed to heed the observations of Dr. Dean Burk and has, in the main, conducted a witch hunt against those who use megavitamins and nontoxic substances to curb cancer. But the pioneering work with vitamins B^{15}, B^{17}, C, and E by medical mavericks—and heretics—as the Krebses, the Shutes, Linus Pauling, Irwin Stone, and Ewan Cameron, is not only holding the line but pointing to the future. Their vindication, and that of Warburg and Burk, is now only a question of time.

Peter DeMarco And Procaine PVP

Patients of Peter DeMarco, M.D., could hardly believe their eyes. Pennsylvania health officials strode into their physician's office in Morrisville, containerized and sealed all of the medicine he had developed to treat the ills of upwards of 800 patients, and said they would have to do without.

That was in January 1978. Just ten days before, DeMarco, a

quiet, pipesmoking doctor who is revered in almost godlike terms by patients who believe he has at least mitigated their suffering and, in many cases, saved their lives, had lost his license to practice in neighboring New Jersey. Health authorities there claimed there had been an outbreak of hepatitis among DeMarco's patients. The number of such patients was variously estimated at seventeen to ninety-five, but as far as I was able to determine, no list of them was ever produced.

In Pennsylvania, the press reported that "the state embargoed the drug"—a substance developed by Peter DeMarco himself and called *procaine polyvinyl pyrrolidone*—Procaine PVP for short—"after health officials learned that the federal Food and Drug Administration had revoked permission for DeMarco to administer the drug more than 10 years ago." Pennsylvania grabbed his license, too.

Thus began chapter two of a story that had begun earlier when patients by the dozens testified in favor of their doctor at hearings in New Jersey. They now embarked on a crusade not only to defend him in Pennsylvania but to regain his license. About 500 of these grateful patients of the vascular surgeon, whose controversial serum has indeed achieved notable responses in a very wide gamut of maladies, grouped themselves into an organization called SOS—Save Our Shots—then hired an attorney and prepared to do battle.

Had it not been for this move, I suspect Dr. DeMarco, a softspoken loner of the quiet laboratory variety, would have gone down to defeat. He had run afoul of pharmaceutical companies and of their policing force, and was expected to pay the price—isolation, neutralization and, for all intents and purposes, elimination. In fact, the discovery of something useful backed by a lone innovator who rejects overtures made by drug companies and/or the medical monopoly is redolent of the Koch and Hoxsey "unproven cancer remedies" (see chapter six). But his patients would have none of it.

As this book was completed, legal maneuverings had only partially carried the day. Dr. DeMarco had for a time been restored to the good graces of Pennsylvania officialdom, but his license there was under attack as this decade began. He told me in December 1980 that he had treated "thousands of people successfully" with PVP for a broad spectrum of ailments.

Peter DeMarco, accused by a New Jersey official of being "unfit to continue to practice medicine," a man who has "engaged in the most flagrant and gross form of malpractice and neglect," took the criticism matter-of-factly. "The monkey isn't on my back, it's on theirs," he said. "The largest drug companies in the world are right here in New Jersey. They all know about my serum. You'd think, if they were the great humanitarians they are supposed to be, that they'd be down here, offering, say, even a penny a bottle. They aren't. It may be that drug companies don't want people throwing their pills away. Nobody has ever regenerated cells in vertebrate animals before"—which DeMarco shows by slides of patients that Procaine PVP has indeed done. "And there hasn't been one drug discovered that has come from outside the established drug industry. They've all come within." Of his discovery, DeMarco says tantalizingly, "I've solved the problem of novocaine. You can turn on or off protein synthesis until a certain stage in healing is reached." One version of the drug is available in Europe, he adds.

DeMarco is hardly the picture of a con man. Tall, athletic, in his midforties, informally attired, he exudes more economic necessity than affluence. His personality has not been designed to win friends. He is succinct, abrupt, taciturn; but his patients swear by him. They have claimed stunning responses to everything from arthritis, scleroderma, gangrene, and lupus to heart disease, back pain, eye hemorrhage, blindness, diabetes—and even cancer. I have spoken to a dozen or so of them. None has expressed anything but respect and admiration for DeMarco, and all are certain they have been effectively treated with their intravenous injections of Procaine PVP. By 1979, SOS spokesmen were certain that at least ten patients had died because of the embargo of their doctor's material—which had never been shown to be toxic.

A graduate of the prestigious Hahnemann Medical School, DeMarco has been involved in the research and development of Procaine PVP since his student days. He told me that he has treated thousands of patients with it over an eighteen-year span. "Extensive animal work has been done, including 10,000 slides on nmimal experiments," he added. As early as 1963, he and his associates, in conjunction with the drug firm Philadel Labs, sought a license from the FDA for Procaine PVP. Two weeks after meeting with FDA officials, he said, he and his colleagues were contacted by a major pharmaceutical house, whose vice-president and two researchers took him and a partner to dinner.

"We asked, 'How did you get our name?' " DeMarco recalled. "And they just smiled. They offered us a contract. It couldn't have been too good because we turned them down. Two weeks later the FDA turned *us* down." DeMarco filed for patent rights in 1963 and they were issued in 1967—but all to no avail, since the FDA construed the substance as an unlicensed drug "in interstate commerce" when patients crossed a state line to secure it. The *Journal of the American Medical Association* twice refused to publish DeMarco's articles on the use of Procaine PVP.

Nonetheless, he continued to use the drug, with ever-growing success, until the investigation of him by New Jersey in 1977, a probe he and his patients feel was only a thinly veiled maneuver of government bureaucracy and major pharmaceutical firms to "get" him. The claim that an unusual number of DeMarco's patients came down with hepatitis from unsterile clinical conditions is at best a murky argument. "The whole state of New Jersey had had a rise in hepatitis," DeMarco told the press. "And those people who came down with it are from Trenton. That water is polluted. Even before the filtration plant broke down last year those people were drinking water with sewage in it. Some of these people could be coming to me with hepatitis already."

I have spoken to no patient who feels either that he was conned or poisoned by Peter DeMarco. All of them have expressed a sense of outrage that they have been denied their shots of something which they are certain helps them. Helen Pesce, a prime mover of SOS, put it this way:

> Peter DeMarco's patients have banded together and have tried to fight a frustrating battle to regain their right to freedom of choice so they can have available the much-needed drug. Two patients have died [this was in early 1978], several of them have been admitted to hospitals and many have suffered regression and are deteriorating rapidly. You understand, those patients who are now under the stress of losing their lives are those who came to Dr. DeMarco near death and under his care did in fact lead reasonably healthy lives....
>
> [One] allegation is that Procaine PVP is not effective, yet documented cases prove that blindness in diabetic patients with Procaine PVP [is ended], patients whose gangrenous limbs were to be amputated as directed by other physicians now use those limbs, heart-diseased patients now have stronger heart muscles and all traces of painful angina are erased and those "sick" people work and lead normal lives.

The patients found they were not acting alone. Both editorialists and county government figures wanted to know of just what "crime" Dr. DeMarco had ever been found guilty. Had Procaine PVP killed anyone? Was there any real evidence linking his practice and hepatitis? If Procaine PVP were only a placebo—the same argument hurled at laetrile—how could it possibly hurt to make it available to patients who, by the hundreds, swore they were receiving some efficacy from it? The mayors of Trenton, Lawrence, and Hamilton townships in New Jersey quickly sprang to DeMarco's defense, but at the same time there was no budging the Club from going after this unwanted maverick.

DeMarco philosophized to a reporter, "Many scientists pray that what they discover is of no economic value. If it is, God help them. They receive nothing for it. If they go it alone they will be crucified. Most of them wind up in the insane asylum and are made heroes of only after they are dead." Others, as we shall see, confirm this harsh appraisal.

The Heirs Of Max Gerson Fight Degenerative Disease

I had seldom seen a happier group. On 2 July 1978 nine patients who months before had been in the terminal throes of degenerative disease—principally cancer, but also heart disease, rheumatoid arthritis, and multiple sclerosis—were presented to the media in Los Angeles by Norman Fritz and Charlotte Gerson Straus, the daughter of Max Gerson.

Mrs. Straus and Fritz initiated the Gerson therapy physicians' training program and are heirs to the therapy pioneered decades before by Dr. Gerson (chapter six). They were marking a year of work at a Gerson therapy center in—of course—Tijuana, Mexico, which was rapidly becoming a major medical refuge in North America as unproven remedies are chased out of this country but continue to gain American support because they *work*.

The patients that Mrs. Straus and Fritz presented to the media hardly looked seriously ill—yet all were documented cases of cancer and other diseases. All had been on the modified Gerson program, an intensive, nontoxic therapy involving a vigorous detoxification regimen, fruits and vegetables organically grown mostly in the United States, and the ingestion of thirteen or more freshly pressed raw juices at hourly intervals.

There were six cancer cases, one "MS", one rheumatoid arthritis, and one heart case among them. To keep the record straight, it is true that a 55-year-old patient, suffering from angina and atherosclerosis since 1960, and under drug therapies of all kinds since then, died after only a month on the program. But during that time, he had been able to walk with freedom (whereas before he had hardly been able to cover short distances), his blood pressure was back to normal, the pains in his ankles had gone, and his energy level was higher.

The other smiling patients had survived as of this account. Gary Heaton, diagnosed with multiple sclerosis in 1973, had reached such a point by 1977 that he had extensive numbness in the arms and legs, poor coordination, occasional falling spells, inability to walk a straight line, double vision, hypersensitivity to pain, and loss of bladder control. His physician had told him, "Learn to live with it"—frequent "advice" to sufferers of MS. After he began the Gerson therapy in March 1977, Heaton quickly noticed a tingling sensation replacing the numbness and a return of bladder control. When I met him in Los Angeles there were absolutely no outward signs that he had been pondering life in a wheelchair months before.

Eric Goodman, a sixty-four-year-old patient, had had a malignant skin cancer removed in 1967 and a diagnosis of sarcoma in 1975, when he refused surgery for the removal of his jaw and the roof of his mouth. He also suffered from severe heart fibrillation, low energy, sinus trouble, arthritic back pain, sleeplessness, and hemorrhoids. He had been on the Gerson therapy since August 1975. By 1978 his heart had become normal without drug therapy, his energy level was high, he slept well, reported no back aches, and said he had no hemorrhoids or any visible trace of cancer.

John Ashbaugh, who was case number thirteen in Dr. Gerson's *A Cancer Therapy—Results of Fifty Cases,* was on hand to say he had been in good, cancer-free health for twenty-seven years after having been diagnosed with malignant melanoma. He had lost one arm to earlier treatment. The surgery had not "gotten it all" and metastasis was diagnosed in 1951, when he began the Gerson program. His tumors diminshed in the early portion of the treatment and he had been free of them ever since.

Physicians had said things like "no more than two months to live" and "death will be swift and certain" to Jacquie Davison, who was diagnosed with widely dispersed melanoma in June 1975. With nowhere to turn, she tried the Gerson program. By mid-1978 she was in excellent condition and had abundant energy—without a sign of cancer.

Tests and exploratory surgery in Oregon in 1974 showed Della Robinson to have a grapefruit-sized inoperable tumor mass in her liver. In January 1975, down to sixty-seven pounds, she was given from three days to three weeks to live and sent home with a supply of morphine for her severe pain. She began the Gerson therapy right away and claimed that she was free of pain in three days and was able to leave her bed in three months. After six months of treatment she was back to her normal weight, 125 pounds, and was able to take a tour. As of 1978 she was working ten hours a day, five days a week, as an accountant.

A December 1977 leg operation on Marilyn Swanson, diagnosed with a tumor invading the fibia, tibia, and muscle tissue, failed to "get it all." New tumors had appeared by January 1978, her right leg was swollen, and her toes and foot were turning a bluish purple. A surgeon recommended leg amputation, but also warned that the cancer might spread elsewhere. Miss Swanson refused the amputation and switched to the Gerson therapy instead. Within five days the incision was closed and healing, the tumors had softened, and the leg swelling was gone. By mid-1978 she was virtually free of all signs of cancer.

One of Mary Lee Rork's eyes was removed in 1972 for lachrymal carcinoma—tear-duct cancer. In spring 1973, 6,000 rads of cobalt were administered to her head. By September 1975 nodules appeared in both lungs, and two months later a biopsy confirmed inoperable metastasized lachrymal carcinoma. She was told that chemotherapy offered little hope and was given four to six months to live. She did not begin the Gerson program until October 1976. A year later she was told her nodular densities had calcified, and in 1978 she claimed to have more energy than at any time since her teens.

Rheumatoid arthritis was diagnosed in the case of Deanna Powell in February 1970 when she was only eighteen. By 1976, she was bedridden for the summer, and her doctors were treating her with gold and Prednisone, standard—if only palliative—therapy in rheumatoid arthritis. By May 1978 she was in constant pain, with stiffness and swelling in all joints. Her ankles were swollen, she could only walk with great difficulty and a pronounced limp and suffered from heart palpitations. She began the Gerson program on 13 May 1978. As of July 2 of that year, when I saw her, her pain was gone, movement was returning to her wrists, elbows, and fingers, her ankles were normal, her circulation had improved, and the heart palpitations had ceased.

The attempt to treat cancer, multiple sclerosis, rheumatoid arthritis, and heart disease by all-nutritional means is, of course, unorthodox, and hence the need for Gersonists to set up shop across the border. There, they were by 1979 claiming "routine recovery" in 90 percent of early to intermediate cancer cases and 50 percent recovery when the disease has been termed "incurable."

Rene Caisse, Essiac, And The Indian Herbals

If investigation and research now under way in Canada, with the approval of the Ministry of Health and Welfare and several well-moneyed backers and the Resperin Corporation, is successful, an underreported half-century battle for an Indian herbal remedy for cancer will have come to a successful conclusion and will have helped vindicate herbalism in modern medicine.

Nurse Rene Caisse was 90 years old when she died in the late 1970s, the eve of the beginning of renewed serious interest in "her" Indian remedy. She had claimed for decades that the herbal preparation cures cancer. Hundreds of patients, and the work of several scientists, supported her claim, even though she was cold-shouldered by Canadian and American medical bureaucrats, who have usually operated in lockstep in fighting "unapproved" or unwanted remedies—laetrile and Koch compounds being particular cases in point.

However impressive Rene Caisse's discovery is, it is only one of *many* herbals for cancer used by Indian tribes over the years. And the Indian herbals are in themselves only North American versions of other folklore-herbal remedies that have been known for centuries on all other continents, their benefits largely excluded from Western orthodoxy primarily because the *synthetic* drug industry is the purveyor of toxic, expensive drugs to fight cancer even when some of these drugs (such as vincristine) were discovered in plants.

As late as 1979, Dr. Charles Brusch of Cambridge, Massachusetts, who treated patients with the Caisse preparation twenty years earlier, was quoted as saying he was still "one hundred percent for it." And he added: "They stopped sending it to me from Canada because if it was picked up at the border Rene Caisse would have been in trouble."

"It" refers to Essiac—Caisse spelled backwards—and the controversy is redolent of laetrile and unproven remedies in general in this country. And, as in the case of laetrile, it has had both research and use in Canada as well as the United States to back it up despite its bum's rush by the health authorities.

Miss Caisse said she ran across the "cure" in 1922, while working in another Ontario hospital where an elderly woman patient with a strangely scarred breast turned over to her the formula of an ancient Indian remedy that the woman said had cured her of cancer.

While ancient Indian remedies may sound like the stuff of quackery, it is to be recalled that long before the White Man's medicine invaded Indian America, this continent's natives were practicing preventive medicine and nontoxic therapies with all manner of plants. Later, as we will see in chapter nine, they actually taught French explorers the answer to scurvy before anyone had ever heard about vitamin C. Indian teas and herbal preparations have been used for centuries to cure or manage many disease conditions, and it is easy to forget that many drugs are plant extracts.

The Canadian said she altered the original herbal formula and, aided by a physician, she began treating dozens of patients suffering from cancer with remarkable—and documented—results. But no sooner had she announced that she had a treatment for cancer than her problems began.

In 1926, eight physicians petitioned the Canadian government to let Miss Caisse test the cancer treatment on a large scale. They claimed at the time that Essiac relieved pain, reduced the size of tumors, and prolonged life. For a time, while Miss Caisse was treating patients at Bracebridge, Ontario, the town became a medical mecca. Patients arrived from around the world, and the king of England is reported to have written encouragement. Miss Caisse commuted weekly to Northwestern University Hospital in Chicago, where she assisted five doctors in treating thirty volunteer terminal cancer patients. After eighteen months, they generally concluded that Essiac prolonged life, broke down nodular masses to more normal tissue, and relieved pain.

She recalled that a Chicago hospital offered her laboratories and a residence if she would move to the United States. A group of Buffalo, New York, businessmen offered to put up a million dollars in cash to control the world marketing of the product, but she turned them down. Reporter Ron Laytner wrote that "she wanted Essiac used immediately on suffering cancer patients—authorities demanded prior testing on animals. She wanted recognition of Essiac as the cure for cancer. The laboratories wanted her formula."

Prompted by petitions bearing more than 50,000 names of patients, their relatives, friends, and physicians asking the provincial government to allow the treating of patients with the material, the Ontario government in 1939 set up a commission to investigate the claimed cancer cure. Nurse Caisse brought along 380 Essiac-treated patients who believed they had been cured. The commission heard 49 of them. Even though Essiac was credited with a number of possible cures, the evidence was not enough. Morover, Miss Caisse committed the heresy of not telling the probers what Essiac was. They concluded that either the patients had never had cancer or their cures had been brought about by some previous standard treatment—the ever-recurring Catch-22 argument against laetrile, Krebiozen, Glyoxylide, the Hoxsey treatment, and other "unproven remedies."

Rene Caisse's cancer clinic was shut down. But for years after she secretly administered the remedy to cancer patients. Some of them are still alive after forty years.

Miss Caisse explained to reporter Laytner her reason for keeping the formual secret: "Some say I've been cruel holding it back. They don't understand that if I gave it up to the researchers Essiac would have been shelved in favor of present-day treatments. As long as the authorities didn't know what it was they couldn't condemn it. Every cancer cure they researched has disappeared once they got its formula.... They wanted to test it on mice first. I knew it was good. I didn't want it wasted on mice but used immediately on suffering humans."

Both Dr. David Wauld of Sault Ste. Marie, a cancer specialist, and K. J. R. Wrightman, director of the Ontario Cancer Treatment and Research Foundation, reported that tests on the substance refuted claims as to its worth—but don't tell the patients that.

Indian herbal remedies did not begin and end with Essiac.

Dr. Wilburn Ferguson (chapter six) developed several extracts from the head-shrinking plants used by the Ecuadorean Jivaro Indians and with them established a rather astounding record of use in human cancer and in animal tests, lines of research which temporarily had the support of the Club. In fact, the Ferguson compounds were probably among the best-tested, best-documented of the substances later to be quietly dropped as "unproven" by the American cancer establishment.

In 1982 the Bradford research group brought to national attention the half-century use of Indian salves or poultices which had been quietly utilized in the direct "pulling" of tumors by a handful of doctors in this country. One of the primary users of the "black and yellow" salves originally developed by North American Indians claimed that by 1982 he had "pulled" 100 tumors non-surgically with these preparations. These were mostly of breast malignancies, but lung and brain tumors had also been liquefied by the applications of the poultices, he claimed.

I was made privy to many cases of "pulled" or liquefied tumors by these salves the same year. It was obvious that much more research was needed, but there was no doubt that a combination of plant compounds from many sources do have cancer cell-destroying properties. The Ferguson compounds alone have been documented as anti-inflammatory, antibiotic, mood-elevating and analgesic as well as antineoplastic, and point to a profoundly important line of research either dropped or ignored by the American cancer establishment.

As this decade began, fresh interest was stimulated in North America over the use of extracts from the bark of an Andean tree for their use in cancer, particularly in leukemia. The herbal medicine extracted from the *tajibo* tree, known also as *pau d'arco,* is another line of research known to—but dropped—by American cancer orthodoxy, despite solid cases and credentialed research in Argentina and Brazil.

The Callawaya, descendents of the ancient Inca of Peru, have used the *quechua* extract from the bark for centuries not only for leukemia but also for the treatment of anemia, arteriosclerosis, asthma, bronchitis, colitis, diabetes, skin sores, gastritis, and a number of infections.

Drs. Theodore Meyer and Prats Ruiz introduced tajibo extracts into contemporary cancer treatment in Argentina, Dr. Meyer has found within the extract anti-bacterial and anti-viral properites, such as Dr. Ferguson found among some of the eight plants he used in the tumor-destroying Jivaro extracts.

Indian folk medicine has resulted in a host of herbal remedies for cancer in North America, just as folk medicine from around the world has emphasized the use of herbs in natural therapies elsewhere. The unresolved medical controversy over chaparral tea, whose apparently active cancer ingredient, nordihydroguaiaretic acid, (NDGA), was subjected to partial, and somewhat conflicting, studies at the Universities of Utah and Wisconsin, brought a fresh wave of interest in herbals during the 1970s.

Medical anthropolgist John Heinerman has reported how an anti-cancer formula using herbs (chaparral, blood root, red clover blossoms, burdock roots, echinacea root, goldenseal root, comfrey leaves, ginseng root and greater celadine) along with several other ingredients, secured anti-cancer results but landed its purveyor in legal trouble because the herbal combination was promoted as a cancer cure.

Some of the ingredients are among the thirty-nine herbs listed by Dr. Jonathan L. Hartwell of the National Cancer Institute (NCI) in 1960, all of which have rendered some evidence of anti-cancer or anti-tumor effects. That is to say, as late as 1960, the NCI was aware of a rich and varied folklore, with some supporting evidence, of the usefulness of herbs in malignancy. The list includes such notables as garlic (listed at the time as used in Texas and California for lung cancer, leukemia, and "general cancer") to cranberries, a poultice of which was said to be used in Arkansas for skin cancer.

Comfrey, goldenseal, and other important herbs have been referred to by naturopaths, herbalists, and folk medical practitioners for decades. Their counterparts exist throughout the world and reflect a vast treasure trove of natural remedies that are useful not only in cancer but in the whole spectrum of human ailments. Much of herbal medicine is being resurrected in China (see Heinerman), the ancient motherland of laetrile or amydgalin. (American scientists who visited the communist country in 1974 found, among natural therapies in experimental use, amygdalin from the dwarf flowering cherry, American plum, and Japanese apricot in addition to other herbal treatments.)

There is, thus, a great body of evidence to suggest that the American orthodox Club is well aware of the great promise of herbal remedies in cancer in particular and medicine in general, but the vast majority of the American population has little access to the products or the information. The reasons for this are varied, but they again indicate the overwhelming reality that cancer treatment investigation has largely been determined in the modern era in this country by the vested interests of the major drug companies, particularly of the synthetic drug industry.

Too, American scientists point out that the legalization and marketing problems with herbal remedies derive from the pharmacological nightmare implicit in such substances. Literally hundreds of thousands of compounds may be involved in herbals. Under the parameters of American oncology, which primarily are established for the testing of *poisons,* the technology required to run through all the possible combinations until a single, useful drug is extracted from a common herb, or combination of herbs, is an awesomely expensive enterprise, let alone a scientific challenge.

Due to the law, which again *only* favors the huge drug companies which can foot the multi-million-dollar bills for "new drug" development and lay claim to patent rights on these new, synthetic drugs, unidentified or unclassified substances used in therapy, however successful they may be, technically are "unlicensed new drugs" and are suppressed as such, most particularly when they are mentioned in regard to cancer, that greatest of the research and treatment gravy trains in America. This is a key reason why folk medicine and folk remedies, however much of demonstrable benefit they are, cannot legally "make it" through the

American legal maze. The American public, of course, is the great loser in this, as usual, as the soaring cancer rates show.

We will never know how many useful teas, salves, poultices, and herbal applications are known to small groups of people but cannot be known to the public at large in cancer-stricken modern America because of the unholy convergence of vested interest, bad science, and bad law.

Multiple Sclerosis Pioneers

For AMA doctors, the rapid spread of multiple sclerosis (MS) is the proliferation of an incurable disease. MS sufferers are basically told to get used to the idea of the disease's incurability and to adjust their lives accordingly. The gathering nutritional/metabolic evidence points to a single assessment of this belief: Phooey.

Take the case of Bill Morse, Jr., a Texan who, as assistant attorney general, once helped state authorities harass "wayward" practitioners who espoused metabolic/nutritional—and other offbeat therapies, the very ones which would later bring his advanced case of MS under control.

When I talked with him in 1981, he had been fighting the ravages of MS for 18 years, but only in the last eight had he made, not only progress, but *real* progress. In 1973 he lay dying—bedridden, almost blind, virtually helpless, unable to care for himself. A neurologist had told him he would never recover from the condition. "I was completely out of it. I couldn't get out of bed. I couldn't see," he remembered. He had enough vision left to learn from what he read and what was read to him about MS.

"I learned MS was a hypo-allergic reaction to stress that could be prevented or cured with exercise or nutrition," he remembers today. By 1981 he was not only sharp of vision but was able to walk and lead a normal life, including fishing and appearances before the Texas legislature to argue against the Medical Practice Act, designed to renew orthodox, AMA-style medicine's stranglehold on Texas.

Before the legislature and in the media Bill Morse explained that with nutrition, hyperbaric oxygenation (oxygen treatments), stress reduction techniques, and acupuncture, practices all variously described as unproven or illegal or unethical, he had literally risen from his deathbed to be restored to virtually full health by age forty-three. He was not alone. A growing number of Americans have learned that nutritional manipulation and natural therapies are at least of help in MS. In one case, injections of laetrile or amygdalin brought about a significant turnaround in an MS woman patient.

Much of the interest in treating MS with metabolic/nutritional therapies springs from the work of Dr. Frederick Klenner, a medical maverick from Reidsville, North Carolina. Dr. Klenner has put together regimens consisting of major vitamins and minerals, including the Warburg "active respiratory groups," and dietary manipulation. The total metabolic/nutritional approach he developed included virtually every known non-toxic food factor found of benefit in preventing and treating cancer and cardiovascular disease as well as premature aging and of any known use in any way in strengthening the damaged myelin sheath, the special tissue around nerves whose deterioration marks the onset of MS. He has also achieved responses in the nutritional treatment of myasthenia gravis, an ostensibly incurable disease related to MS, and has shown that megadoses of vitamins C and B complex help patients "beat the blues."

In 1977 the Victoria, B.C., Canada, *Victorian* reported that more than 200 people throughout Canada had been returned from the ravages of MS to health through the Klenner approach and cited the case of Colleen Leek as a graphic example. By September 1976 Miss Leek suffered from blurred and double vision, a lifeless right arm and severe balance impairment. Hospitalized that month, she was given ACTH (cortisone) treatment and was discharged twelve days later after noticing only minor improvement. She then began a new round of deterioration in her diagnosed MS, became almost totally blind, experienced a great deal of pain, and was told by her physicians that nothing could be done for her. "I was told to take up a hobby," she recalled. Luckily, she heard of the Klenner program and that other Canadians were seeing fabulous results with it. "When I asked my neurologist about it, he just went 'snaky'—he told me I was to take nothing but the treatment I was already receiving," she said.

Miss Leek luckily rejected that idea and joined the Klenner regimen. One year later, she was dancing, running, and laying claim to "more energy than I've had in a year." Her treatment: four daily injections of vitamins B^1, B^5, B^6, and B^{12} and raw liver, and oral ingestion of vitamins B^1, B^2, B^6, calcium pantothenate, magnesium oxide, lecithin, and vitamins C and E.

It is too early to announce total victory over MS or any of the other rapidly rising mystery cripplers which accompany the industrialized/technologized West. But it is apparent that nontoxic food factors and natural substances, involving the "active respiratory groups" and free radical scavengers, have genuine roles to play in them all and that such approaches are *not* "nutritional quackery."

Drs. Burton, Livingston, Maruyama, And The Anti-Cancer Vaccines

While at least a part of the now badly splintered cancer Establishment in America is pressing ahead for a cancer vaccine—and finding none so far—there have been several promising avenues developed that are either unorthodox or simply befouled by the bureaucratic spawn of the Food, Drug and Cosmetic Act.

Efforts to stimulate the body's immune system in the fight against cancer, while considered quackery little more than a decade ago, are finding adherents within the Club as more about the body's self-defense system becomes known. Since diet is a major influencer of the system, the immune-system-stimulation school of research and therapy may be regarded as a bridge between unorthodox nutritional therapy and orthodox drug-based treatment.

Ponder the plight of Dr. Lawrence Burton. The Long Island, New York, researcher, a zoologist by training, claimed in 1977 that ninety hopeless cancer patients of 150 he had treated with an immunity-stimulating serum during the foregoing three years were alive because of the therapy he developed. Also, he said, he had been able to arrest cancer in 100 percent of laboratory mice bred to develop spontaneous cancer.

As he told *Midnight/Globe* at the time, "This is not the cure-all to cancer. We have had our miracles and our disappointments. I don't have all the answers. This serum, when it's right, is the gosh-awfullest miracle that you have ever seen—a tumor is gone like that! But it doesn't always happen that way."

Without using the word "cure," Dr. Burton claimed triumphs in halting and/or eliminating cancer of the brain, lungs, breast, liver, lymph glands, stomach, bladder, and bones—but no thanks to the FDA. He had to make his claims from a clinic in Freeport in the Bahamas, where he moved in 1978 after his research program ran into difficulties and finanical support dwindled.

The initial group of Burton patients received treatment at the Immunological Research Foundation (IRF) in Great Neck, Long Island, with special FDA approval. But the federal agency refused to let Burton broaden his experimental therapy to other human patients without tests that he said would have been pointless, time-consuming, and far too costly for the nonprofit IRF to fund.

Based on the doctor's earlier twelve years of experience studying the immune systems of mice, the Burton "immuno-augmentative" approach involves the use of several protein molecules produced by the body. One of these is an antibody that kills tumors, another is a molecule that triggers the action of the former, a third can ostensibly block the action of either the tumor-killer or its trigger, and a fourth is a "de-blocker" that can stop the action of the blocking molecule.

Burton and fellow scientists, who continue to get highly encouraging results, believe that if the molecules are present in the right proportions the body can fight cancer on its own. He and his staff analyze a patient's blood and separate out elements of the blood in order to put together a serum tailor-made for the individual patient, based on the amount of the key molecules he needs to bring his immune system to full capacity. When the serum matches exactly what the body lacks, Burton has argued, results are immediate and astounding. Journalists in Long Island reported tumors seeming to "melt away" within minutes and hours of treatment.

In the Bahamas, the Burton method has since turned in hundreds of impressive responses. By 1982, so great had the popularity of the approach become that legislation was passed in Florida and Oklahoma to allow the use of "blood fractions" for immune treatment as an experimental cancer therapy.

It will be remembered that several unorthodox therapies that date back to the last century were actually based on stimulating the body's own immune defense system. These include the revolutionary achievements of Coley, Doyen, and Deaken (chapter six).

The use of a vaccine of live tuberculosis bacilli—*bacillus Calmette-Guerin,* or BCG—is slowly coming into its own as a cancer treatment. The tuberculosis BCG vaccine has been demonstrated effective in cancer cases in the United States, Canada, France, and several other countries, either by itself or in combination with other therapies. The notion that by giving someone the bacilli of a disease another may be brought under control is only the modernization of the thinking pioneered almost a century ago by Coley. It is ironic that while BCG is routinely used in most of the world as a protection against tuberculosis it was for a time rejected by medical orthodoxy for that purpose in this country.

Very likely of equal importance to the BCG vaccine treatment in cancer is the vaccine developed in Japan by Chisato Maruyama of the Nippon Medical School in Tokyo, who has tested his discovery on 140,000 cancer patients for fifteen years. He developed the current product from an effort mounted in 1944 to find a vaccine useful against tuberculosis and leprosy, during which he discovered that patients suffering from these diseases almost never had cancer. The Maruyama vaccine is, of course, opposed in the United States by the FDA.

So great has the popular response to the Maruyama vaccine been that it has created a political furor in Japan along the lines of the laetrile and DMSO controversies in the United States.

In 1981, after years of hedging on the issue, the Japanese Health and Welfare Ministry announced its recognition of the vaccine as an experimental treatment in human cancer patients, even though, under Japanese law, it had been allowed at the Nippon Medical School under the personal responsibility and supervision of Dr. Maruyama, a dermatologist by training, and his colleagues.

The decision by the Japanese governmental body had reversed as earlier ruling against the vaccine on the basis of "insufficient evidence," a charge which many Japanese doctors and patients took virtually to be a joke, since thousands of them have seen positive results from the medication, one of the natural substances used in the treatment of actor Steve McQueen (chapter one). The bureaucrats explained their about-face as a way of staving off what they termed "social unrest" caused by further proscription of the remedy from general use.

Dr. Maruyama has explained to me personally on several occasions that the real opposition to his medicine is very similar to that against amygdalin and other natural substances in America: It is inexpensive, it is not a synthetic drug, and it clearly flies in the face of major pharmaceutical interests involved in the development and marketing of expensive, patented, toxic drugs.

But in Japan, despite pressures against natural substances, the law allows limited use of experimental drugs under personalized supervision of proponents, and thus that country at this time has far more medical freedom of choice than does the United States, from which Japan takes its cue in a great deal of cancer research.

For years, Dr. Virginia Livingston of California has been breaking ground with the development of "autogenous" (self-made) vaccines, based on her own bacterial theory of cancer. She postulates that a bacterium that she calls *Progenitor cryptocides* ("ancestral hidden killer") may be found in all cancer tumors. Similar to the tuberculosis bacillus, it can change form and, in one manifestation, may appear to be a virus. Unlike viruses, it can be cultivated in nontissue cultures and be killed by antibiotics.

Dr. Livingston makes the autogenous vaccines from the urine of cancer patients. The cryptocides killer constitutes, as a vaccine, a central part of a treatment program also involving Otto Warburg's "active respiratory group" vitamins, other vaccines, antibiotics, gammaglobulin, and glandular extracts. She has claimed some spectacular controls of "hopeless" patients. Some other metabolic/nutritional therapists use autogenous vaccines and BCG as part of their overall program as well.

Dr. Livingston has also championed the use of abscissic acid—a plant growth regulator—as an anticancer substance. Abscissic acid *may* account for cancer regressions after the consumption of certain vegetables, regressions often attributed to the possible action of vitamins, minerals, and other substances.

The Breakthrough Of Selenium

Metabolic/nutritional therapists have for several years known that the trace mineral selenium, in combination with vitamin E, helps maintain cellular integrity and helps the body metabolism produce antibodies to ward off invaders. They have also known that too much selenium can produce toxic effects. But in 1978 several researchers announced that an increase in the ingestion of the mineral could cut the mortality rate from cancer by 80 to 90 percent in the United States and that selenium may be a cure for cystic fibrosis. The early information points to a likely selenium deficiency in the American diet.

Foods rich in the mineral include fish and other seafood, liver, garlic, onions, kidneys, mushrooms, eggs, and whole-wheat breads and cereals. It can also be purchased as a supplement in health food stores. Too, 1980 research showd that apricot kernels contain about 35 micrograms of selenium.

Dr. Gerhard Schrauzer, professor of chemistry at the University of California-San Diego and a nationally prominent expert on selenium and cancer research, said that epidemiological evidence from twenty-eight countries and nineteen U.S. states makes the case for the preventative role of the mineral. "The results show the higher the selenium intake, the lower the cancer mortality rate, and vice versa," he said. He estimated the average American diet contains 50 to 150 micrograms of selenium and that 200 to 300 micrograms are needed for maxium cancer protection.

Dr. W. L. Broghamer, associate professor of pathology, Louisville University School of Medicine, has said that recent research has shown that selenium "tends to protect animals against development of tumors."

As interest in "free radical pathology" develops in the resolution of the cancer problem, it has been noted that selenium is a "scavenger"—a destroyer—of "free radicals," the heavily damaging products which result from improper metabolic oxidation of fats and proteins. Free radicals are linked to cancer and indeed most of degenerative disease. Selenium has been shown to be an essential component of the enzyme glutathione peroxidase, which "bonds" with, or deactivates, free radicals.

Selenium also "scavenges" toxic, carcinogenic chemicals and plays a role in boosting body immune mechanisms.

Research by Drs. J. E. Spallholz and Douglas V. Frost has shown that selenium is crucial in developing antibodies and ubiquinone (or "coenzyme Q") which ward off both infectious diseases and cancer.

Selenium and vitamin E seem to work synergistically in preventing heart disease and stroke. Indeed, Dr. Curtis Hames of Claxton, Georgia, demonstrated that the soil of counties of Georgia in which hypertension and cardiovascular disease appeared at rates many times higher than the national average had two-thirds less selenium than elsewhere in the country. (Though some thirty other vital trace elements are also deficient in the soil of the so-called "heart disease belt" of the South).

Selenium and vitamin E have long been used to treat arthritis in dogs. The same combination is now achieving positive benefits in humans. Selenium also acts as an anti-inflammatory, and selenium deficiency has been implicated in sudden infant death (SID) syndrome and male sterility.

In late 1978, a St. Louis veterinary pathologist claimed that cystic fibrosis, a deadly disease of children long thought to be a genetic disorder, is actually a nutritional deficiency disease and can be cured. Dr. Joel D. Wallach, who said he had been called a "snot-nosed horse doctor" by geneticists because of his attempts to refute the forty-year-old theory that cystic fibrosis is caused by genetic disorders, claimed the disease is caused by a lack of selenium during the first three months of pregnancy. It can be prevented by proper diet and can be cured by surgery in some cases and with selenium in others, he said. "It's mind-boggling that this is true," he said in announcing the discovery. "But nothing has said tilt. Everything keeps reinforcing this."

In 1981 Dr. Daniel Medina, associate professor of cell biology at Baylor, told the Medical Cancer Society writers' seminar that in a test in which selenium was added to the drinking water of mice, it led to an up-to-60-percent decrease in the incidence of mammary cancer.

Mental Visualization And Cancer. The Simonton Method

Dr. O. Carl Simonton, former chief of radiation therapy at Travis Air Force Base, California, and his colleagues have come a long way since 1973 when word of an intriguing new approach to cancer was first published. For the first time in a coordinated way, the harnessing of mental attitude as an anticancer weapon was enunciated and demonstrated by credentialed researchers.

Dr. Simonton's method, now usually described as a kind of "biofeedback" program, is a natural parallel to the growing evidence that attitudes play a role—though the magnitude of the role is still a subject of much debate—in the induction of cancer, and that indeed there is a psychological "cancer profile" that a majority of patients seem to fit. For those of us just kooky enough to believe most of everything is in the mind anyway, Dr. Simonton has probably provided the jump between mind and matter. If so, the ultimate future of cancer research—and indeed of medicine itself—will more and more lie in the mental realm.

In 1973, the results of a two-year study in which cancer patients were asked to use mental visualization techniques and meditation as part of the fight against cancer were published. The general conclusion from these tests, reported Dr. Simonton, was that with the exception of two cases in which some improvement was noted even though attitudes remained negative, there was improvement or a lack of same in correlation to mental attitudes and degrees of participation in the program of positive thought. Twenty showed "excellent" results.

Dr. Simonton was not by any means substituting mind therapy for standard modalities; he was simply bolstering the latter with the former and asking his patients to, for example, visualize their lymphocytes as an organized army, surrounding and decimating the invading forces of cancer.

Since the 1973 study, he and his colleagues have worked out more routines for mental visualization relaxation to allow the mind to be a major weapon in the anticancer arsenal. Much more work needs to be done in the field, but it is a wide-open one.

What Simonton and his group have shown is the validation of

an opinion long held by many physicians—a postive mental attitude reinforces and is utterly essential to good health. It has already been scientifically insinuated that negative thought interferes with metabolism and the delicate enzyme-hormone balance. If this is so, then the reverse—that positive thought must be good for it—is almost certainly true. This is why the majority of metabolic/nutritional therapists not only do not oppose prayer and faith in combatting degenerative disease, but actively encourage them.

DMSO And Dirty Work At The Crossroads

By 1982 it appeared that the pitched battle over dimethyl sulfoxide (DMSO) had at least temporarily replaced amygdalin (vitamin B^{17}, laetrile) as the major, ongoing medical controversy.

In battles similar to those earlier waged around amygdalin, the fight for DMSO involved science, politics, and the media. Here again was a war in which an unwanted or "orphaned" drug of essentially inexpensive manufacture and useful in a wide gamut of degenerative disorders was being opposed by a suspicious combination of interests.

Going into 1982, ten states had in whole or part "decriminalized" the use of DMSO, federally accepted as "legal" solely in the treatment of a single human condition (interstitial cystitis, a painful bladder disorder), and 28 state legislatures had had some kind of legislation before them during the previous two years dealing with DMSO.

Political leaders, actors and athletes were on hand to tout the value of the solvent for everything from tennis elbow and ankle sprains to arthritis and cancer. Metabolic/nutritional therapists, already aware of DMSO's demonstrated efficacy as a free radical scavenger, were rapidly incorporating it into their total programs for many diseases.

The FDA, stimulated to do battle by the aroused Club, moved viciously against distributors and medical users of the substance. Confiscations and raids occurred in New York and Washington in 1981. In the former state, federal marshals even confiscated a book touting the merits of DMSO, claiming its mere presence constituted "labelling." This action was later legally reversed.

Furthermore, the government, clearly reaching for ways to "get the goods" on DMSO's major modern-era proponent and champion, the widely respected Dr. Stanley Jacob of the University of Oregon, had indicted the scientist and a Food and Drug Administration official on "illegal payments" charges, a move which, Dr. Jacob said, would allow him to help "completely vindicate" himself and DMSO in a court of law. (See *note*, page 209.)

In October 1980, FDA officials claimed that they had turned up "disturbing" indications that the most important scientific studies on DMSO were misleading and that adverse effects had been covered up.

FDA representatives were also on hand before a Senate hearing to claim that DMSO's major proponent owned $600,000 worth of stock in a company that manufactured the chemical and that certain information between DMSO researchers and the government had strangely disappeared.

Vague accounts of missing reports and deficiencies, let alone the thought that DMSO might somehow be harmful to people because of a report that some test animals underwent eye lens alterations, served to help muddy the waters of a relatively simple compound which was getting a laetrile-style runaround. DMSO had suffered a bumpy history already.

Earlier in 1980 the House of Representatives, responding to complaints from constituents, particularly elderly citizens who have found that topically applied DMSO is a marvelous pain-killer in arthritis, introduced a bill to mandate DMSO approval for certain ailments and to circumvent the Food, Drug and Cosmetic Act, which had already served as an easy way to keep cheaply produced DMSO in legal limbo. Legislators in the House Select Committee on Aging attacked the FDA for blocking approval of the substance in light of studies showing it to be both safe and effective.

The widespread use of the compound, already made famous by athletes who had found it useful for a number of maladies, ballooned after the popular television program *Sixty Minutes* aired a segment on DMSO in March 1980. The FDA, as policeman for the drug trust, was, once again, between a rock and a hard place. Thousands of Americans wanted the legal right to use the stuff; it had not cleared the various redtape loopholes of the amended Food, Drug and Cosmetic Act; it obviously "worked" for thousands of people; it was getting plenty of media attention; and it was becoming a political hot potato. The FDA had to do something. It reacted in its time-honored way, awkwardly and clumsily, but with brute strength.

None of this was fooling Dr. Jacob, associate professor of surgery at the University of Oregon's Health Sciences Center. He told the media that DMSO is "the most thoroughly investigated drug in the history of medicine," that there is "no evidence of ocular toxicity," and that "a pseudo-scientific game is being played with the American public."

Dr. Jacob has told the press that it is not just the FDA, but major drug companies (which fear they may not make a huge profit from DMSO's manufacture and sale) which have "neglected" the compound. He has stated that a drug company executive told him, "I don't care if it is the major drug of our century—and we all know it is—it isn't worth it to us." At least not at a cost of about $4 a quart to produce.

After all, the "arthritis industry" does not trail far behind the actual killer diseases as a major concern of Americans, particularly elderly ones, many of whom live lives tortured by arthritic pain. There is a veritable multitude of ointments, creams, and drugs for arthritic pain and for relieving symptoms of tendonitis, bursitis, and acute spinal injury. All of these conditions have responded favorably to dimethyl sulfoxide, a byproduct of the paper pulp industry.

It was in 1963 that Dr. Jacob and chemist Robert Herschler announced the discovery of DMSO's analgesic properties. DMSO, derived from lignin in trees, has been around since its discovery in Russia by Alexander M. Saytzeff in 1866 and was first used in a variety of ills, including scleroderma. Metabolic/nutritional therapists have also used the compound intravenously in cancer therapy, and it is considered useful by some in treating stroke.

The FDA, empowered by the amended Food, Drug and Cosmetic Act, stepped in shortly after word of the Jacob/Herschler findings were released and halted clinical testing, even though no cases of eye toxicity had occurred in some 100,000 people treated with the substance.

In 1978, the FDA ruled that DMSO was "legal" for use in chronic interstitial cystitis. It was already used as horse liniment. But word of DMSO's broad-spectrum use, particularly in arthritis, was already out and a flourishing "underground" operation of DMSO preparations got underway.

Enthusiastic endorsements of DMSO by former Alabama Gov. George Wallace, the Oakland Raiders' Daryle Lamonica, Atlanta Falcons' June Jones, and other people in the public eye helped bring DMSO to the fore with a popularity among "unproven remedies" second only to laetrile.

Drs. Jacob and Herschler found that DMSO creates a reversible electro-chemical block around nerve endings, hence jamming pain signals that would otherwise be sent to the brain. Dr. Jacob has subsequently fitted DMSO use into four categories, treatment of injuries such as bruises, strains, and sprains; arthritis; severe head injuries; and certain kinds of skin infections.

Metabolic therapists have used DMSO, a fast-acting absorption agent, to help flood the tissues with needed nutrients. Aside from occasional itchiness and rash from topical injections, the only side effect of DMSO reported so far is the garlicky odor of the recipient.

Drs. Jacob and Herschler were issued patents for the uses they had discovered for DMSO—patents that were shared by the University of Oregon and Crown Zellerbach, one of the nation's largest paper manufacturers. But that was in DMSO's "good old days" before much attention was paid to the compound.

Now, with the FDA claiming missing, or covered-up, or misleading information and issuing vague remarks ranging from "nobody's died from using DMSO" and "it's a relatively safe drug, as drugs go" to "there is no evidence that DMSO has altered the course of any disease," the legal future of DMSO remains murky as this is written.

But, as in the case of other useful remedies cold-shouldered by the Club, DMSO is clearly an idea whose time has come. The American people will continue to demand access to it, FDA or no.

Bruce Halstead, M.D., a veteran cancer researcher, toxicologist, pioneer in chelation therapy, and metabolic/nutritional physician, finds that DMSO "is unquestionably one of the safest drugs available in the field of medicine when properly administered by a physician. No deaths have been reported by the use of the drug.... If the FDA were to apply the same drug standards to drugs now approved and in use as they have been applied to DMSO, there would not be a single drug available in the United States today. The same standards that are imposed upon DMSO would also eliminate table salt, aspirin, alcoholic beverages, and cigarettes. It is now estimated that over six million persons have used DMSO in one form or another as a therapeutic. Thus far no significant toxic side effects have been documented in humans that remotely [justify] the suppressive action taken by the FDA."

Robert W. Bradford And Dr. Denham Harman: "ROTS Pathology" And Free Radicals

The chief pioneer of "free radical pathology" research in 1982 presented to the National Academy of Sciences (U.S.A.) his theory, with supporting arguments, that the manipulation of free radicals could add up to ten years or more to a person's life. At the same time, independent research on two different fronts was linking free radical pathology to cancer. The areas of research into these breakdown products of "toxic oxygen" increasingly indicate the links between natural substances, cancer and aging, and have opened a whole new dimension in prevention and treatment.

I have before alluded to free radicals—a term I once jokingly considered to mean a non-dues-paying member of a leftist organization. Indeed, the rapidly growing research into these strange substances suggests a thorough revolution in treatment, prevention, and the monitoring of a vast range of pathological conditions. The universe of free radicals helps explain the unexpected successes of selenium and DMSO in degenerative disease, creates a new role for amygdalin or laetrile (as a "scavenger" par excellence of the most dangerous of the free radicals, hydroxyl radical) and gives additional backing to the concept of nutritional and metabolic management in chronic, systemic, degenerative disease, since "scavengers," or destroyers, of free radicals abound in many natural foods and some vitamins are suspected of serving, or helping to serve, as free radical scavengers themselves.

Dr. Denham Harman, the primary proponent of free radical pathology in the U.S.A., who began this vital research at the University of California (Berkeley) and continued it at the University of Nebraska, has emphasized the link between the decline in free radical scavenging substances and the aging process, and has stressed that dietary ways to introduce the scavenging or blocking substances into the body include making sure we get enough of vitamins C and E and the trace mineral selenium.

As suggested in the theory propounded to the NAS, free radicals are *the* basic cause of aging in man, animals, and plants. Damage caused by these altered or toxic forms of the oxygen molecule accumulates day after day and becomes the basis for aging, the Harman work suggests.

In one experiment on mice, NAS was informed, the reduction of free radicals in the body resulted in a 30 percent increase in life span, equivalent to raising the American median age from seventy-five to ninety-five years.

In the meantime, researchers at the University of Iowa who studied fifty different "forms" of cancer found a breakdown in cellular defenses against superoxides, a kind of free radical. All the cancer cells tested had little or no manganese superoxide dismutase (SOD), the enzyme which protects cellular mitochondria from superoxides. The fastest-growing cancers seem to have the least SOD, research shows.

Also in the meantime, the ground-breaking research by the Robert W. Bradford interests (Bradford Research Institute in California, American Biologics-Mexico Hospital in Mexico) continues to affirm the efficacy of adding free radical scavengers to virtually *all* treatment protocols for degenerative disease, and using the effects of such substances on blood as an easy detection and monitoring device for all stages of all conditions in which free radicals play a role.

This line of research, and its considerable successes so far, are most infuriating to the Club because it is Bradford, the physicist-engineer originally associated with Stanford University, who set up the Committee for Freedom of Choice in Cancer Therapy, Inc., which led the fight to decriminalize laetrile (amygdalin) in 24 states and conducted independent research on vitamin B[17]. He is regarded as an arch-heretic whose mere association with the laetrile controversy is consistently used to besmirch his scientific sorties into areas far beyond amygdalin and cancer.

Adding such free radical scavengers as SOD and catalase to nutritional and metabolic treatments at the Bradford-directed American Biologics-Mexico Hospital in Tijuana, Mexico, Medical Director Rodrigo Rodriguez was able to secure startling positive effects in lupus, asthma and multiple sclerosis as well as terminal cancer, in cases treated in 1981. In a case of multiple sclerosis, a disease still regarded by American medical orthodoxy as incurable, striking positive effects were secured from intravenous amygdalin, a response in line with the determination by an earlier Rutgers University study that amygdalin is a scavenger of the hydroxyl radical.

Working with biochemist Henry W. Allen (and outside consultants to his own research institute), the iconoclastic Bradford developed the theory that modifications of the normal oxygen molecule, including but not limited to free radicals, and hence primarily encompassing superoxides, hydroxyl radical and hydrogen peroxide, may cause distinctive patterns to appear in coagulated blood. He and Allen baptized the oxygen products as "reactive oxygen toxic species" (ROTS, a seemingly appropriate acronym) and postulated that distinctive patterns in dried blood were the effects of ROTS pathology and could be used to diagnose and monitor the entire range of chronic, systemic, degenerative diseases.

Bradford's first interest was focused on cancer and in resurrecting the little-known and controversial Bolen blood test in this endeavor. It was while in effect re-discovering the Bolen test and researching free radical pathology that the ROTS concept and the significant discovery that ROTS pathology produces markers in the blood which can diagnose and monitor many diseases arose.

The Bolen blood test itself is another one of those medical mysteries in which significant new information or research lines were either covered up or ignored. In 1942 H. Leonard Bolen, M.D., then head of proctology and gastroenterology at Fall River General and St. Anne's hospitals, Fall River, Massachusetts, while working with the Goldberger blood "sedimentation" test, found that blood clot patterns seemed to parallel different stages primarily of cancer and also of pregnancy. His research led to a line of investigation taken up by other scientists which tended to confirm that cancer could be detected at stages ranging from incipient to advanced by examining a number of markers. O. C. Gruner, M.D., confirmed the general approach at McGill University. In 1950 N. Philip Norman, M.D., and Anna M. Slicher found a diagnostic accuracy range of 97 percent by examining some 4,000 blood drops from 350 patients.

It is true that Bolen's early research found that blood clot markers could indicate several other maladies, including ulcerative colitis, tuberculosis, acute bronchitis, and arteriosclerosis as well as cancer—but most of his findings dealt with cancer, as did the work of Gruner. Hence, the Bolen test became fairly established with the notion of cancer detection. This work occurred during and after World War II, and spanned the Atlantic. In France it was taken up by Dr. Henri Heitan of Germany, who emigrated to Paris in 1934 and became a major medical figure in postwar Europe. While American medical orthodoxy moved to snuff out the Bolen test, Dr. Heitan kept it very much alive and helped add the dimension of *color* as a major component of analyzing distinctive blood clot markings. The Club's assault on Bolen occurred in the *American Journal of Surgery* in September, 1952, when Beverly H. White, M.D., *et. al,* found in Veterans Administration Hospital tests that the Bolen approach was accurate "only" in 68.4 percent of cases in 303 cancer patients. They also found that several blood clot patterns from differing conditions were indistinguishable, and that in one case a stomach cancer was indistinguishable from a blood clot reaction from hemorrhoids. A U.S. Public Health Service study at Tufts College Medical School also found the test's cancer accuracy range from a low of 15 percent (for skin) to 83 percent (for lungs).

Because of confusing findings and an accuracy rate well below that shown by such investigators as Norman and Slicher, the Club promptly moved to indicate disinterest in an intriguing analytical technique which, in essence, means that with a five-minute test consisting of pricking the skin, drying the blood, and analyzing drops under a microscope cancer can be detected and monitored.

Dr. Heitan continued using and updating the test and, with disciple Phillipe LaGarde, M.D., eventually came up with the Heitan-LaGarde Color Microphotographic Test. Even so, this test was aimed essentially at diagnosing and monitoring cancer. Several other European investigators and a handful of American doctors continued to utilize the Bolen test as a way to look at cancer in various stages.

Only when the Bradford Research Institute got involved was a new horizon created for the assay. The BRI scientists found that where Bolen and others had probably gone wrong was in their reliance on the test primarily for cancer. They also realized that none of the early researchers knew much about free radicals.

Suspecting that what was really being seen in the coagulated blood were the effects of ROTS pathology and that each condition was displaying varying patterns, the BRI in 1980 launched an international metabolic research project together with a specially outfitted microscope aimed at easily determining the primary characteristics of toxic oxygen products and biochemistry in the blood—the translucent masses or gaps, the integrity or lack of same of the fibrin net around clumps of red blood cells, the distinctive colorings of the cells and gaps, and the tiny, buckshot-like particles which also showed up in the masses, as well as flaking and flecking within the cellular clusters.

The evolution of the HLB (for Heitan-LaGarde-Bradford) Test thus led to a rapid proliferation of interest in the modified test and in the whole scope of ROTS pathology. By 1982, 250 physician-participants in eleven countries had helped confirm that the HLB test effectively diagnosed and monitored more than a score of conditions, ranging from cancer, tuberculosis, asthma, and arthritis to mental stress, bursitis, and the effects of smoking.

There is a suspicion now that the toxic oxygen breakdown products—the free radicals and hydrogen peroxide (ROTS)—are involved in almost every pathological condition, and hence that their biochemical interplay in the body provides the clues in the blood which can lead to early, and very inexpensive, diagnosis and also allow clinicians to monitor the progress of treatment.

The Bolen test is still listed as an "unproven" or "ineffective" diagnostic tool for cancer.

Note: The initial trial of Dr. Jacob on an alleged "illegal payments" scheme involving an FDA researcher, Dr. K. C. Pani, resulted in a hung jury—and considerable expense for the defendants. The government, incredibly, decided to drag Dr. Jacob through a second trial. This ended in October 1982 with all charges dropped against the surgeon as long as he admitted in a statement that the payments made to Dr. Pani had been "inappropriate." Dr. Jacob had indeed made loans to his friend, Dr. Pani, to assist the latter in paying bills for his dying wife's cancer treatments. Dr. Jacob believes the second trial was probably the last vestige of judicial moves against DMSO, which is currently being investigated by several universities and is on the way to full acceptance. Dr. Jacob stated in November 1982 that DMSO almost certainly would have been crushed out of existence by the Club had it not developed within a university setting.

Chapter Eight
Vitamin B^{17} and Metabolic Therapy

The Real Story: Prevention

On a spring afternoon in 1978 three giants in the laetrile movement sat around the living room of the Krebs family home in San Francisco—a Queen Anne mansion designated a state landmark—and signed their names to a historic document. Ernst T. Krebs, Jr., the "godfather" of vitamin B^{15} and vitamin B^{17}, signed for the John Beard Memorial Foundation. Andrew R. L. McNaughton did so for the McNaughton Foundation. Robert W. Bradford, founder of the Committee for Freedom of Choice in Cancer Therapy, did so for the Bradford Foundation. Approvals were to come from Dean Burk, Ph.D., for the Dean Burk Foundation, and from cancer researcher Bruce W. Halstead, M.D., for the International Biotoxicological Center, World Life Institute.

The document was succinctly entitled "Technical Identification Specification for Amygdalin (Laetrile)" and months later would be filed with the U.S. District Court for Western Oklahoma as part of the ongoing efforts to secure legal sanction for the use of laetrile for cancer patients.

The historic importance of the document, however, was that it constituted the first agreement among the laetrile forces on exactly how to differentiate, semantically, the words *laetrile* and *amygdalin,* for both were and are used synonymously, and usually along with *vitamin B^{17}* and *nitriloside,* to designate the anticancer substance.

In essence, these long-time battlers for the vindication of the theory and use of laetrile agreed that, despite the confusion among all these terms that occurred during laetrile's turbulent history, *laetrile* should rightfully be regarded as a specific breakdown product of the common compound amygdalin, even though the term *laetrile* had already entered into the picture statutorily, being used by California law to designate the class of chemicals called beta-cyanogenetic glucosides, particularly amygdalin and prunasin.

Officialdom had been able to score points off the laetrile proponents by correctly insisting that there was such a confusion in terms that it could not be determined exactly what laetrile really *was*—even though, as officialdom also had to admit, all the liquids, powders, and tablets seized by the government for review over several years had always turned out to be refined amygdalin.

The laetrile proponents had not been without sin during the years of agitation and propaganda, for sure—for Laetrile, with a capital L, a trademarked term, had entered the Merck Index as a name for a theoretical synthetic product never marketed commercially. Too, Laetrile (again with a capital L) had been used in patents as refinements of amygdalin, which has appeared in the Merck and pharmacopaeias for over a century. Arguments over the "right" to the use of the capital-L Laetrile are still unresolved.

Not until biochemist Ernst T. Krebs, Jr., elaborated the theory of the "nitrilosides," or vitamin B^{17}, in the 1960s did the semantics war break out in full force. A big part of the problem of course, was the confusion over the terms *drug, food,* and *vitamin*—for the designation of laetrile or a similar product as a food factor could keep it out of the grasp of the "new drug" provisions of the Food, Drug and Cosmetic Act as amended in 1962—and the opposition consistently accused Krebs and his collaborators of advancing the vitamin theory as a way to get around these provisions. This charge, I came to realize, was false, since Krebs, Jr., had been leaning toward the vitamin theory well before its expostulation in 1969, and the evidence on which he based the vitamin identity of the B^{17} compounds has been consistently growing.

Whether the refined, purified extract of amygdalin put up in vials for injection purposes or sold in tablets for oral use was a food rather than a drug became a key point in litigation, but as a journalist and delver into semantics it became clear to me that, like so many things, laetrile is both of these. That's because, under the broadest possible use of the word *drug,* anything used to treat a pathological condition, and this might even be a crust of bread for a man dying of starvation, can be construed as a drug. That does not make it less a food, and by the mid-1970s the realization was rapidly growing among the nation's metabolic/nutritional therapists that by providing laetrile in cancer therapy they were not giving a drug to "treat" a tumor, but adding a vital nutrient to the body's metabolism so that the body itself could "treat" the cancer, whether the "treatment" immediately translated into a tumor reduction or not. The entire concept of providing nutrients in the form of vitamins and minerals to nourish the body, rather than administering specific drugs to treat the symptoms of specific diseases, is still a minority one *vis-a-vis* drug-based allopathic medicine, which has long constituted the medical Establishment in this country.

A primary piece of evidence in Krebs' lifelong battle for the vindication of vitamin B^{17} comes in the salty person of Dr. Dean Burk. In 1978, "the Dean," as the laetrilists affectionately styled the then seventy-four-year-old biochemist, told me once again, as if there were any doubt in my non-biochemically-oriented mind, "The evidence is overwhelming that laetrile—or, rather, the laetriles—constitute a vitamin, and an anticancer vitamin at that, and will be so recognized by a majority of scientists."

Burk, whose entire professional life has been devoted to cancer research in this and several countries, has a tediously lengthy, academic track record to prop up such sweeping statements. "I've been into vitamins since 1918, even before they were recognized as such, and they all go through the same business," Dr. Burk analyzed. "Their effects are observed, the substance is analyzed, its mode of action is not at first well appreciated, but eventually there is a clear-cut fitting of it into the vitamin picture, including its catalytic value in the enzyme process. Amygdalin is a vitamin, and will be increasingly recognized as such, and an anti-cancer vitamin at that, in the same sense that vitamin C is both an anti-cancer and an anti-scurvy vitamin." As we note in chapter eight, Dr. Burk was an early supporter of the concept of ascorbic acid, or vitamin C, as an anticancer fighter, too.

To Ernst T. Krebs, Jr., the fourteen or so substances variously referred to as beta-cyanogenetic glucosides, cyanophoric glycosides, and similar designations, *are* vitamin B^{17}. The most medically prominent of these compounds are amygdalin and prunasin, but linamarin—the presumptive anticancer agent in bitter cassava—and dhurrin, in certain grazing grasses, also figure in the picture. Krebs coined the term *nitriloside* to cover these designations, and the simpler term *vitamin B^{17}* to stand for them all.

Chemical designations aside, the vitamin B^{17} compounds are all sugar compounds—that is, they bear one or more units of sugar and may be attached (as is amygdalin) to a benzene ring or an acetone. They also carry a cyanide radical, that is, *bound* cyanide which, when locked within the B^{17} compound, is harmless. Upon hydrolysis, or breakdown, they yield one or more sugars and cyanide. In the case of amygdalin, whose chemistry is particularly historic and well-known, the breakdown results in sugar, cyanide, and benzaldehyde. One specific action of cyanide against cancer is known. It is also speculated that the "synergistic" action of cyanide with benzaldehyde is involved. Dr. Burk and others have postulated a number of ways the compound becomes an anticancer agent under the appropriate conditions.

Dr. Burk waxes less enthusiastic about the Krebsian hypothesis that cancer is, more than anything else, brought on not only by unchecked trophoblast cells but also by a near-absence of vitamin B^{17}

in the "civilized" diet. And yet it is *that* hypothesis which *ought* to be the "big story" about laetrile. It is a measure of the brainwashing of the Western mind by allopathic medicine that emphasis on the *treatment* of cancer remains ever so much more exciting than the outright *prevention* of cancer in the first place.

I have followed Dr. Krebs—the "doctor" is honorary—around the country for years, and I have never heard him deviate from the central thesis I first heard him propound in 1971: cancer is essentially a vitamin-deficiency disease, the deficiency is of vitamin B^{17}, and a disciplined effort to restore this natural food factor to the diet could eventually mean the elimination of cancer in a single generation. Despite all the attacks made on Krebs as a presumptive profiteer (though "neither I nor my family have ever made a dime off laetrile," vitamin B^{17}'s guru ever intones), a man claimed to be merely pushing a product, the fact is that the Krebs message was always the same: ingest *natural* vitamin B^{17} and cut your chances of ever developing cancer. Period.

This was by no means the point of view of some of the people interested in drumming up laetrile sales, and even today is by no means a universally accepted notion among the hundreds of physicians who have incorporated amygdalin into their treatment programs. It is by far the most astounding aspect of the whole laetrile controversy, yet one which seems forever muted in the clamor over how effective or ineffective laetrile, the pharmaceutical preparation, is in the treatment of desperately ill cancer patients. And in my peripatetic probe of laetrile in many countries over several years, it has never failed to capture far more of my interest than do the recovery stories, however dramatic, of laetrile-based metabolic/ nutritional therapy.

It is the Krebs hypothesis that any population that consciously or unconsciously is ingesting adequate amounts of vitamin B^{17}— though what constitutes "adequate" is not agreed upon—will have marginal to very low rates of cancer. And, by golly, that just happens to be true, even if there are also *other* variables that must be taken into account.

It is not only early on-site observers by UNESCO investigators who have found the natives of Hunza, an isolated region of Pakistan, to be virtually free of cancer. It is also true that the mostly vegetarian diet of these frequently centenarian people, their hard work and mountain existence, must also have something to do with their radiant health and notable longevity. But their cultural attachment to apricots—the eating of the seed or kernel as a common snack, their ingestion and use of the rest of the fruit, and their measuring of personal wealth in terms of apricot trees—must be regarded as a statistically impressive variable. For apricot seeds are, by historic coincidence, the chief source of the product laetrile (see my *Vitamin B^{17}: Forbidden Weapon Against Cancer* for the intriguing history of the early development of laetrile).

Manuel D. Navarro, M.D., of the Santo Tomas University Research Center, Manila, has been using amygdalin in cancer therapy for more than a quarter-century, as well as researching natural sources of vitamin B^{17} in the lush islands of the Philippines. By 1977 he had linked the very low incidence of cancer in the native populations of Mindanao to the continual ingestion of many sources of vitamin B^{17}. That rate, about 1 per 100,000, is even smaller than the low rate of cancer in the nonurban Filipino north, where generations of Filipinos have subsisted on diets of cassava, wild rice, wild beans, berries and fruits of all kinds, and even regional dishes such as one favored by the Ilocanos of northern Luzon, a rather unpleasant-tasting concoction prepared from the semi-digested plants and grasses (most of them containing B^{17}) from the rumen of goats.

In Zamboanga City, Mindanao, a city official gratuitously pointed out to me that the young children who dive for pearls from colorful *vintas,* and who will spend most of their lives doing this, are naked most of the time, do their job under a tropical sun, and yet virtually never show up with skin cancer. Their staple is *camote encajoy,* or the regional version of the cassava root, richly endowed with the vitamin B^{17} compound linamarin.

When E. T. Krebs, Jr. wrote of the vitamin B^{17} theory (in the *Journal of Applied Nutrition* in 1970 and in several monographs for the McNaughton Foundation), he noted that both the mostly vegetarian Hunzakuts and the mostly carnivorous "primitive" Eskimos of the Artic Circle, at least earlier in this century, were essentially cancer-free populations, with the major linking element in their otherwise widely varying diets being vitamin B^{17}. He found, as did later researchers, abundant evidence of low cancer incidence in tribes of American Indians, which rose only after the Indians' exposure to the White Man's eating habits. I bore that in mind in Canada as I quaffed glasses of chokecherry juice, widely consumed by Cree Indians and other populations that, until recently, reported low levels of cancer. The chokecherry, of course, is abundantly blessed with vitamin B^{17}. Various Indian teas made from the seeds and pits of fruits are well-known to students of indigenous populations in the American Southwest, among whose peoples cancer was also virtually unknown until the advent of food stamps.

The Loma Linda studies of Seventh Day Adventists in the Los Angeles basin, and the subsequent study of Mormons in Utah (see chapter four) were doubly important to the partisans not only of vitamin B^{17} but to vegetarians as well; both subverted the view that primitive peoples may be more free of cancer simply because they live in less polluted environments and have less stressful lives. The presence of a population within one of the earth's most polluted areas with an appreciably lower cancer incidence can be explained *only* on the basis of dietary habits, and champions of vitamins B^{17}, C, and A in cancer prevention all had ammunition for their points of view in such research.

Other vitamins, minerals, and enzymes in a "natural" diet cannot be overlooked in any population so studied, and it is probably safe to say that a wide range of factors is involved in cancer prevention, but the Krebs hypothesis on the need for vitamin B^{17} as a centerpiece in this universe of factors, far from weakening during the more diet-conscious seventies, was strengthened.

Additional evidence for the prevention theory was developed in East Germany and in Maryland, just a few years apart. Save for the possibility, which must not be discounted, that there are other factors at work in those natural foods that contain vitamin B^{17} compounds, these two sets of evidence strongly suggest the correctness of the Krebs hypothesis. In 1974, the Manfred von Ardenne Research Institute in Dresden, a center of pioneering work in cancer in many areas, reported that the simple addition of bitter almonds—which bear the highest known concentrations of vitamin B^{17}—to standard chow in a free-food choice caused "a significant prolongation of survival time, which is associated with inhibition of tumor growth" in mice bearing the cancer "form" known as Ehrlich ascites carcinoma.

In 1977, Dr. Vern L. van Breemen of Salisbury State College, Maryland, reported that the addition of apricot kernels to standard food in pilot experiments with special strains of mice bred to develop breast cancer and leukemia showed impressive differences both in terms of developing the disease and increased survival times between the animals that had an opportunity to ingest the kernels and those that did not. When he reported his early findings to the Maryland state legislature, seven animals in the leukemia control group and five in the breast cancer control group—that is, mice that had not been given apricot kernels—had died, while *none* of the mice on the kernels had. Ultimately only one of the mammary cancer mice developed a slow-growing tumor, and, while the leukemia results were less impressive in terms of total symptoms, leukemia-prone mice that ate apricot kernels enjoyed life extensions of up to 50 percent over what would normally be expected.

In fact, the rapid rise of cancer among *domesticated* animals, particularly dogs and cats, also bolstered the vitamin B^{17} deficiency hypothesis, for man's favorite house animals are as exposed to unnatural diets as is man himself, and the variety of animals—and eating habits—on American farms makes an interesting laboratory in which to test the central thesis. It is intriguing to note that range animals do not normally develop cancer, but cats and dogs, particularly those up in years, do. On a farm, it can be argued that *all* the life forms thereon are exposed to the same polluted water and air, but once again what varies enormously is their diets. The nitriloside—

that is, vitamin B¹⁷—content of pasturage, fodder, and silage is usually high, particularly in white clover, alfalfa, lucerne, vetch, the millets, the sorghums, Johnson grass, Sudan grass, arrow grass, lupines, broad beans, velvet grass, wild berries, and the leaves of all members of the *Rosaceae*. Most of the animals grazing on these sources are statistically not apt to develop cancer, though cancer in horses, the third most domesticated animal, is significantly higher than among other grazing animals. There is, however, an epidemic of leukemia among cats, and canine cancer has been on the rise for years.

Krebs states that man evolved in an environment in which vitamin B¹⁷ was as abundant and natural to his diet as was vitamin C. But, just as civilization has tended to take much of vitamin C away from him and he may be paying for this with what the vitamin C pioneers call "chronic subclinical scurvy" (see chapter nine), so also is Western man paying for a deficiency in vitamin B¹⁷ through the whoslsale development of cancer. However, Krebs and other collaborators have speculated that vitamin B¹⁷ may be implicit in many conditions other than cancer. It would seem to be involved in vitamin B¹² metabolism, and is a hypotensive agent—as thousands of loyal apricot kernel chewers can attest.

Such researchers as Dr. L. K. Oke of Nigeria have drawn parallels between the high consumption of nitriloside-bearing cassava and markedly lower rates of cancer. In some of these same populations, hospital admissions for sickle-cell anemia are also much lower, even though the sickle-cell genetic trait is common among them. Several B¹⁷ researchers believe the rise in sickle-cell anemia among American blacks, for example, is more due to their predilection for Western European and American diets than anything else. I reported in my first book the scattered evidence for control of the sickle-cell anemia hemolytic crisis through the use of laetrile tablets. Vitamin B¹⁷ seems to have an effect on rheumatoid arthritis, and is probably useful for a wide range of conditions. However, since there is no official recognition of a "vitamin B¹⁷ deficiency syndrome," it is routinely denied that vitamin B¹⁷ can even be considered a vitamin. Dr. Burk points out that the nitrilosides do in fact fall within a normal definition of a B-complex vitamin because of their essential ubiquity in nature, their non-toxicity, and their water-solubility. What remains to be demonstrated to the satisfaction of the orthodox mind is the *necessity* of vitamin B¹⁷ in the body. Krebs feels this is established, however subtle the deficiency state may seem to be at the outset. The American Cancer Society's argument that vitamin B¹⁷ cannot be a vitamin because its absence does not seem to cause anything founders in general on the rapid rise in cancer statistics in the "civilized" world and such vital experiments as those by van Breemen.

By 1980, the Bradford research group had added important new dimensions to the vitamin B^{17} theory.

Their researchers suspect that *thiocyanate,* which is formed in the body by cyanide in the presence of thiosulfate and rhodanese, the classic detoxifying enzyme for cyanide, may indeed be the "surveillant, antineoplastic" factor from ingested nitriloside compound-bearing foods.

Thiocyanate, not amygdalin itself—which is a compound which introduces a thiocyanate-building factor into the body—is absolutely necessary for proper body function, affecting both anabolic and catabolic functions, blood pressure, iodine storage, the pH of cellular mitochondria, hydrochloric acid content in the stomach, the action of thyroxin, the thyroid stimulating hormone (TSH), muscle contraction, blood vessel tone, renal functions, the activity of ATP enzymes, and other functions.

While thiocyanate is found intact in certain foods, the body derives most of it from nitrilosidic food (vitamin B^{17}).

The Bradford group pointed out in research in 1980 that it is known that cancer patients have about one-tenth the "normal" blood serum thiocyanate level, and that Western peoples—that is, those who no longer consume abundant amounts of nitrilosidic foods—have very low levels of thiocyanate. The average blood serum thiocyanate level in Americans (and, by inference, most of the Western world) ranges between 2 to 5 milligrams percent, they found, against a "normal" which should be in the range of 8 to 13 mg. Again, "primitive" peoples have much higher blood serum thiocyanate levels. These are the same peoples who are associated with much lower rates of cancer.

The Bradford group also added information which was in a sense heartwarming to the Establishment—at least in terms of the overemphasis on the cyanide problem in B^{17}: thiocyanate, like everything else, has a toxic level, too. Hence the Bradford group began insisting on the necessity of monitoring amygdalin intake with blood serum thiocyanate (BST) levels and argued *against* the reliance on amygdalin tablets for the remainder of a cancer patient's life.

In the meantime, the rekindling of interest in thiocyanate also points the way for the *natural* control of high blood pressure.

In 1980, Rutgers University tests demonstrated a whole new role for amygdalin—scavenger—or destroyer—of the deleterious free radical called the hydroxyl radical. Researchers Richard E. Keikkila and Felicitas S. Cabbat of the Rutgers College of Medicine neurology department, writing in *Life Sciences,* were agonizingly careful to note that the research had nothing to do with cancer or the laetrile controversy.

They simply found that the amygdalin given intraperitoneally to mice was able to block the development of diabetes induced by the drug alloxan. They wrote: "The data are consistent with the concept that the protection by amygdalin is due to its scavenging of the deleterious and highly reactive hydroxyl radical which was generated from alloxan.... We were drawn to consider amygdalin ...as an agent that might potentially protect against alloxan [because] amygdalin most likely was a good hydroxyl radical scavenger since amygdalin contains both a benzene ring and a sugar moiety...and... amygdalin...can be tolerated by experimental animals at rather high doses."

Aside from the analgesic properties of amygdalin and its anti-cancer properties from cyanide and benzaldehyde singly and in synergism, as well as its other properties derived from conversion to thiocyanate (which itself is suspected of an anti-cancer effect), the addition of free radical scavenging adds more strength to the vitamin concept of the compound and its relatives.

It is true that Dr. Krebs tends to be dogmatic in his utterances about B^{17}, but no revolutionary movement was ever accomplished without occasional sledgehammer rhetoric and sweeping statements. On top of that, I have yet to hear of an instance in which the disciplined and routine ingestion of vitamin B^{17} for several years was ever followed by a case of cancer. I am not saying there will not be any such cases, or that there has never been any such case, it is simply that I am unaware of any after hundreds of interviews with cancer patients and extensive correspondence and research on the subject. I share Dr. Burk's feeling that it seems almost too simple to suggest that the mere addition of vitamin B^{17} in the diet is a sure block to cancer, but ultimate truths usually turn out to be simple, and I have yet to have any personal knowledge of an exception to what Krebs first told me in 1971.

(The belated discovery of elevated selenium levels in apricot kernels, and the presence of abscissic acid and other key substances and vitamins in many foods which are abundant in vitamin B^{17}, point to a universality of anti-cancer factors in them and help explain actual cancer victory cases through the use of certain dietary manipulations *alone,* without the addition of pharmaceutical products.)

Vitamin B^{17}'s major champion claims simply and straightforwardly that the willful addition of major sources of vitamin B^{17} into the diet—in this country, that would normally mean the seeds of apricots, peaches, pears, plums and prunes (but virtually *every* black, bitter seed bears the vitamin, as do the seeds of essentially all fruits except the citrus fruits)—means prevention of cancer. There is no "recommended daily allowance," but since a number of populations, such as the Hunzakuts, take several hundred milligrams of the substance *per day,* whereas an American is lucky to get that amount in a full year, surely 100 mg. per day cannot be too much.

Indeed, the very ubiquity of vitamin B^{17} in nature makes it hard to realize why there is so *little* of the material in the standard American diet. The reasons are primarily cultural and historic, not common sense. Most of us have been told to spit out the seeds of apples, watermelons, and the like that we might eat. And it takes an effort to break open the pits of apricots, peaches, and pears to get at the seeds, or kernels within, so that source is removed from us. By switching from millet to wheat for bread production, the West also deprived itself of a major source of vitamin B^{17}. We characteristically do not eat grazing grasses, but would be lucky if we did. If we live on farms, we might occasionally consume wild berries and receive amounts of vitamin B^{17} that way. As it is, we're lucky to get trace amounts in a year's time by consuming the bamboo shoots, lentils, and sprouted alfalfa we might get at a health food store or in a good Chinese dinner, or by eating enough lima beans or taking in enough buckwheat.

The greatest concentrated amounts of vitamin B^{17} are available to the West in the form of seeds of apricots, cherries, nectarines, peaches, pears, plums, prunes, and apples, but, as we have seen, the FDA has intermittently made the interstate shipment and sale of packaged apricot kernels difficult, and bitter almonds—an even better source of B^{17}—while sometimes available in stores in Chinatown, are technically banned from this country.

The encroachment of civilization on primitive—and rational—eating habits has simply removed vitamin B^{17} from easy access one step at a time. It is part of what Krebs calls "our profound deviation from biological experience," and we are paying the price.

Since the most persistent question asked by Krebs and most of the laetrile proponents around the country is, "How many seeds should I take to prevent cancer?" they came up with two answers, both being rules of thumb and not scientific statements: one seed of the aforementioned fruits per ten pounds of body weight (fifteen for a 150-pound individual, for example) *or* the ingestion of all seeds in the B^{17}-bearing fruits a person might normally eat. That is, a person might eat two or three apples a day (rather than ten or twelve) so his consuming the *whole* apple in each case would include all the seeds from those two or three apples.

Levels of consumption have become critical inasmuch as the laetrile opposition has devoted so much time to proving the "danger" of laetrile through the release of cyanide and, as we have seen, construed the overconsumption of nitrilosidic foods with "poisonings from laetrile" as a fiendish scare tactic, one which reached its most vicious level with the University of California at Davis dog studies. The fact is, overconsumption of the vitamin B^{17} foods can, like the overconsumption of anything, including water and air, be toxic and even fatal. Also, the reliance on monodietary items, such as cassava, can result in *other* deficiency states and the symptoms of malnutrition, including a number of dangerous reactions. There have been deaths attributed to cassava in Nigeria, the Philippines, and elsewhere, but they have always been due either to the consumption of irrationally high amounts or sole dependence on the stuff. There have been reported cases in this country of poisonings from consuming slurries of apricot kernels in water, but these again have been, in each instance, from unusual or abnormal ingestion practices. Dr. Mas Goenawan and his colleagues in Indonesia, who have been using bitter-cassava-based cancer therapy for more than seventeen years, have *never* seen a case of fatal poisoning from their therapy, and have reported that a cup of tea with a lump of sugar in it will head off any toxic reactions from cassava. What all of this points to is the reality that normal, reasonable amounts of foods rich in vitamin B^{17} are no more dangerous to the body than the normal, reasonable ingestion of lettuce. And, as cancer researchers of the calibre of Dr. Bruce Halstead have reported time and again, the active ingredient involved, amygdalin, is less toxic than most drugs in use, and vitamin B^{17} itself, in any rational portion, is certainly safer than refined sugar and refined salt.

University of California chemist James Cason was one of those openminded scientists willing to take an objective look at the possibility of *prevention* through vitamin B^{17}, and he was equally smitten with the idea of an adequate level of vitamin C being essential for the same thing. As he summarized it for the June 1978 *Vortex,* a publication of the American Chemical Society:

> If I believe that eating 100 mg of nitriloside and 2 g of vitamin C per day will prevent me from becoming a cancer victim, and I live according to my stated convictions, and *I am wrong,* I suffer no penalty for my poor judgment, because I am doing nothing other than eating food that is commonly regarded as nutritionally beneficial.
>
> If one who believes that all this stuff about cancer resulting from nutritional deficiencies is nonsense, lives by his convictions, and *he is wrong,* that individual stands a very good chance of paying an awesome penalty for his faulty judgment.

In my mind, the "scoop" on vitamin B^{17} lies in the very exciting likelihood that it is directly involved in cancer prevention, if it is not itself the specific preventative of cancer. But any such argument is, at this writing, still regarded as the most extreme and silliest of the postulates of the laetrile champions. It is also, not so parenthetically, the most terrifying concept that seeps into the allopathic mind, for what it really means is that, in the long run, there would be practically no need for cancer *treatment,* including even the use of synthetic "laetriles."

Amygdalin In History

Assuming, again, that it is vitamin B^{17} that is the active ingredient in the nitrilosidic foods that are connected with cancer prevention, by far the best researched of these compounds is amygdalin—technically, D-l-mandelonitrile-beta-D-glucosido-6-beta-D-glucoside. It is the *rediscovery* of the therapeutic use of amygdalin wherein lay the primary contribution of the Krebses, father and son, to the development of laetrile. But labeling all the related compounds as vitamin B^{17} and noting their roles in cancer *prevention* is, as far as I am concerned, their greater contribution.

Researching the history of amygdalin, Dr. Bruce Halstead found the earliest mention of the nitrilosidic seeds (bitter almonds, apricot kernels, etc.) in the *Great Herbal* of China (ca. 2800 B.C.), wherein it is noted that a paste made from them was useful in breast cancer.

It is also true that ancient Egyptians used the force-feeding of apricot kernels with water to administer the "apricot death" to prisoners. On the other hand, for centuries the Romans used "bitter almond water"—*aqua amygdalarum amarum*—as an elixir.

Medical anthropologist John Heinerman has written that the ancient Sumerians "employed an effective poultice of dried wine dregs, crushed juniper berries and prune pits" (probably amygdalin) for a disease which may have been malignant melanoma. Too, the Assyrians used the pits and kernels of various unnamed kinds of fruit for the treatment of "swellings" or "growths." English herbalist John Gerarde referred to the healthful properties of peach and apricot kernels in his classic herbal work in 1633.

It was not until 1830 that Robiquet and Boutron-Charland prepared amygdalin in its pure state from plants, and not until 1837 that two German scientists, Justus von Liebig and Freidrich Wohler, discovered that amygdalin is split by an enzyme complex into sugar, cyanide, and benzaldehyde. But even as early as 1833 amygdalin appeared in the *United States Dispensatory* as a common treatment for several disorders. It is also mentioned throughout the nineteenth century as a useful expectorant and we know at least anecdotally that it was used by some physicians as an analgesic. Not until the 1970s was it discovered that in Russia two cases of cancer had been "controlled" successfully—one for over eleven years, the other for three—through the use of amygdalin. The citations on the cases appeared in an 1845 edition of the *Gazette Medicale de Paris*.

Heinerman notes that during the Civil War the value of fruit kernels against cancer-like infections became more important. It was an herbalist surgeon employed by the Confederate Army, Dr. Francis Porcher, who pointed to the hydrocyanic acid within the fruit kernels as responsible for whatever medical virtues they contained.

In 1924 Campbell and Haworth accomplished the chemical synthesis of amygdalin, whose physical and chemical properties have been reported in the *Merck Index* for over eighty years.

Ernst T. Krebs, Sr., the pioneering San Francisco physican who actually began work—in the 1920s—on what would become laetrile, initiated the extraction process of the substance from apricot kernels under the theory he was treating cancer with an enzyme complex. In the 1930s and 1940s Krebs and several other American and foreign researchers successfully used the early seed extracts on patients. It was not until the 1940s, however, that the local toxic reactions they sometimes observed were determined to be due to the presence of cyanide—information that led Ernst T. Krebs, Jr., to work on extracting a purified, crystallized amygdalin from the kernels. The result of this work was said to be refined amygdalin. It is probable that the early efforts in laetrile manufacture and use were along the lines of the development of a drug to treat a disease, but even so, the younger Krebs had, by updating an earlier theory on the nature of cancer, brought into play what may be one of his major contributions in the overall cancer field, the "unitarian," or "trophoblastic" thesis. Further work with laetrile ultimately convinced him of its vitamin nature, one increasingly bolstered by broad epidemiological studies. It took other researchers in other areas of metabolic/nutritional therapy to begin fitting the substance known as vitamin B^{17} into a general, overall attack on cancer, for laetrile alone proved disappointing as a "magic bullet."

Vindicating The Trophoblastic Thesis

Ernst T. Krebs, Jr., has drawn the wrath of the cancer Establishment not only for his codiscovery of laetrile and daring to author the theory that it is vitamin B^{17} and that vitamin B^{17} is a naturally selected preventer of cancer, just as vitamin C is the naturally selected preventer of scurvy, but also by daring to argue that cancer is not hundreds of diseases, but *one*.

It is the accepted "line" that cancer is a complex of diseases with hundreds of variations, and that the "causes" of these many cancers vary. However, as of 1982, and despite combined private-public expenditures in the war on cancer of well over $10 billion in ten years, orthodoxy was consistently forced to admit that it does *not* know what the real cause of cancer is, let alone how to "cure" it.

Efforts to put all "forms" of cancer into the same basket and to come up with the "magic bullet" to eradicate them all—let alone prevent them—are regarded by the American Cancer Society as sure signs of cancer quackery. However, time is once again on the side of Krebs, who has stuck by his guns on the trophoblastic thesis just as vigorously as he has adhered to the vitamin B^{17} prevention hypothesis.

Taking its cue from Scotch embryologist John Beard (1858-1924), the unitarian, or trophoblastic, thesis of cancer, which a number of researchers in the 1940s and 1950s helped elaborate and with which they still agree in whole or part, is, in summary, this: cancer is the appearance of trophoblastic cells at the wrong time and/or place. This being so, whatever inhibits trophoblast cells must also inhibit cancer. Hence, the internal answer to cancer should be pancreatic enzymes and the body's immune system.

Arising from human germ cells, the trophoblast is as essential to the life cycle as oxygen and blood sugar. It is the trophoblast that, being invasive, destructive, and metastatic—that is, rapidly spreading—eats out a niche in the uterine wall in which the fertilized egg is nestled and ultimately derives nourishment from the mother. The attacking trophoblast, should it continue to grow, would eventually kill the embryo and the mother, but, as Beard noted at the turn of the century, there is a fail-safe mechanism in the life cycle that inhibits the trophoblast when it has performed its utterly necessary function.

Comparing the characteristics of trophoblast cells and cancer, Beard came to the felicitous conclusion that they are one and the same—except that cancer at some point is regarded as an "invader," whereas the normal trophoblast is not. Marshalling the body's defense system should inhibit the extrauterine cancer. If the unitarianists are correct, cancer is *necessary* to life, and, ironically, is ultimately linked with death.

Under the Beard theory, since greatly expanded and modernized by Krebs, pharmacologist Charles Gurchot—who stimulated Krebs to pursue an active interest in the Beardian postulates—and several others, *all* manifestations of cancer are simply variants of the original problem—trophoblast running unchecked within a given tissue and/or spreading from tissue to tissue. Originally, it was thought that cancer could only arise from residual primitive germ cells, "leftovers" so to speak, which might be found anywhere in the body. But it puzzled Gurchot for years that cancer seemed to arise also from "normal" tissue. He may have closed the gap with research published in *Oncology* in 1975, which in essence indicated how the presence of cancer-causing substances might alter the genetic machinery of cells to convert them into trophoblastic—or trophoblast-like—cells. The process whereby a cell switches over to a fermentation process for energy, or the mirror-image opposite of oxygen-based energy (the "Warburg principle") might also explain the "trophoblastization" of a cell. A number of biochemists, by no means champions of the trophoblast theory, have theorized approximately the same chain of events as suggested by Gurchot.

Krebs drew more evidence for the trophoblastic character of *all* cancer by noting, through the 1970s, that more and more researchers were discovering the presence of HCG—human chorionic gonadotrophin, a hormone elicited in the birth process *and* in cancer cells— in various "forms" of cancer. Indeed, Dr. Navarro in the Philippines had refined an earlier HCG detection test, originally based on pregnancy tests, to identify the presence of cancer before it ever came to clinical attention. The connection between elevated HCG levels and cancer is becoming ever more obvious, with numerous researchers, either ignorant of, or even hostile to, Beard and Krebs making that very connection. Dr. Navarro stated the case best of all in a research paper entitled "Why Are Cancer Patients 'Pregnant'?"—in which he poined out that males who were "positive" on the refined pregnancy test for HCG were not, of course, pregnant—but they *were* cancerous. He has reported cases in which the actual clinical signs of cancer did not appear for months and even years after a positive reading.

Nonetheless, American cancer research until recently has brushed off the unitarian thesis and the HCG test as either quackery or unreliable or both. But it is slowly beginning to take another look, and in doing so is once again vindicating the aphorism that today's quacks are often tomorrow's pioneers. In 1978, researcher Herman F. Acevedo, Ph.D., of the Department of Laboratory Medicine at Allegheny General Hospital, had a surprise for the Sixth Pan American Cancer Cytology meeting in Nevada. "Pieces of the puzzle are slowly coming together, and the trophoblastic theory will, bit by bit, gain acceptance, but so far the scientific community has been reluctant to accept what this evidence implies. But they will—they'll have to," Dr. Acevedo told his audience, most of whom had never even heard of the theory.

In covering the Acevedo presentation, the Establishment-oriented *Medical Tribune* headlined its coverage, "One-Mode Cancer Theory Makes Comeback" and assessed, "[The theory] has been roundly discredited in recent years by the American Cancer Society. But it has been revived by strong biochemical evidence."

Using such sensitive techniques as immunoelectron microscopy, Acevedo and his colleagues examined over forty different normal and malignant cell types and identified a specific antigen found only in the membranes of the cancer cells. They determined that the antigen was similar biologically but not chemically identical to the trophoblast hormone. It reacts specifically with HCG "and so is related to proteins found heretofore only in normal embryonic tissues, spermatozoa, and some cancer-associated bacteria," they reported, adding that the HCG-like protein "appears to be the chemical denominator among cancers."

Summarized the *Medical Tribune,* in what for patient unitarianists and laetrile proponents constituted yet another rung up the ladder from quackery to credibility as viewed by the Establishment, "The accepted view is that the word 'cancer' is a poorly defined clinical concept useful for classifying hundreds of malignant diseases. If these diseases stem from different causes, a general immunological approach would be impossible. This common antigen, however, could open the way to a vaccine or *general treatment for cancer."* (Emphasis mine.).

The medical journal went on to say that because of the presence of the "HCG-like protein," normal cells "transformed into cancer cells" have a charge 10 to 100 times greater than normal. Since like charges repel, the scavengers of the body's immune system—the macrophages—and the immune system's destroying troops, the lymphocytes, cannot approach close enough even to recognize, let alone destroy, cancer cells. The *Tribune* added that the "trophoblastic hormone" operates in the same way in the fetal environment to protect the blastula—the cellular cluster—from which the microscopic embryo "buds." That is to say, the body does not identify the new growth as an "invader"—*because, after all, it isn't!* Only when the growth remains unchecked does the body belatedly respond with the mimicking tissue and encapsulation that will ultimately, in cancer, become a tumor.

By using isolated cancer-cell systems from human and animal cultures, Dr. Acevedo showed that the cancer antigen is synthesized in each transformed cell. "Every cell has the genetic information to synthesize the [H]CG-like protein," Acevedo reported. "Its synthesis by cancer cells can only be explained through depression or activation of the genetic control, but we don't yet understand how to operate that control."

In a statement redolent of the observations made decades before by champions of the Beardian theory, Dr. Acevedo added, "But life itself is a random process—and cancer is part of life. It is poetic that the protein that allows life to thrive in the womb is the one that kills you."

It is important to realize that HCG has the dual effect of destroying rhodanese, an enzyme that detoxifies *cyanide,* and or providing a protein shield for the developing trophoblast—or cancer—thus conferring protection against the body's immune system, which otherwise would identify the new growth as an invader and destroy it.

In this decade, the Club is by no means united against the theory that cancer is a single condition with multiple forms. No less a scientific/intellectual light than scientist-author Lewis Thomas, M.D., chancellor of Sloan-Kettering Cancer Center, is quoted as saying: "I regard cancer as one disease. I do not beleive that there is any evidence whatever for the often-expressed view that cancer is perhaps 100 diseases and the answer will have to come down piece by piece for each. No doubt the way a virus *initiates* cancer is different from the way the chemical carcinogen initiates cancer. But the central mechanism that transforms a cell and triggers the cancer will turn out, in my opinion, to be the same...."

Intrinsic Defense—Extrinsic Defense

Two of the Krebses' multiple contributions to medicine and

science are thus brought to the fore in the development and use of laetrile—the identification of the unitarian nature of cancer, and the administration of a "missing" nutrient to "control" it.

The early champions of Beardianism knew, from new research, that what specifically inhibits the further growth of trophoblast after it has accomplished its purpose in the life cycle are pancreatic enzymes. Further studies showed chymotrypsin and trypsin to be the major elements in this inhibition. Hence, for Beardians, the challenge in cancer therapy lay in developing proteolytic (protein-digesting) enzymes and synthetic versions of pancreatic enzymes for cancer treatment.

Yet the development and use of such enzymes as magic bullets in cancer, while successful in some cases, was marked by years of frustration. Beardians came to realize that enzymes *alone* are normally not the answer to cancer, at least when it has reached the clinical stage. It was due in part to that frustration that Krebs Jr., who had bounced around academically between medicine, biology, biochemistry, pharmacology, and anatomy, took up a renewed interest in the apricot kernel extract originally pioneered by his father and ultimately developed laetrile.

In so doing, he put together this general theory of cancer: the "first line of defense" against cancer (that is, trophoblast at the wrong place and/or time) is the totality of the body's immune system and pancreatic enzymes. Due to a host of factors, prominent among them the animal-protein-rich diet of Western man (pancreatic enzymes being used exhaustively in the digestion of such food), this first line of defense may be faulty, depleted, or weakened.

Mother Nature has provided a "second line of defense," however, in the nitrilosides, or vitamin B^{17}, to do the same job through cyanide release (and probably that of benzaldehyde as well) in suppressing cancer, while also causing other positive metabolic responses in the organism. That is to say, the pancreatic enzymes and the body's immune system are the *internal* factor in cancer-inhibition and the nitrilosides the *external* one.

But in "civilized" man, not only may the first line of defense be weakened or not present, there is virtually no second line of defense either. Under this theory, the thousands of carcinogens in the environment, X-rays, sunshine, and the like, are not *causers* of cancer—only "organizers," for they set up a situation in which either germ cells are triggered into division or otherwise "normal" cells revert or change to a trophoblastic nature. While the triggering of estrogen in the body's tissue-repair mechanism seems to be a central factor, *anything* might "insult" the tissues enough to provoke the chain of events which only later will be called cancer. But as long as the intrinsic and/or extrinsic defense factors are at work, no clinical cancer will manifest itself.

Also in this view, since cancer is a "natural part of the life cycle," it is safe to say that everyone has cancer many times in his life. But the healthier and, to some extent, the younger, he is, the *ultimate* exhibition of cancer, the lumps and bumps, "specks on the lung," etc., will not appear until it is "too late."

Both Krebs and most of the metabolic/nutritional therapists—and many of the latter do not agree with Krebs on the universality of the trophoblastic thesis or on the prevention aspects of vitamin B^{17}—hold that what is meant by the metabolic/nutritional management of cancer is the "control"—not its "cure." Simply stated, if cancer is a deficiency of vitamin B^{17}, then it is necessary to increase and maintain the level of vitamin B^{17} forever, just as one would increase and maintain any nutrient forever. This maintenance and holding in check of a natural part of the life cycle that is *not* a problem until it goes awry is control—not cure. Hence, save for the earliest days of laetrile, the proponents nowadays seldom discuss laetrile in terms of curing cancer but of controlling it. Their parallel is diabetes, which *may* be controlled adequately by insulin and diet, bit is not cured by them.

Since Krebs has devoted far more of his public time to arguing for the prevention of cancer than treating it, it is appropriate to point out that prevention is a lot easier than treatment. He and other laetrilists argue to the point of exhaustion around the country that laetrile, let along the whole program of metabolic/nutritional therapy, is not a magic bullet—it cannot restore tissues already destroyed either by cancer or by the destructive orthodox treatment for it. Many patients may ultimately bring their cancers under control and still die from the earlier effects of the disease and/or its treatment. And, too, for several reasons we explore below, laetrile does not always work at all.

Krebs, Jr. has pegged his defense of laetrile on the adage that "that which cures also prevents"—curing at least in terms of the early onset of the disease. It is true that advanced, terminal cases of identified nutritional deficiency states may *not* always be saved by the administration of the missing nutrient. The same is true, of course, for cancer.

But no matter what Krebs might say, the unitarian thesis, the vitamin B^{17} prevention hypothesis, the intrinsic-extrinsic theory was cold-shouldered for years by American medicine, and the San Francisco biochemist was given the same treatment accorded Andrew Ivy, Harry Hoxsey, William Koch, and others who dared to take on the cancer Establishment. But unlike others, Krebs' defense succeeded, not only because of the increasing scientific evidence that most of his views are somewhere close to target, but because his substance "went political."

Even so, it has been an uphill battle all the way, with the Establishment trying to prove that the scientific validity of laetrile could not be demonstrated.

A Biochemical Mystery Thriller

Several hundred physicians around the world are now using amygdalin in the treatment of cancer, and most of these are now in the United States, whether the FDA, the American Cancer Society, and the AMA like it or not. Many physicians use laetrile together with standard therapies, a few use it alone, others use it with a full metabolic/nutritional program. Others, such as West Germany's Hans Nieper, use it in conjunction with other experimental therapies. By no means do all the physicians who use it agree with the vitamin B^{17} prevention theory of the trophoblastic thesis.

They use laetrile because it often "works"—that is, somehow, some way, it is exerting some form of positive effect, whether that effect be measured subjectively (and hence subject to an attack of being a simple placebo) or objectively. By no means is there agreement as to why and how it works—but the questions are beginning to be answered.

It is also true that laetrile alone is of only limited use against cancer, and that even the expanded laetrile-enzymes-diet program championed by Krebs, Jr. and the McNaughton Foundation-era laetrilists is disappointing in offering anything like guaranteed success in cancer therapy.

It is not the province of this book to get into the fascinating if laborious controversies over the biochemical actions of amygdalin/laetrile or their various theories. Suffice it to say that in the present era work on synthetic laetriles is continuing, that "second-generation" laetriles are being looked at. Nieper in West Germany and, for a time, Israeli researchers, have done important work in the further research of the nitrilosides and their use. The Bradford group has done the most exhaustive and dogma-free research in this area and produced precise information on the varying biochemical pathways of the oral and injectable compounds.

Too, much to the chagrin of the once-burgeoning laetrile underground, the Bradford line of research pointed to numerous production problems which tended to undercut the therapeutic strength of, or greatly alter the effects from, a wide variety of products sold as "laetrile," but more importantly elucidated that for the classic action of laetrile to occur—the release of cyanide and benzaldehyde in the cancer cell—a whole host of biochemcial actions and interactions must take place.

For the orthodox side, it can be said that laetrile or amygdalin has failed in some genuine tests simply because the parameters for testing cancer drugs are those used for testing poisons, which injectable laetrile simply is *not*.

However, the unyielding opinions of the late Dr. Kanematsu Sugiura at Sloan-Kettering, and the existing studies of amygdalin/laetrile at recognized cancer centers in several countries continue to speak for its usefulness in cancer as a single modality—*not* as a magic-bullet drug to cure, but as an important food factor which has a range of properties varying from definitely anti-cancer to causing subjective feelings of well-being. The analgesic and free radical-scavenging effects from amygdalin, and the multiple physiological effects of the thiocyanate whose presence is owed in the main to the vitamin B^{17} substances, add to its usefulness.

The testimony of the current era is that amygdalin or laetrile is best used within a total holistic framework—within a universe of vitamins, minerals, enzymes, dietary manipulation, vaccines, biologicals, detoxification programs. This does not undercut the strong suggestion of cancer *prevention* from the normal ingestion of nitrilosides. And, it must be understood within the reality that there are obviously any number of substances which can attack and destroy cancer cells—but in terminal cancer, the simple destruction of cancer cells is just half, and not even always half, the therapeutic job involved in attempting to save the patient. It has been the failure to recognize this central fact which has turned in so much disappointment for the adherents of single-shot "magic bullets" in cancer therapy—be these nostrums from the "orthodox" or the "unorthodox" side.

Robert Bradford, who ruffled the amygdalin manufacturing world by his group's disclosure in 1979 that many, if not most, amygdalin pharmaceutical compounds on the flourishing "gray" and black markets were decomposed and degraded compounds—not actually amygdalin itself—led to a review of the effects on cancer patients who were on "laetrile shots." Bradford argued that the difficulties with the pharmaceutical preparations of the unstable amygdalin compounds in solution were more state-of-the-art manufacturing problems than willfully sloppy procedures by profit-hungry manufacturers, whose market, truth to tell, did indeed boom after the mid-1970s. Too, the Bradford group noted that even *if* the anti-cancer effects by amygdalin-*like* products were not being achieved because of cyanide, whose presence was not detectable in many degraded or decomposed products, there might still be some anti-cancer effects from benzaldehyde. This, he and other researchers have noted, would come about through interference of the cancer cell's fermentive or anaerobic mode of metabolism. The presence of benzaldehyde products in the system would also acount for the oft-reported improvement in patient well-being and might also explain why many physicians and patients were confusing the sudden improvement in well-being with presumptive (but by no means always genuine) anti-cancer effects *per se.* All such speculations did not deviate from the likelihood that the synergism of cyanide *and* benzaldehyde—unleashed by the metabolites of pharmaceutically proper amygdalin under the appropriate physiological conditions of patients—is still by far the more potent of the vitamin B^{17} attacks on cancer.

That benzaldehyde itself can be effective against cancer became a line of research advanced primarily in Japan by Mitsuyuki Kochi, M.D., a former professor of bacteriology at Yokohama Medical School and owner-operator of the Ichijo-Kai Hospital and Kochi Tumor Center in Chiba, near Toyko. He announced in 1979 that in three years' time, some 200 cancer patients, most of them "terminal," and all of whom had failed on earlier therapy, had been treated with benzaldehyde-based compounds, and some 50 percent had had positive responses. He had achieved total recoveries from pancreatic cancer and myelogenous leukemia with his CDBA (benzaldehyde-beta-cyclodextrin inclusion) compounds.

News of the Kochi advances broke in the United States within the context of the laetrile controversy, though Dr. Kochi was by no means a part of the laetrile movement and did not involve his benzaldehyde study with metabolic/nutritional therapy. However, the synchronicity of his discovery and its background with the laetrile story was apparent.

A student of the Bible as a Seventh-Day Adventist—the same denomination whose members report far less cancer and from whose ranks some of the primary amygdalin research has gone on—Dr. Kochi reached the conclusion that the cure of the "boil" of Hezekiah by Isaiah by a "cake of figs" in II Kings, 20:1-7 was actually the therapy of a form of cancer.

Only after years of animal experiments did Dr. Kochi determine that the anti-cancer activity he was seeing from a fig extract preparation was actually due to benzaldehyde. He then undertook a ten-year program of work with human patients which led to the advanced experimentation today.

Because of Dr. Kochi's own unblemished credentials and the scientific method pursued in his research, even Western orthodoxy took a seemingly unbiased interest in his work—chagrined, obviously, by the parallel fact that benzaldehyde constitutes a third of most vitamin B^{17} compounds.

In the meantime, continuing amygdalin research suggests that the anti-cancer effects from *oral* amygdalin derive primarily from benzaldehyde and the thiocyanate formed as cyanide is detoxified. But other modes of operation are also being explored.

Too, work at the Bradford Foundation and Research Institute, and other research centers, has not only pinpointed the cyanide attack on cancer from the *injectable* route, but has strongly emphasized the absolute relevance of nutrition as to whether the compounds "work." In the injectable mode, for example, nutritional conditions are implied in these areas:

• "The glucose metabolic pathway," or the route of utilization of blood sugar, is the pathway from which both glucuronic acid and uridine diphosphate (UDP), essential in the detoxification of toxic substances such as mandelonitrile, arise. Imbalance in this pathway is of key importance, and helps explain why individuals with a glucose metabolism dysfunction, usually expressed as diabetes, have a 30 percent greater likelihood of developing cancer.

• The acidity of the cancer cell cytoplasm, the alkalinity of the mitochondrion's plasma, the swelling of the mitochondrion and the permeability of its membrane, are all dependent on specific nutrition. Low-protein ingestion, for example, tends to generate the ideal conditions of mitochondrion membrane permeability and the correct alkaline-acid balance within the cancer cell and its mitochondria.

It has also been shown that the passage of needed substances through cell membranes is closely linked to nutrition—whether, for example, there are adequate "transporter" minerals present.

Hence, it is possible to administer relatively high doses of laetrile without any specific anticancer activity being noted. But it is also possible to provide relatively low levels of the substance and see, as the early Krebs researchers saw, dramatic effects.

The controversy over the proper pharmaceutical preparation of amygdalin was far from resolved as this book went to press. Some researchers suspected that the earlier products turned out by Krebs, Sr. were far more effective at much lower doses when a handful of investigators were overseeing the limited production. Massive-dose amygdalin did not begin until after production changed from Krebs-directed production in experimental laboratories in the United States and Canada to the Mexican manufacturers.

Ironically, the development of an alleged "stabilized" aqueous-solution laetrile and a synthetic laetrile occurred just as the entire laetrile movement in the United States was under the threat of being driven back underground—and also as information developed, geometrically, that the nontoxic answer to cancer lay in far more than amygdalin alone.

**Metabolic/Nutritional Management Of Cancer:
The Developing Evidence**
Vitamin B^{17}'s history has been long and troubled, marred by claims and counter-claims as well as vested interests, but its therapeutic form, laetrile, has been the Marine Corps of the metabolic/nutritional medical revolution. The battles over laetrile/amygdalin, in both the scientific and political realm, have served to catalyze the entire movement for alternative cancer therapy in this country—and to no small extent, throughout a good deal of the world.

A handful of physicians, particularly in laetrile's earlier era when Ernst Krebs, Sr. probably thought he had an anti-cancer drug, have indeed found anti-tumor effects from laetrile alone. There is, too, the suspicion that Krebs, Sr. took with him to the grave some secrets about laetrile extraction and manufacture. The reality in this decade, however, is that laetrile, as a treatment—again, separating this vital area from the realm of *prevention*—does much better when it is a part of a total program. Interest in laetrile has served, across the board, to expand interest in the whole field of nutritional therapy in cancer, and it is safe to say that without the laetrile controversy the nutritional and food factor manipulation of cancer in particular and degenerative disease in general would be nowhere nearly as advanced as it is today.

This new, total approach, which some prefer to call holistic, and which Europeans aptly style "biological," is, I am fond of saying, the discovery of a new continent. The mapping of this continent continues as new information comes in. Laetrile is, in effect, a planet joining a galaxy of therapies which includes approaches to cancer that range from the old to the new.

Indeed, "laetrilists" in the seventies, to some extent, were playing catchup ball with exponents of other nontoxic therapies working quietly on several fronts. The "whole-body" treatment of cancer, exemplified in the work of Joseph Issels and other European specialists, was based on information and routes of work and research many decades old. Several of the therapies of natural management of degenerative disease were already well within the province of naturopaths and homeopaths, whose work had long been obscured in America by the brutalizing power control of the allopathic, or drug-based, schools of medicine. And proponents of the chiropractic and osteopathic shcools, thought systems which had won grudging acceptance by the medical community throughout years of conflict, found it ideologically tenable to make common cause with the amygdalin proponents, the megavitamin ("orthomolecular") researchers, and others. It was the *politicization* of laetrile, a relative johnny-come-lately in the universe of natural, holistic approaches, which helped galvanize all the non-allopathic tendencies into a generally united front, one which is now mounting a unified final assault on the bastions of drug-based crisis medicine and its abysmal failure to come to grips with the killer degenerative diseases.

Each area of nontoxic metabolic therapy has its adamant champions. The vitamin C activists are convinced that the answer to the cancer puzzle lies in the judicious use of ascorbic acid as the *sine qua non* in treatment. The European specialists in enzymes and vitamin A make the same case for their favorite substances, and so do the vitamin B^{17} theorists. As we have seen, Dr. Max Gerson broke new ground by controlling cancer with nutrition alone and by emphasizing the utter importance of detoxification. The 1970s brought mental visualization techniques and "mind control" into the total picture. What we are now seeing is a union of nontoxic approaches and disciplines aimed at the substitution of toxic drugs, system-destroying radiation, and mutilating surgery in the management of cancer, save in those ancillary areas in which some form of surgery is still necessary.

There are several hundred American physicians, and several score foreign ones, using laetrile openly in cancer management. Some use it strictly as a backup for, or adjuvant with, standard therapies..A few use it alone. Most are blending it in with one or more parts of the metabolic/nutritional program, and those who conscientiously do this are, by and large, seeing the best results.

Confusion arises, however, on defining what the phrase *cancer treatment* really means. If the simple removal of a localized tumor mass means that cancer has been treated, then metabolic therapy may fail as many times as it is successful. But if overall patient improvement, including a variety of subjective signs and feelings, is measured, then metabolic therapy already is far and away better than orthodox therapy. In other relevant terms, such as life-extension, the metabolic/nutritional approach is also a winner.

Further, the use of laetrile and/or enzymes locally may also account for rapid tumor diminution. Dr. Paul Wedel, originally of Oregon, a laetrile-controlled cancer patient himself, showed how massive doses of locally applied laetrile do have a local effect on tumors. There is also evidence that a laetrile salve is extremely useful in eliminating skin cancer. But the local application of laetrile, however useful it may be in local masses, is not the usual administration of vitamin B^{17}, for in most cases physicians are not faced with a strictly localized problem but with a chronic, systemic, metabolic malfunction of which lumps are only symptoms

A blending of nontoxic therapies—nontoxic in the sense that they do not involve poisons or immune system depressers, even though their megadoses can indeed produce toxic effects—has thus arisen to constitute, in general terms, the metabolic/nutritional management of cancer as understood in the 80s.

The programs involved may or may not use laetrile as a centerpiece. The basic constituents of the program, first and foremost, include the manipulation of eating habits, detoxification (and, usually, colonics), the administration of food factors as intravenous and/or oral substances (vitamins A, C, B^{15} and B^{17} and frequently E), trace minerals, protein-digesting enzymes, free radical-scavenging enzymes and related substances, immune system enhancers, and may include vaccines and biologicals. Musculoskeletal manipulation, herbal teas, ointments, poultices and capsules may be part of the program, along with mental-visualization techniques and, recently, "free-form" amino acids.

The addition of cellular (or "live cell") therapy is frequent in such programs—a therapy that is in itself not new and has a pioneering group of champions who see in it the single major factor in building the immune system and rejuvenating the body. Cellular therapy brings into focus a frequently missing part of metabolic programs: manipulation of the endocrinological/hormone system, the key to a vast array of biochemical processes. It involves the injection of cells from the endocrine glands of animal embryos (and, experimentally in some countries, human fetuses) under the empirical evidence (but as yet scientifically unexplained) reality that proteins from a gland in an animal stimulate the human counterpart.

While this line of European research has essentially been pooh-poohed in America along with a number of other novel biological approaches, in extreme instances it has been turned to, and with impressive results, even by American orthodoxy. A case in point are the seventeen responses (reported in 1981) in a severe immune-depressing disease called histiocytosis. The cases, at Boston University Medical Center, involved shots of extracts of calf thymus glands, a method which was successful where chemotherapy had failed.

Wolfram Kuhnau, M.D., a primary disciple of the late Paul Niehans, pioneer of cellular therapy, and at this writing involved in individualizing live-cell programs with a total metabolic/nutritional program with the Bradford group in Mexico, has noted that the human brain may be considered the greatest of the endocrine glands. Information within orthodox science continues to pinpoint new secretions from the brain only a few of which are understood but most of which are surely involved in the biochemical symphonic interplay of hormones/vitamins/minerals/enzymes whose manipulation and supplementation comprises the physical part of holistic medicine.

Metabolic/nutritional therapists are aware that their program in cancer has broad and fundamental applications in the whole of chronic, systemic, degenerative disease, rejuvenation and the slowing of the aging process. They recognize that the nature of cancer is inextricably interwoven with the immmune system and aging, and research on many fronts is tending to bring these disparate issues together and pointing to new treatment techniques—as, for example, the discovery that the hitherto unsung steroid hormone dehydroepiandrosterone (DHEA) has anti-cancer effects in laboratory animals and is almost certainly involved both in obesity and the aging process.

Going into this decade, the crux of virtually every alternative program (with the exception of some single-shot vaccines, promoted by their developers as literal magic bullets) was dietary manipulation, an area which most enraged American medical orthodoxy and also continues to cause doctrinal grief between the various facets of the alternative medical movement. Suffice it to say that, taking their cue primarily from Max Gerson's mostly-vegetarian and juice-centered degenerative disease diets, metabolic/nutritional therapists have in essence agreed that the addition of more natural fruits, organic vegetables and their juices, and the ingestion of natural whole, unrefined grains with the removal or vast reduction in animal proteins and the banning of processed foods, refined carbohydrates, alcohol, and stimulants (most particularly caffein and nicotine) are in general dietarily "good" for patients.

American medical orthodoxy has focused on the eating plan primarily for cancer patients as the worst form of quackery, even though information on many fronts tends far more to substantiate it than to detract from it.

The advent of cytotoxic allergy testing, to determine to what extent patients are allergic to certain foods, represented a great leap forward in metabolic therapy going into this decade. It paralleled the rapidly rising reality that, among all the negatives of the industrial/chemical age, Americans and other dwellers in the technologized West are increasingly allergic, most of them completely unaware of it, to many foods, including such common ones as carrots and lettuce as well as the gluten in wheat. These hitherto undetected or unknown allergies could, and doubtless did, spell biochemical disaster for people earlier treated with dietary regimens.

The Kelley program, emphasizing "metabolic typing" of people, and the Bradford group's development of "individualized, integrated metabolic programs" (IIMP) represented advances in the dietary manipulation area, but in both cases they represent beginnings of knowledge, not end-products. In the meantime, the spokesmen for American allopathic medicine, engaging in frequent intellectual dishonesty, utilize single snippets of animal work in all-out efforts to block, thwart or criticize eating habits as primary therapeutic tools in cancer.

It is beyond the scope of this volume to deal with attitude adjustment and to examine the role the mind seems to exert both in the causation and control of cancer. Suffice it to say that the "complete metabolic therapist" sees in cancer and its natural therapy a unity of mind, soul, and body—hence the holistic nature of the metabolic/nutritional modalities involved in cancer management.

The great majority of physicians whose interest in and curiosity about laetrile were aroused by the controversy concerning it are AMA-lining, orthodoxy-trained allopathic physicians who still perceive in cancer a specific disease to be treated by one or more specific drugs. They are not interested in, and usually know nothing of, nutritional and metabolic therapies, which generally are relegated *in toto* to the category of quackery in the minds of local medical boards. However, these physicians are impressed by even a ray of evidence from a single use of a single nontoxic agent as long as this ray can seem to be elevated beyond the placebo or spontaneous remission arguments, which constitute allopathic medicine's own fail-safe defense against unwanted evidence.

The "bridge" between allopathic physicians and those of metabolic orientation in the use of laetrile has been established by those who have had experience with both the so-called proven and the so-called unproven remedies by mixing them. In this regard, the work of Mario Soto de Leon, formerly at the Cydel Clinic in Tijuana, is of paramount importance. Even as the laetrile controversy was breaking white-hot, Dr. Soto, a U.S.-trained physician who had been instrumental in achieving the legalization of laetrile use in Mexico (under the name *amigdalina*), was still on the books as a foreign researcher of the National Cancer Institute. His credentials to make statements about cancer research and therapy were, then, a cut above those of many practitioners.

Shortly after the Cydel Clinic—part of the complex owned and operated by the Del Rio family, which at the time had a near-monopoly on the Mexican production of laetrile—opened in late 1975, Dr. Soto began experimenting with the mixing of therapies. Visitors to Cydel might receive standard therapies along with elevated levels of laetrile, a fact which greatly disturbed the more hardcore laetrile proponents and all of those in the movement for the legalization of laetrile.

But time has tended to bear out much of Dr. Soto's work—at least in terms of the effect of amygdalin on the *symptoms* of cancer. Dr. Soto several times reported to Mexican officials, and in a cluster of cases to the NCI, and in information prepared for the Committee for Freedom of Choice, that he could give up to double and triple the recommended amounts of dangerous, toxic chemotherapeutic agents —such as 5-FU—*as long as* they were given with increased doses of amygdalin. He found pronounced anticancer effects achieved this way, normally with a total elimination of, or at least a diminution in, the side effects that usually result from chemotherapy.

What Dr. Soto's work in hundreds of cases has shown is that the use of laetrile can eliminate or reduce the side effects of chemotherapeutic agents, while allowing either the conventional chemotherapeutic agents and/or the laetrile (which is, of course, a chemotherapeutic agent, too) to exert a specific anticancer effect. This reality was also found in the carefully watched cluster of 4,800 cases at the nearby Clinica del Mar, the fifteen-year-old cancer treatment facility of Dr. Ernesto Contreras, who for years has been one of the few M.D.'s in all North America who used vitamin B^{17}. In both the Cydel and Del Mar caseloads—as in every other caseload I was able to examine over the period of several years—what was evident first and foremost was the analgesic effect of amygdalin. In case after case, the patients involved could go off morphine and a host of other painkillers and rely solely on laetrile shots to curb or eliminate completely the pain associated with cancer. In fact, it was this first evident reality that enraged me, as a newspaper reporter-editor. If laetrile *did no more* than cut pain, why should it be construed as "illegal?"

Dr. Soto was one of the first physicians to devote and implement the administration of high doses of amygdalin in general cancer therapy—going swiftly from six to twelve to eighteen and more grams per patient per day. As long as these levels were intravenous, not oral, the only problems that arose from time to time were "anaphylactic shock" from impure vials and/or the body's reaction to building up the kind of tolerance for the dose levels. Dr. Navarro in the Philippines also occasionally gives dozens of grams of intramuscular laetrile, and Israeli cancer researcher David Rubin, M.D., around whom a mini-controversy swirled, used up to seventy grams per day in a "drip," or intravenous, infusion. That is to say, amygdalin is used at levels that for toxic chemotherapy are simply unthinkable.

Dr. Soto was able to achieve the complete reduction of certain forms of lung cancer and several other tumors by the use of amygdalin alone, without reliance on a metabolic program. The Contreras staff also achieved similar results. Again, what was being looked at were tumors, not an assessment of the health of the entire body. But by 1978, when Dr. Contreras had compiled the results of 4,800 cases in separate five-year periods, he took into account the entire span of results, both subjective and objective, to indicate that laetrile, and usually its attendant metabolic program, achieved sweeping results in both areas in a majority of patients.

In fact, the statistics that Dr. Contreras developed—and was barred from presenting at the Twelfth International Cancer Congress in Buenos Aires in 1978—were similar to those developed by all practitioners around the world who had appreciable caseloads and adequate time for follow-up. These included Dr. Wedel of Oregon, Dr. Phillip Binzel of Ohio, the late Dr. Helen Calvin of Indiana, Drs. James Privitera and Stewart Jones of California, and very much the burgeoning caseload of Dr. John A. Richardson, who recorded his results in *Laetrile Case Histories,* the Cydel Clinic load, that of the Fairfield Medical Centre in Jamaica, the Navarro experience in the Philippines, and a few others.

These pioneers have come up with between 65 and 70 percent "positive response"—this phrase including everything from a patient's simply feeling better, to those 3 to 4 percent of cases in which all signs and symptoms of cancer vanished and had disappeared for at least five years. This general figure is far from a perfect record for amygdalin-based metabolic therapy, since it implies that 30 to 35 percent of patients received no appreciable effect. Yet the importance of the numbers is that the vast bulk of patients seen by all these physicians had already been declared "terminal," and usually came to the clinics with but weeks or months to survive. They were, indeed, looking for a miracle, and none of the therapists referred to here have ever promised miracles.

In terms of laetrile, a few surviving patients originally treated by Ernst T. Krebs, Sr., M.D., and Dr. Navarro constitute the "recordholders" for survival—a handful, admittedly, but impressive nonetheless. The most frequently monitored case is Mrs. Carmen Gutierrez of Manila, the former terminal (metastasized) breast cancer case who (as of 1982) had completed twenty years of recovery—by most accounts a "cure."

At this writing, Mrs. Gutierrez is not on a specific supplemental program *per se*, though she does watch her diet and intermittently takes laetrile. Many patients, for example Glen Rutherford in Kansas, for whom the Supreme Court case involving laetrile affidavits is named, have continued on rigorously-adhered-to regimens of supplements and dietary changes.

By 1982, and in no small part due to the continued U.S. District Court affidavit process for the legal importation of amygdalin and the "decriminalization" of laetrile in twenty-four states, laetrile was available for use on a per-patient basis in a score of clinics across the United States. Metabolic/nutritional therapies were available in these and in other clinics, but it was quite difficult for a complete program to be achieved in the United States alone because some of the substances used, and the uses of other substances, and many of the diagnostic techniques involved, were regarded as illegal or unethical. Hence, "alternative clinics" continued to flourish in Mexico and several other countries primarily for American patients who could afford to leave their homeland. Hoxsey-centered, Gerson-centered, amygdalin-centered, enzymes-centered, vaccine-centered and general holistic clinics and hospitals exist for the refugees from American medicine.

While in earlier days most laetrile-using patients represented the flotsam and jetsam of orthodoxy and had been cut, burned, and poisoned all to no effect, in the past few years a growing number of "virgin cases," that is, patients with no prior orthodox treatment, have successfully been controlled with the metabolic program. It is also true that some of these have failed. Outrageously, medical orthodoxy was always quick to write off failures in the previously treated group as "failures for laetrile." For those who seemed to respond to the metabolic/nutritional program, orthodoxy was always quick to argue that it had been due to "previous treatment." For those who obviously felt better but still had tumefaction, orthodoxy could claim a "placebo effect" was underway, or—and this was quite correct in many cases—that simply by removing patients from chemotherapy and/or radiation they might undergo a short-term period of "feeling better." For those who had the records to prove that they had indeed responded to laetrile, vitamins, minerals, enzymes, and the diet and had *not* received prior treatment, the unarguable concept of "spontaneous remission" was reserved. For those who were responding, however dramatically, but who did not have a full-scale medical records workup to document their improvement over their conditions under earlier therapies, the insulting analyses of "prior misdiagnosis" or "the patient never had cancer in the first place" were often made.

Some of the most exciting work I came across in the natural approach to cancer through the use of presumptive vitamin B^{17} compounds is in Indonesia, where Dr. Goenawan and his staff in a converted tuberculosis sanatorium have been using bitter cassava as the basis for a metabolic program for cancer for more than seventeen years. Aside from a carefully watched diet and adjunctive vitamin therapy and the occasional use of immune stimulants, the patients at Goenawan's Cisarua Sanatorium are fed up to ninety grams of Sao Pedro Petro—"bitter"—cassava a day. This strain of cassava was originally grown in Brazil and is cultivated in the benign climate of the Cisarua area between Jakarta and Bandung, Java, Indonesia. The patients also take hot baths in water filled with cassava leaves, and the cassava may be used as poultices and tampons. The active vitamin B^{17} compound is linamarin.

Dr. Todotua Simandjuntak, a Goenawan disciple who authored several papers on the program, noted that the SPP variety of cassava has approximately 200 mg of cyanide per kilogram of raw cassava, as opposed to approximately 25 mg in common cassava. The abundance comes in the 1,830 mg of linamarin per kilogram of SPP cassava. No cases of cyanide death or extreme illness have occurred at Cisarua.

In 1977, Dr. Goenawan, one of Indonesia's grand old men of medicine, and also highly respected in military circles, told me that of 3,500 people on whom he had records from their treatment at Cisarua, he had seen 10 percent surviving five years or more—the record so far in a metabolic therapy caseload. Also, of the thousands of patients—whose total therapy cost in 1977 was six dollars a day—he had never seen one who failed to respond at least in some subjective way to his program. Some 85 percent of the patients referred to Cisarua are "terminal," he noted.

I found the Goenawan technique and results to be the most under-reported caseload in cancer therapy. Among other things, they bolster both the prevention and treatment aspects of vitamin B^{17} and suggest that the development of a synthetic linamarin could be one of the most promising avenues in cancer therapy.

Harold Manner And The Loyola Mice

A major touchdown for amygdalin-based metabolic therapy was scored in late 1977 when the chairman of the department of biology at Loyola University in Chicago made a startling announcement. He and a team of graduate students had achieved 100 percent positive responses, and 89 percent total regressions, in mice specially bred to develop breast cancer by treating them with a combination of vitamins B^{17} and A and protein-digesting enzymes. Moreover, Harold Manner, Ph.D., was to announce months later, more than 100 women with breast cancer were responding to the same approach, with vitamin C and dietary manipulation added.

Dr. Manner's announcement caught the opposition off guard. Working quietly for several years on the theory of action of amygdalin, combining it with other vitamins, and gathering information from laetrile-using clinics, this department chairman of a prestigious university was not suspected of being part of the "laetrile apparatus." He made his announcement at a meeting of the National Health Federation and continued to repeat it, with a recitation of facts and figures, at public meetings around the country. While his report was submitted to regional scientific academies later, his open airing of the Loyola tests was the only evidence that they had ever taken place.

But rather than the Establishment seizing on the announced protocols and seeking to replicate them, its spokesmen criticized the Loyola biologist for not having published his results in a "learned" journal. In self-defense Dr. Manner argued that he did not believe American women should have to wait eighteen to twenty-four months before such promising work appeared in the pages of a scientific journal.

Extrapolating his findings to humans, Manner and his research team argued that a daily regime of twelve grams of intravenous amygdalin, a million units of emulsified vitamin A taken orally, and a minimum of fifteen grams of vitamin C per day, together with the injection of twenty-five grams of proteolytic enzymes in a tumor, would bring about its destruction. The tests he and his students ran on mice also included toxicity studies and a series of combinations of agents until the B^{17}-A-enzymes formula proved successful.

Dr. Manner was careful to point out that the long-term effects of the treatment in humans could not be estimated at such an early date, "but in the meantime, while they wait, these women have not lost their breasts."

The Manner research was criticized by officialdom on the grounds that it relied too heavily on enzymes and that the animal studies were wanting in several areas. Nonetheless, a number of clinics and doctors by 1980 had adopted "the Manner program" of combined enzyme-vitamin-amygdalin therapy and were reporting heartening results. (The "Manner program," the "Kelley program," or any program along similar lines, are stylized versions of general parts of the entire metabolic/nutritional galaxy. All have a place in the final victory over cancer and probably of degenerative disease in general.)

Dr. Manner has detailed in his own book *(The Death of Cancer,* Advanced Century Publishing, Chicago: 1978) how word that he was legally buying pure amygdalin from a U.S. company for use in cancer experiments greatly increased the red tape generated for such purchases. Although he had long been licensed to receive, store, and use drugs and pharmaceuticals in the state of Illinois and had done so repeatedly, he had never before encountered so much difficulty as he did in securing supplies of amygdalin, he said.

Many metabolic therapists did not perceive that the Manner trials meant the last word in cancer therapy—indeed, some of them also criticized the excessive use of enzymes—but the tests provided one more big piece of evidence for the validity of the overall metabolic/nutritional approach.

The Future Of Amygdalin In Metabolic/Nutritional Therapy

The future of amygdalin in cancer therapy seems assured if only because the concept of *treating* cancer will continue, for a long time, to take precedence over *preventing* the malady outright. And amygdalin's role in the treatment process will be along two lines:

• Its continuing role in metabolic therapy as a primary ingredient in that therapy, even if it is demonstrated that other substances may be of greater importance.

• The development of a laetrile "drug" based on its glucuronide structure. Indeed, as this was written, something of a race seemed to be on in the ranks of both orthodoxy and unorthodoxy to come up with a synthetic laetrile—that is, a laetrile artificially produced outside the body and in its glucuronide form, a fit target for the beta-glucuronidase elicited in the cancer process.

The exploitation of beta-glucuronidase activity through linking toxic compounds with glucuronic acid was well underway by 1981, with the Japanese announcing that a 5-FU-glucuronide compound had achieved antitumor effects in test animals.

The scramble for "second-generation" laetriles, that is, synthetic equivalents or derivatives of amygdalin's breakdown products, is underway. In fall 1978 Dr. Hans Nieper of Hanover, West Germany, who helped vindicate the vitamin B^{17} principle in Germany with the development of "B^{17} orotate," and who is well regarded by American orthodoxy, told me, "Mother laetrile had laid her eggs, and boy, does she have a brood!"

The American cancer Establishment had earlier been shaken by conclusions reached by Israel's Drs. Rubin and Myron Issahary, who had visited the Mexican laetrile-using clinics. These two researchers had found that laetrile has merit, is not quackery, and should be used in all stages of cancer treatment. Contradictory statements attributed to others in Israel that "laetrile has never been used" there (even though laetrile was indeed the subject of ongoing investigations there in the mid-1970s), were used against the laetrile movement. The Israelis, however, were only being precise. Laetrile as described in the *Merck Index* (a synthetic) had indeed never been used in Israel. Or most anywhere.

Semantic precision became doubly important as this decade began, for with the development of synthetics would come patent rights, and profits. Amygdalin itself could never be patented, for it has been "grandfathered" by being in existence for ages, one of the chief reasons why the laetrile proponents, even if they *had* considered amygdalin to be a drug, were not willing to risk millions of dollars in research to vindicate the substance.

The onrush of evidence to support the theory and action of amygdalin has at least opened up a whole new dimension of research, and has led, inextricably, to Establishment efforts to co-opt it, a damning with faint praise for which a generation of cancer sufferers can only be thankful.

All such enthusiasm, of course, still deflects from the central reality of the vitamin B^{17} controversy, that cancer is probably preventable through the willful addition of the substance in the diet. This, not the securing of patent rights to a truly effective new drug, would be the *real* revolution in cancer.

In the meantime, the laetrile-stimulated advances in metabolic/nutritional therapy have underscored the realities of the chronic, systemic, metabolic nature of cancer. They have forced a whole new look at all aspects of nutritional causation and manipulation of the disease. They have focused heavily on the reality that to shrink or destroy a tumor is *not* in itself a victory over the disease of cancer, or of the disease-proneness of the individual.

They have brought to the fore a host of novel approaches, including the exciting promise of endocrine system stimulation by live-cell therapy, the integration of chiropractic (from the West) and acupuncture (from the East) in both treatment and diagnosis, the experimental use of everything from hyperbaric oxygenation to kinesiological (muscle acceptance-rejection) and irrodological evaluation (reading whole-body health through changes in the iris) in diagnosis. They have, of course, likewise attracted the camp followers, hangers-on, offbeat theorists, and general excess baggage that any great movement inevitably attracts. But out of all the mishmash of ideas, movements, research, and theories, the effort at whole-body evaluation and whole-body treatment is advancing geometrically.

The interlocking strands of research and advocacy in all aspects of metabolic management of cancer are leading to non-toxic, non-invasive, natural modalities for all of degenerative disease and its *prevention*.

Dr. Sattilaro And The Macrobiotic Diet

The September 1980 *Saturday Evening Post,* as a mainstream reflection of the times, heralded the advent of new thought in cancer with the stirring account of how Dr. Anthony Sattilaro, president of Philadelphia's Methodist Hospital, had seemingly "cured" himself of widely disseminated cancer simply by practicing the "macrobiotic" diet, one composed chiefly of whole grains and vegetables.

The diagnoses—and the confirmed absence of cancer in Dr. Sattilaro after fifteen months of "unorthodox" or "unproven" *natural* therapy—were of extreme significance because they were made in the United States on a U.S.A.-credentialed physician, and because Dr. Sattilaro had originally been given just a year and a half to live.

As the *Post* put it:

> The impact of Sattilaro's recovery is still being felt at Methodist Hospital. Several doctors and other staff members at Methodist have already changed their diets. His secretary... is now practicing macrobiotics, as are other staff members. But what is most apparent, according to Sattilaro and the hospital staff, is that his recovery has caused an important reassessment of diet's role in the treatment of disease.

Dr. Sattilaro, certainly no quack, had earlier gone the route of orthodoxy for prostatic cancer—a needle biopsy of the prostate which left him with an infection, followed by three operations (including removal of his testicles); administration of the female hormone estrogen, which provoked severe nausea; and the use of a morphine-cocaine-compazine combination to control his pain. He rejected the suggestion of cobalt. Only by coincidence did he, in an emaciated and fatigued state, make contact with the Philadelphia East West Foundation, where he learned of, then followed, the macrobiotic diet—50 percent cooked whole grains (brown rice, wheat, barley, millet, *etc.*), 25 percent locally grown vegetables, 15 percent beans and sea vegetables, the remainder condiments, seeds, and nuts.

As. Dr. Sattilaro later described his response to this "unproven remedy" (and vitamin B[17] proponents would be remiss in not noting the B[17] contents, among many other good things, in the diet), "Everything that I knew in terms of my Western training as a physician argued against continuing this approach. And yet, what was happening was that I basically had never felt better in my whole life...."

Four months after Dr. Sattilaro went off estrogen, and fifteen months after he began the macrobiotic diet, bone scan and gamma camera showed him free of cancer. But he remained on what metabolic/nutritional physicians call the "transition" and "restorative" programs—altered, carefully monitored eating habits being central to them.

There will have to be many more Sattilaros, many more Carmen Gutierrezes first overcoming the life-threatening "crisis" phase of cancer management and going on to survive through the "transition" and "restorative" phases, before the majority of American oncology looks seriously at these flings with "unorthodoxy." But the evidence is mounting. Its message is simple—you don't *have* to die from cancer.

Note: New aspects in the metabolic/nutritional management of cancer to develop monthly. Going into 1983, there was increased interest, primarily from Soviet research, into hydrazine sulfate as a major contributor to resolving the cancer question.

In Mexico, the Bradford Research Institute-American Biologics complex was pioneering "free-form" amino acids and microwave hyperthermia as vital adjunctives to its metabolic programs. Development of several formulations of "free-form" amino acids was also proceeding almost surreptitiously in the U.S.A.

In June, 1982, the most important bombshell dropped by the Establishment—reflecting the externalizing of internal struggles within the Club—came in the form of a 400-page report released by the government's National Research Council (NRC). The report, including extensive documentation and a compilation of research in many areas, found "increasingly impressive" evidence of the links between diet, nutrition, and cancer. It found cancer-inhibition links to vitamins A and C and foods which contain them and even parenthetically referred to widespread evidence of cancer inhibition by "aromatic isothiocyanates" and their components—a frightfully complicated way to say "vitamin B^{17}."

The report, by this nation's blue-ribbon scientific advisory body, also argued to dietary changes along the lines of those previously advocated by the metabolic/nutritional mavericks. This impressive *volte-face* from within orthodoxy is a sign of the times. The report was titled, appropriately enough, *Diet, Nutrition and Cancer.*

Chapter Nine
Suppressed Nutrients

Are We Chronically Deficient?
The metabolic/nutritional medical revolution is shedding light on every nutrient that goes into the body, and along the way is bringing new vitamins to the forefront (B^{15} and B^{17}, for example) while exonerating and expanding the claims made for the "traditionals."

It is also probing the role of minerals and the application of enzymes, and seeing in the vitamin-mineral-enzyme hormone-machinery intricate interlocking parts of the holistic totality of health, a mechanism grievously disturbed by the artificial environment and artificial food that civilized man has created.

The Club has paid little attention to the role of nutrients in disease prevention and treatment, but the sheer force of evidence, let alone political success as in the laetrile movement, has caused it to undergo what an earlier era would call an "agonizing reappraisal."

It is still heresy in American orthodox medicine to claim that there can be a general nutritional therapy, other than in those specific deficiency states that orthodoxy agrees *do* exist. It is commonplace now to regard rickets, pellagra, beriberi, night blindness, pernicious anemia, and scurvy as specific vitamin-deficiency diseases, yet the manner in which each of these states was ultimately linked to the appropriate vitamin is a story, usually slow and agonizing, in and of itself.

What the new wave of physicians is suggesting is that modern man has likely created a whole conglomeration of deficiency states of which he is not directly aware. If the Krebses are anywhere near the mark, for example, Western man has a chronic, unrelieved vitamin B^{17} deficiency whose most notorious manifestion is cancer. For some of the vitamin C partisans, as we shall see, Western man also suffers from chronic, subclinical scurvy. A number of researchers with impeccable Establishment credentials have argued that there is at least an insinuated vitamin A deficiency among civilized peoples. Indeed, due to the absence of many vital nutrients because of the multiple procedures of food processing and the milling of grains, there is a potential series of deficiencies of major vitamins and minerals. It is these deficiency states that, when *compounded* by the assault of synthetic and toxic chemicals, ultimately lead to one or more degenerative disease conditions that are not only treatable through recourse to natural, nontoxic substances—the vitamins, minerals, and enzymes themselves in graduated doses—but preventable through changes in diet and life style.

It is not the scope of this book to make a case for each of the nutrients whose use is being discovered or rediscovered. Information is now coming in from many areas on a variety of these.

In this chapter I call attention to four promising vitamins, each of which has stimulated its own controversy, and each of which is being demonstrated as useful, indeed vital, in helping curb the plague of degenerative disease. The *acceptance* of vitamins A, C and E is not itself a controversy—it is the *applications* of these substances over which a major rumpus with orthodoxy has occurred and will continue to occur. In the matter of vitamin B^{15}, as in the case of vitamin B^{17}, securing a fair hearing for the nutrients *as* a vitamin—a catalytic factor necessary to human life itself—has been almost as big a fight as the debate over its use.

It is generally held that, save in those specifically identified vitamin deficiency conditions for which A, C, D, E, and certain of the B vitamins have been demonstrated to be the answer, Americans generally do not need vitamin and mineral supplements. We get all we need, we are told, by following a more or less "balanced diet." As we have seen, the concept of the "balanced diet" in our technological society is essentially a myth, and the "recommended daily allowances" of nutrients do not relate to reality.

It *is* true that the individual who lives on his own "organic" farm hundreds of miles from a center of human habitation will have an excellent chance to provide himself with enough of the natural nutrients he needs to approach an optimum situation in which he may stave off degenerative disease and live in relative good health till the time of his passing as ordained by his genetic material. But such a scenario does not pertain to 99.9 percent of Americans—and it is for them, the metabolic physicians say, that at least some form of supplementation is called for.

The natural diet—good health—longevity link is anecdotally, and empirically, obvious from the informal studies of primitive populations. It is intriguing to note that in those groups already defined as either cancer-free or at least statistically close to that happy description, degenerative disease in general is less reported.

This includes the highly touted Hunzakuts of Pakistan, the Vilcabamba Indians of Ecuador, several peoples of Southeast Asia, Abkhasians of the Soviet Union, and, indeed, tribes in the Americas and those particular religious sects and denominations that, for whatever reasons, are more (but by no means exclusively) vegetarian in their diet and shy away from stimulants. It is also true that most of these populations work harder physically and that their lives are not dominated by the automobile. It is almost axiomatic that the harder they work and the poorer they are the better their chances of survival to "ripe old age" often are. Literally forced to live off the land, they are continually ingesting whole fruits, vegetables, and grains in a natural, raw and/or sprouting stage before these foods have been stored, frozen, cooked, canned, buffered, emulsified, flavor-added, or preserved. These people are indeed getting "recommended daily allowances" of vitamins and minerals, and they also are bringing in the enzymes that go along with them.

In 1965, researchers of the Vascular Research Laboratory at Maimonides Hospital in Brooklyn advanced the theory that primitive men in Africa, consumers of whole grains, were free from noninfectious heart disease. In 1959, two researchers at Makerere College Medical School, Kampala, Uganda, found much the same evidence by examining the present-day population of Uganda.

At the time, half the population of Kampala consisted of poor blacks, the other half relatively prosperous Indians—later to be expelled from the country. The researchers noted that the staple of the poor blacks was hulled millet with maize. It is common for them to boil the millet and use with it a sauce made of fibrous plants and fruits. They eschew eggs and milk products as well as meat. The Makerere researcher found them to be free of heart attacks involving myocardial infarction (clotting or blockage in the heart muscle) and free of diseases involving clotting in the circulatory system.

The Indians, who were vegetarians by religion, nonetheless ate "differently." Wayne Martin records it this way, "These Indians like their food swimming in fat. The Kampala Indians, in common with Americans, got 50 percent of their calories as fat. While the blacks consume high-fiber-food...the Indians liked white rice, which is almost fiber-free, and refined sugar, they consumed many eggs and butter fat...and they used large quantities of hydrogenated cottonseed oil."

The result—while virtually no blacks died of diseases of veins and arteries, half the deaths of Indians were attributed to such ailments.

The "poor" people of Kampala, then, forced to rely on the food at hand and tampering with it only little, have been getting most of the nutrients they need to stay free of most forms of cardiovascular disease. Their more affluent neighbors, at the time, were able to afford a "richer" diet. Not only did they deprive themselves of some of the nutrients they needed, but by adding refined carbohydrates and excess animal fats, they were loading their bodies with elements antagonistic to their own evolutionary, biological experience.

Such scattered reports should not, however, fuel a back-to-nature movement by overglorifying what the "noble savages" do. Some forms of malnutrition and chronic deficiencies in one or more vital substances, along with parasites and infections, also plague primitive peoples. The healthy reliance on cassava, for example, however great a block to cancer it may be, may also lead to other deficiencies when intake of protein is not adequate.

What the Kampala and similar studies point to is the biological wisdom of whole-grain diets and natural vegetables with a small intake of animal protein and an avoidance of refined carbohydrates. They do not signal the need for a crash or fad regimen that totally removes vital nutrients from the diet.

Vitamin B^{15}: The Unsung Miracle

No sooner had the vitamin B^{17} controversy broken full force upon the American governmental-medical-pharmaceutical Club than it had its hands full combating another nightmare, vitamin B^{15}, which had actually been developed before laetrile was put on the market.

Much to the chagrin of the American Establishment, however, vitamin B^{15} was solidly accepted in a number of foreign countries, very much including the Soviet Union, and even by a modest if growing number of American scientists. Worst of all, its codevelopers were the Krebses, father and son.

Vitamin B^{15} was rapidly making inroads into the American market under various forms and labels by 1979 and was routinely used by metabolic/nutritional therapists. It was much harder for the FDA to attempt to "control" it because no specific therapeutic claims were ever made for it. It was not a "drug" to "treat" a specific disease. Nonetheless, by 1978 the FDA had made seizures of the material and it was banned by court order in New Jersey. Similar action followed in 1980.

Unfortunately for the Krebses and laetrile, had the attention ultimately given vitamin B^{17} and cancer first been accorded vitamin B^{15} (pangamic acid, pangamate, etc.), it might possibly have found its way into acceptance by orthodoxy on such a vast scale that when vitamin B^{17} came along, it would have had fewer credibility problems. For vitamin B^{15} had no cancer Establishment to fight. It was not being used as one-shot, single-modality treatment for anything. It was just *there*. Alarmingly and gnawingly *there*. And *working*.

As in the case of laetrile, a tawdry battle over patient rights, real and imagined, has surrounded vitamin B^{15}, with various companies and promoters sniping at each other and arguing over who had the "real stuff" among several dozen formulations promoted as "vitamin B^{15}"—but that market battle in no way undercut the validity of vitamin B^{15} in theory and in practice. As is also the case with laetrile, vitamin B^{15}'s history is tangled, and seems to have originated along entirely separate paths of research. Moreover, there is controversy even among some major proponents of the substance as to whether it is specifically a vitamin or a preparation—or preparations—of what some see as the only really "B^{15}" active ingredient, a nutrient called N, N-dimethylglycine (DMG), whose existence was first reported in 1941. Research into DMG continued by American, German, and Japanese scientists before the Krebses actually proclaimed "vitamin B^{15}." Stories in *New York* magazine and the *Wall Street Journal* in 1978, combined with the FDA's confiscations of the material, all of which only served to expand interest in pangamic acid, zoomed the vitamin from comparative obscurity to open-throttle national furor. The half-dozen or so shipments of the vitamin that the FDA had seized in 1978 did nothing more than whet the nation's demand for more information, and this at a time when the laetrile fever was at record high.

About the same time, the B^{15} craze hit Canada, not only because of the propaganda in the United States but because of persistently good reports on the substance from Soviet scientists—who admit the Russians got the original idea from Krebs ("a prophet is without honor in his own country"), and because of the known use of the vitamin by Russian and other Eastern Bloc athletes. Soviet research, supported by scattered reports from other countries, gives the substance high marks for its effects on heart disease and allied states. It has been prescribed in the USSR for senility, autism, gangrene, alcoholism, allergies, schizophrenia, neuritis, neuralgia, emphysema, liver problems, and syphilitic lesions, and was found useful in diabetes.

Nutritionally-minded physicians in this country have used it in the above conditions as well as a speculated block to air pollution and for its probable role in the prevention of cancer as a B vitamin. Orthodoxy has, in the main, not yet agreed that this ubiquitous, water-soluble food factor is itself a vitamin, even though it has been listed as a vitamin in such prestigious indices as the *Merck Index*. Health-food faddists had long been interested in pangamic acid, simply on the basis of the known Soviet research, but when *New York* reported that former heavyweight boxing champion Muhammad Ali, runner Dick Gregory, and medical writer Dr. Robert Atkins routinely used it, interest blossomed geometrically.

The English-language *Moscow News* reported in April 1978 that "an important feature of this vitamin is that, to all intents and purposes, it is completely non-toxic.... Soviet doctors often prescribe calcium pangamate [a frequent designation of vitamin B^{15}] alongside corticosteroids or sulfanilamide preparations since it considerably reduces the toxic effects of the large doses of these drugs."

The Krebses developed pangamic acid from apricot kernels, the same providential material from which purified amygdalin (laetrile) was originally extracted, but it is also found in many other fruit seeds, in cereals, rice hulls, yeast, shoots, ox blood, and horse liver. Its near-ubiquity in seeds gave rise to its designation ("pan-gamete") and provided one argument for its proper classification as a B-complex vitamin.

But its early isolation and identification as a vitamin received about as much favorable attention in its country of origin as did laetrile. The Russians, however, picked up on the Krebs work (dating from 1951) with a vengeance. After experimenting with the original Krebs formula and using it on animals and a thousand patients, Soviet scientists introduced it into pharmacies in the 1960s, with Prof. Yakov Shpirt of Moscow Clinical Hospital No. 60 predicting it would eventually become as common as table salt.

The *Moscow News* reported its synthesis by the A. Bakh Institute of Biochemistry of the USSR Academy of Sciences. It has been produced in conjunction with the Moscow Experimental Vitamin Factory by the Russian pharmaceutical industry under the trade name Calcium Pangamate, and its official description is "an active substance that can improve the lipid metabolism, increase the oxygen takeup by the tissues, remove the effects of oxygen insufficiency, and also diminish the side effects caused by other drugs."

Used in capsule form, vitamin B^{15}—when available—has become a standard part of metabolic therapy in America and, since it apparently facilitates oxygen uptake at the cellular level, it seems to complement the action of vitamin E.

New York reported that "Soviet athletes eat B^{15} like candy, and Russian experiments on swimming rats and human rowers showed a decrease in the buildup of lactic acid, the cause of muscle fatigue. Thus the appeal to long-distance runners like Dick Gregory." Indeed, vitamin B^{15} as a stimulator of cell respiration—essential to the life and health of the cell, and whose blockage helps set the stage for cancer, in conformity with principles laid down decades ago by Otto Warburg (but long opposed in this country)—*should* be a metabolic agent par excellence.

Dr. Shpirt has encapsulated vitamin B^{15} indications this way:

> Moreover, it has been found...that vitamin B^{15} restores impaired metabolism in the myocardium [heart muscle] by increasing its creatine content while simultaneously dilating the venous vessels of the heart. At the same time vitamin B^{15} exhibits a lipotropic action [preventing the accumulation of excess fat in the liver]. When it is added that

vitamin B^{15} has no undesirable side effects and that its toxic dose for man is 100,000 times the therapeutic dose...the interest in the drug displayed by clinicians is understandable.

He also reported on the first confirmation of the use of vitamin B^{15} in diabetes mellitus and noted its usefulness in combating the ravages of old age:

> Since calcium pangamate stimulates protein metabolism in the myocardium, normalizing lipid metabolism owing to the presence of labile methyl groups and simultaneously enhancing oxidative processes, it is evident that its use in advanced and old age must become one of the most effective therapeutic measures. The expediency of its use with a view to preventing premature aging is hardly subject to doubt when one takes into account the fact that it causes no undesirable side-effects on lengthy administration. The effectiveness of calcium pangamate in diseases such as atherosclerosis, coronary sclerosis, pneumosclerosis and obliterative atherosclerosis of the lower extremities, which often attend premature aging, increases our conviction that calcium pangamate must find extensive application in the prevention and treatment of premature aging.

The Soviets also found vitamin B^{15} effective in a number of cases of mild diabetes, and all manifestations of gangrene disappeared in eight of eleven patients treated with the vitamin.

Stephen King, Ph. D., of the University of Houston Department of Chemistry, a major researcher of the pangamates, reported that "the metabolism of pangamic acid is tied in with the great biochemical cycles that regulate cellular activity." Being such, the net result of vitamin B^{15} administration (or ingestion) is that "pangamic acid serves as a methylating agent, a lipotropic agent, and a precursor of valuable materals for the cell membrane and neurotransmitters." Dr. King did pioneering work in developing vitamin B^{15} products associated with necessary minerals.

The FDA has been quick to put down the extensive Soviet research and the scattered information from other countries as "inadequate." It has not of course found vitamin B^{15} "harmful"' though a study in 1980 suggested that one element in one formulation of B^{15} might be an indirect cause of cancer. All it can claim in attempts to block the American public from access to it is that it *may* be construed in some treatment programs as an "unlicensed new drug" or as a "mislabelled or misbranded" substance under terms of the Food, Drug and Cosmetic Act, under which it is almost certain that aspirin, penicillin, insulin, and digitalis would never have been approved, as we have seen.

And, as in the case of vitamin B^{17} (laetrile), there is little the FDA can do to stop Americans from getting *natural* pangamic acid by ingesting seeds, brewer's yeast, rice bran, wheat germ, barley, corn and oat grits, wheat bran and wheat flour, or even slurping down ox blood.

And the vitamin B^{15} message has a way of sneaking into orthodox thinking despite the taboo nature of the natural food factor. In the 9 March 1978 *New England Journal of Medicine,* Dr. Peter W. Stacpool made the point that a sister compound of vitamin B^{15} is useful in diabetes and other conditions. *NEJM* editor Arnold S. Relman, M.D., even went so far as to call the B^{15}-related compound a "remarkable agent that may have a potentially very important action in lowering blood lipids."

Dr. Stacpool was discussing "dichloroacetate." It should be noted not only that Dr. Stacpool is the stepson of Ernst T. Krebs, Jr., but that the evolution of vitamin B^{15} is intimately linked to that of DIPA (diisopropylammonium dichloroacetate), which was synthesized by Krebs and Krebs subsequent to the discovery, isolation, and synthesis of vitamin B^{15}. Like pangamic acid, DIPA has received little attention in the United States, but has been the subject of studies in the Soviet Union, Germany, Italy, and Japan.

In the meantime, vitamin B^{15} continues to win favor with metabolically oriented physicians and researchers, including biochemist Richard Passwater, who reportedly interested Muhammad Ali in its use; Dr. Carl C. Pfeiffer, a pioneer in megavitamin therapy and director of Princeton's Brain Bio-Center; Dr. Robert Atkins, who said he rated the vitamin "with the upper echelon of nutritional agents—on a par with B^6, folic acid, and paraminobenzoic;" Dr. Alan Cott, who used the substance on children with behavorial problems; Dr. Bernard Rimland, director of San Diego's Institute for Child Behavioral Research, who said the vitamin "makes autistic kids more normal" and Dr. Michael Schachter, New York, the metabolic therapist who treated Joey Hofbauer.

Said Dr. Schachter of American orthodoxy's position on vitamin B^{15} and the stepped-up efforts to combat its use:

> Orthodox medicine is not used to thinking about how nutrients can be helpful. It is very much concerned with deciding which nutritional treatments are called faddism and quackery. After all, nutrition tends to reduce the importance of certain kinds of medical practice. I think B^{17} is part of this...

Here we have a virtually nontoxic substance with no side effects. The drug companies don't want to hear about it and will do anything to keep it off the market.

The Fight For Vitamin C

When, with little fanfare, the National Cancer Institute announced in July 1978 that it was allocating $225,000 in grants for the study of vitamin C (ascorbic acid, ascorbate) in cancer, including a clinical (human) trial of the substance, proponents of metabolic therapy perceived one more sign, they thought, that things were changing at the NCI.

The NCI's belated interest in vitamin C came more than a year after the federally funded cancer research arm began studies of a synthetic derivative of vitamin A in human cancer and the same year the NCI was split virtually in two over plans to go ahead with a clinical trial of vitamin B^{17} (laetrile).

Only the more suspicious figured, in the vitamin C research as in the laetrile program, that there might be dirty work afoot even here. And, indeed, as we will see, they were right.

But, for awhile, it signalled that genuine interest had finally been triggered by two-time Nobel Laureate Linus Pauling, Ph.D., who had been fighting for NCI grants for vitamin C studies for five years and who had been consistently rebuffed by the federal researchers in efforts to secure a clinical trial. As of 1978, and with only one major exception, the only institutional journals where Americans might find the best evidence for vitamin C in cancer therapy were published in Europe.

The laetrilists alone could not take credit for the NCI's sudden interest in the vitamin, even though it is routinely used as a part of the general metabolic/nutritional management program for the disease. Someone, somewhere, had simply felt that there was something to the evidence amassed by a number of researchers, most prominently Dr. Pauling, chemist Irwin Stone, and Scotland's Dr. Ewan Cameron, who has done the major "on-line" work in this regard.

By the late 1970s, aside from the carefully monitored group of Cameron patients and several more in the United States, evidence for vitamin C in cancer treatment and prevention continued to mount in laboratory tests. A Canadian research team found in 1978 that vitamin C was "pretty well 100 percent effective" in preventing cancer from the preservatives found in ham, bacon, and other smoked meats.

Dr. Robert Whiting of the Univeristy of British Columbia's Cancer Research Center reported on experiments of ascorbic acid on laboratory cultures of human cells to which nitrosamines—cancer-causing agents—were added. The vitamin C seemed to block the formation of abnormal cells associated with cancer and the level of nitrosamines decreased. The nitrosamines form when nitrites, which are ingredients of meat preservatives, mix with stomach acids. Dr. Whiting estimated that 50 to 100 milligrams of vitamic C are enough to protect against such preservatives.

Dr. Pauling and chemist Irwin Stone have been the American pioneers fighting a lonely battle for the recognition of vitamin C in cancer (and in the prevention of colds, Dr. Pauling's first major crusade for the substance), while Dr. Albert Szent-Gyorgyi, who won the Nobel Prize for the isolation of vitamin C, has continued to stress the necessity of the nutrient in human metabolism.

The vitamin C pioneers argue that the civilized world suffers from a chronic vitamin C deficiency, with people ingesting only a tenth as much ascorbic acid in their daily diets as is necessary to maintain the body's defense mechanisms in top form. The basis for this supposition is the fact that man, other primates, and guinea pigs are deficient in one or more enzymes necessary for converting the substance gulonolactone to ascorbic acid, into which the latter is biosynthesized—a process normal to all other animals. Animals under stress "create" enormous amounts of the substance. Man, however, is forced to rely on exogenous (outside) vitamin C. Other mammals, for example, are known to manufacture 60 to 300 milligrams of C per kilogram of body weight per day, or the equivalent of a 150-pound human's production of 10 grams a day. Also, gorillas eat foods that contain vitamin C in amounts approximating 5 grams a day, equivalent to about 2 grams a day for a 150-pound human. Just why man "lost" the capacity to produce his own vitamin C is a subject of heady speculation, but the fact is, he does *not* make his own vitamin C, and therein lies very probably one of the major problems facing mankind in general and civilized man in particular, since the latter is apt to consume far less exogenous vitamin C than did primitive man due to the artificiality of his diet.

Drs. Pauling and Cameron have provided the "hard evidence" for the use of the substance in cancer, publishing in the *Proceedings* of the National Academy of Sciences, following earlier rejections by other journals, including the *Journal of the American Cancer Society*. In 1979 they gathered their clinical experience and a fascinating review of the literature in *Vitamin C and Cancer* (Linus Pauling Institute of Science and Medicine, Menlo Park, Calif., 1979).

The earlier Cameron-Pauling study, published in 1976, compared 100 terminally ill patients given ten grams of vitamin C daily to 1,000 other cancer patients, with both groups treated identically and by the same physicians in the same hospital, with the exception of the C administered to the former. By 1977, all 1,000 "controls" had died, but sixteen of the vitamin C-treated patients were still alive, twelve of them completely free of cancer. The overall result of the study was that the C-treated patients on the average lived more than a year, whereas only three of the control patients survived that long. Linus Pauling wrote:

> The vitamin C treatment seems to have some favorable effect for all kinds of cancer.... The 13 ascorbate-treated patients with cancer of the colon lived more than seven times as long, on the average, as their 130 matched controls. The next largest effect, a nearly sixfold increase in survival time, was observed for patients with breast cancer, followed by a five-times increase in survival time for patients with cancer of the kidney.... At the present time the conclusion can be drawn that a high intake of vitamin C is beneficial for all patients with advanced cancer.

Even so, as Cameron and Pauling explained in a second paper published two years later, "Several experienced investigators in this field have expressed to us their doubt as to whether ascorbate-treated patients and their controls comprised representative subpopulations of the same population and whether comparable times of untreatability had been assigned to the two groups. We decided to investigate these questions."

So the two researchers selected a new set of control patients, and essentially the same group of vitamin C patients and the controls were indeed representative subpopulations of the same population of "untreatable" patients. Survival times were measured not only from the date of "untreatability" but also from the precisely known date of the first hospital admission for the cancer that eventually reached the terminal stage.

This second set of findings, reported in the *Proceedings* of the National Academy of Sciences in September 1978, was even more heartening:

> Our conclusion is that the results previously reported are valid, and in fact, the increase in life expectancy of ascorbate-treated patients with terminal cancer is found to be somewhat larger than was previously reported.

The vitamin C-treated patients were found to have a mean survival time about 300 days greater than that of the controls. Survival times greater than one year after the date of "untreatability" were observed for twenty-two of 100 vitamin C patients against 0.4 percent for the controls. Eight of these were still alive in 1978, with a mean survival time after untreatability of 3.5 years. The twenty-two survived, on the average, 2.4 years after reaching the so-called terminal stage. By 1979, some 500 patients had been treated with vitamin C in Cameron's research, with information being developed on them.

Elsewhere, the *Journal of Orthomolecular Psychiatry,* named for a concept coined by Dr. Pauling in 1968 and emphasizing the treatment of schizophrenia by nutrition, published a lecture by Irwin Stone. Stone, who is credited with getting Dr. Pauling initially interested in vitamin C, wrote *The Healing Factor*—a general discussion of ascorbic acid's healing properties—in 1972. His lecture carried a synopsis of the Pauling-Cameron work and also detailed Stone's views on what he called "chronic, subclinical scurvy"—the universal deficiency of humans in vitamin C, a situation leading to the subtle precursor degenerative disease condition "CSS Syndrome." In his book, the California scientist had reviewed work in vitamin C—which he does not place in the vitamin category—dating back to 1936 and which established a definite link between the nutrient and its effect on cancer. A most impressive account of cancer control with ascorbate was published in the *Medical Times,* Stone noted, in which there was a report of vitamin C doses ranging from 24.5 to 42 grams given to a victim of myelogenous leukemia, bringing about complete remission of the disease. That ascorbate was the healing factor was obvious since the physician in charge twice stopped the doses as an experiment and both times the patient's leukemic symptoms returned.

As Stone told his lecture audience, "This case history was published...22 years ago, and you would think that someone in these many years would have tried this harmless megascorbic therapy in thousands of cases of leukemia that appear each year. A search of the medical literature had failed to reveal anyone publishing a check on these exciting clinical results."

In 1969 Dr. Dean Burk showed in a paper published in *Oncology* that vitamin C kills cancer cells while not harming normal ones. The Burk research group indicated that vitamin C at doses as high as the equivalent of three-quarters of a pound in a 150-pound man had been given to animals without "notable pharmacological effects."

They analyzed, "In our view, the future of effective cancer chemotherapy will not rest on the use of host-toxic compounds now so widely employed, but upon virtually host non-toxic compounds that are lethal to cancer cells of which ascorbate....represents an excellent prototype." Burk and his group pointed out that vitamin C had never been tested for anticancer effects by the Cancer Chemotherapy National Service Center because it was too *non*toxic to fit into their screening programs.

In his lecture Stone noted:

> A substance like ascorbate that will kill cancer cells and be harmless to normal cells had been a

long-time goal and dream of cancer researchers, and in 1969 it looked like it had been achieved. One would expect that a crash program would immediately be organized to thoroughly check and extend these observations and obtain clinical data on this breakthrough. That was seven years ago and no further papers could be found that were published by the National Cancer Institute on this important subject. If an extensive crash research program had been instituted in 1969, the cancer problem may have been solved by now or at least we would know a lot more about the role of ascorbate in cancer.

Stone was not, of course, the first researcher to smell a rat, but he was not fully aware of the murky history of cancer research—and politics—in this country. Nor was Dr. Pauling, at least at the beginning of his investigation.

In 1978 the latter told *Bestways* magazine that even though it has never been shown that one might overdose on vitamin C—and the use of vitamin C at up to 150 grams *per day* has been implemented by some physicians—"there is great pressure working to keep people from taking vitamin C in any amounts that will do them some real good." When *Bestways* asked about where the pressure was coming from, Pauling answered, "From the government for one. And there are more powerful groups behind them. Cereal makers like to say they are giving you one hundred percent of the minimum adult daily requirement and they give you just 50 milligrams in a serving. Whereas you really need at least twenty times that amount to start doing you any real good." He advised four grams a day for most people.

But Pauling had already ruffled the feathers of the medical establishment with his earlier work in *Vitamin C and the Common Cold,* which pointed out how megadoses of ascorbic acid could help head off the most common ailment known to man. The espousal of the vitamin theory of colds prevention earned this double Nobel Laureate an attack from some quarters as a crank and a quack.

In 1978, Pauling told the World Congress on vitamin C in Palm Springs, California, that there is enough evidence now to state that vitamin C-treated cancer patients on the average have survived more than five times as long after being pronounced "terminal" as matched controls who have received no ascorbic acid. He also emphasized an apparent analgesic effect from the substance at high doses, and a restoration of the patient's sense of well-being, symptoms observed in the use of laetrile as well.

Dr. Albert Szent-Gyorgyi, who won the Nobel Prize in 1937 for isolating vitamin C, one of the crowning achievements in a life of scientific innovation, informed the world conference that "ascorbic acid gives life—and the more ascorbic acid you have, the more alive you can be."

"It is the major function of ascorbic acid," he told the audience, "that it acts both as an electron donor and an electron receptor. Without this exchange of electrons, which is below the molecular level, there can be no life." And there is a much greater need for the substance than small amounts of it to prevent scurvy, the only role that medical officialdom in this country has assigned the nutrient. It had, of course, taken almost 200 years for Western medicine to recognize that scurvy *is* a vitamin-deficiency disease, despite work generations earlier that proved this connection in the British navy, and even as late as the second decade of this century some medical textbooks still argued that the real cause of scurvy was unknown.

"I think cancer is to a great extent a question of ascorbate," Dr. Szent-Gyorgyi said. "Cancer is a loosening up of the machine. Things go to pieces. Nobody knows exactly what cancer is, but I do know that in cancer tissue the proteins are very poorly desaturated, that the protein in them is very loose, and I felt strongly that by building a healthy cell from the ascorbic acid right from the beginning, you will get no cancer, or much less cancer."

Nutritionally-minded physician Frederich R. Klenner was on hand to say that he had given patients up to 150 grams of vitamin C daily, both orally and intravenously, in the correction of serious cases of encephalitis of the brain, Rocky Mountain spotted fever, snakebite, attempted suicide, and viral infections.

And Pauling has complained that the National Institutes of Health are not interested in the effectiveness of vitamin C against serum hepatitis. He told *Bestways* that in a 1977 visit to Japan he had seen cases of the complete control of infectious hepatitis in a Fukuoka hospital through the use of large doses of vitamin C. Stanford University Medical School has since begun probing this connection.

The best followed cases of vitamin C in cancer therapy are those of the patients in Scotland, all with advanced cancer and all in the work of Dr. Cameron at Vale of Leven Hospital. Some others in earlier stages of the disease have been treated with vitamin C and conventional therapy with good results, Drs. Pauling and Cameron have jointly reported. These results are, of course, a cluster of cases that have no connection with the composite metabolic/nutritional program for cancer being given by metabolic therapists in the United States and Mexico, where megadoses of vitamins A, C, E, B[15], and B[17] are usually part of the program.

Dr. Cameron's Vale of Leven trials started in 1971 with ten grams of sodium ascorbate, usually given orally but sometimes also by intravenous infusion. One of the most illustrative cases is that of a forty-two-year-old truck driver with a diagnosis of malignant lymphoma. He was scheduled to receive the usual "treatments of choice," chemotherapy and radiation, but because of an administrative delay in sending him to the appropriate facility and his rapid deterioration, he was given vitamin C in the hope that his decline could be slowed down until he could receive the standard modalities. He was placed on a regimen of ten grams per day intravenously for ten days and ten grams per day orally thereafter.

In the manner of a laetrile recovery patient, the truck driver responded dramatically in terms of suddenly feeling fit. His enlarged liver and spleen decreased in size and other symptoms of his disease also declined. He continued taking ten grams of oral vitamin C daily for five months, during which time he remained "well" and went back to work. Unfortunately, the doctor in charge of the case believed the man to be "cured" and halted the oral vitamin C.

A month later, the driver was again sick, and at a routine clinical examination it was determined that the disease had returned. This time when the truck driver was given ten grams of oral C daily there was no such dramatic response as had occurred earlier. Two weeks later the disease had so advanced that he was readmitted to the hospital, whereupon he was administered 20 grams per day intravenously for two weeks and then 12.5 grams daily orally thereafter.

"A slow and sustained clinical improvement" followed, and six months later he was normal in all respects. At the time of the report, the driver was completely well, was in "active heavy employment," and continued to take 12.5 grams of vitamin C daily without a trace of cancer.

Drs. Virginia Livingston (see chapter seven) and William J. Saccoman of San Diego have used megadoses of vitamin C for years, with Dr. Saccoman having used up to 120 grams in four liters of drip solutions daily. It was Dr. Saccoman who independently observed vitamin C's analgesic effects, and he was able to take patients off heavy morphine schedules. He and others have used up to 50 grams of vitamin C daily in oral and intravenous combinations to achieve impressive anticancer effects.

Stone reported on a striking Saccoman case showing that vitamin C *and* toxic chemotherapy can achieve anticancer results, a scenario familiar to laetrile physicians who use vitamin B[17] with toxic drugs:

> Shortly after the operations she was started on toxic chemotherapy. Each chemotherapy session made her extremely sick and totally incapacitated her for 12 or 24 hours. She was also told she would lose all her hair, which only further depressed her. On returning home from the hospital, her father put her on a high ascorbate, high vitamin and mineral regime, giving 30 grams of ascorbate as a mixture of

ascorbic acid, and sodium ascorbate each day orally. She did not lose her hair and a thorough examination six months later after her surgery revealed that there were no signs of the active disease, and the best of all, she was feeling fine. Both the ascorbate and the toxic chemotherapy have been continued to the present, and she is now a very healthy young lady....

Strangely enough, the reports of vitamin use in cancer, while ranging back to the 1930s in Europe, are treated as new discoveries in the United States, where vitamin therapy is still essentially ignored when not outright attacked as quackery. Despite world literature published in the 1950s indicating the usefulness of vitamins A and C in cancer therapy, such information was not taken seriously in this country, by then highly dominated by expensive toxic chemicals and radiation in addition to surgery as treatments of choice. Despite the efforts of Stone and Pauling in the 1960s and 1970s to bring vitamin C to the attention of orthodoxy—and of the proponents of A, E, B^{17}, and B^{15} to do likewise—most of these promising leads were never followed up.

Just how vitamin C "works" in cancer is not fully established. But information about vitamin C is now abundant enough to demonstrate that—as any good vitamin—it has a range of metabolic uses. It is essential in the manufacture of collagen, the "cement" between cells. It is known to help maintain the normal permeability of cell membranes, thus enhancing their health, is essential in the formation of epithelial basement membrane, is an anti-flammatory agent, and is almost certainly an immune system stimulator. It is also a free radical scavenger. It turns out that a primary effect of vitamins A, C, and E is their action against the highly reactive molecular fragments called free radicals. These fragments (designated radicals because they are atoms or clusters of atoms with unpaired electrons) can produce chain reactions to alter thousands of molecules and damage cell membranes. They can also damage the DNA (deoxyribonucleic acid), the genetic building block of life, damage to which may cause cellular abnormalities that may eventually become cancer.

Free radicals are normally held in check by the antiradical vitamins A, C, and E and certain minerals. Also, the number of free radicals can increase whenever there is a deficiency in the "antioxidant" elements (the same vitamins) or when too many chemicals and pollutants that produce such free radicals are consumed.

Dr. Pauling has noted (in "On Vitamin C and Cancer," *Executive Health,* January 1977) that:

> There is evidence that a high intake of vitamin

C operates to increase the effectiveness of essentially all of the protective mechanisms in the human body. Its action in strengthening the intercellular cement was emphasized originally by Cameron, who... suggested that it is able to inhibit the action of the enzyme produced by cancer cells to attack the intercellular cement. It is also known that vitamin C is involved in the various immune mechanisms in such a way that an increased intake makes them more effective in attacking and destroying the malignant cells.

The antiviral and antibacterial effectiveness of vitamin C may also be of significance with respect to cancer.... I believe, as does Irwin Stone, that the greater resistance to cancer and other diseases resulting from a high intake of vitamin C is the result of putting the body into the condition that corresponds to *really* good health. The small amount, 45 milligrams per day, that is recommended by the Food and Nutrition Board is said by that Board to be all that people in "ordinary good health" need. I think, however, that these people are in "ordinary poor health," with enfeebled power of resistance to cancer and other diseases.

The announced 1978 vitamin C clinical trial by the NCI turned out to be the umpteenth example of the Club at work.

In the September 27 issue of the *New England Journal of Medicine,* results of a trial of vitamin C in cancer at the Mayo Clinic, the same institution which was a year later to run the first phase of the laetrile tests, were released. Involved were 123 cancer patients, sixty of whom had been given vitamin C and sixty-three of whom had been given sugar pills.

Because both groups lived an average of seven weeks and the study's authors could find no significant difference in how long the patients lived, how good they felt, or in the progress of symptoms, study leader Dr. Edward T. Creagan told the press, "We can find no current role for vitamin C in the treatment of advanced cancer."

The vitamin C proponents quickly cried "Foul!"

To the press, the stately Dr. Pauling pointed out in detail his long battle to get the NCI to look at vitamin C and to attempt to replicate the Vale of Leven trials. He stressed that, when finally Dr. Vincent DeVita, then the chief of NCI's clinical trails section, said he would arrange for a controlled trail, Pauling had written him that in order to follow the Vale of Leven method as closely as possible, it would be necessary that the terminal cancer patients *not* have received heavy chemotherapy.

"In fact, when the paper on the Mayo Clinic trial was published ...it was seen that Dr. (Charles) Moertel, who planned the Mayo study, had ignored this advice," Dr. Pauling said in a statement issued in his name and that of Dr. Cameron.

The only real meaning of the Mayo study, in Pauling's words, is that "the value of vitamin C is much less for patients whose immune systems have been damaged by chemotherapy than for those who have not received chemotherapy."

Despite the essentially meaningless Mayo study, vitamin C is now routinely used in virtually all combinations of metabolic/nutritional therapy for cancer. Its role as immune stimulant and free-radical scavenger are central in the anti-cancer armament. (Too, as of December 1980, a new round of trials with patients on whom chemotherapy had *not* first been used was announced.)

By 1981, a sharp dispute between vitamin C proponents had erupted as to the meaning of vitamin C in animal tests and the relative importance of other nutritional factors aside from vitamin C in the nutritional management of cancer. The controversy cast doubt on the concept of vitamin C as a "magic bullet" against cancer but emphasized its overall role in metabolic therapy.

The dissenting voice against the Pauling doctrine came from none other than Arthur Robinson, Ph. D., a co-founder of Pauling's Institute and usually accepted as the chief disciple of the Nobel Laureate. In essence, Dr. Robinson charged that while vitamin C *and* a raw fruits and vegetable diet caused an astonishing thirty-five-fold decrease in cancer incidence in test mice in a series of experiments carried out at the Pauling Institute of Science and Medicine in 1978, the same tests also showed that the 10-gram daily vitamin C dose recommended by Pauling for humans actually *increased* the cancer incidence in the test mice, and that the raw fruit and vegetable diet was about as effective as megadoses of vitamin C in preventing cancer.

The publication of these animal tests in whole or part, and omission of some of them in one paper "preprinted" for release, brought the battle between Pauling and Robinson (who was stripped of his executive authority at the Institute and, he said, forced to take a leave of absence without salary) into the open, and triggered charges of bad faith by both scientists.

The orthodox Club, maneuvering at all costs, as usual, to "get something" on vitamin C and cancer, used the internal strife to its best advantage, attempting to claim that proponents themselves had shown that vitamin C was not necessarily the answer to cancer and that it might actually *cause* cancer. Of course, this was hardly the case, since all that was at issue were animal tests, one of which suggested that a certain dose level might cause more cancer than it prevented. Robinson told me in several interviews that he very much defended the use of vitamin C, doubted that it was of very much importance in actual therapy but otherwise had both preventive and health-enhancing roles, and stressed that in his years of work with the nutrient he had failed to see its administration ever shrink a tumor.

The importance of the partially reported animal studies, he emphasized, lay in the preventive and life-extension aspects of vitamin C use. Too, they strongly supported the overall nutritional or metabolic management of cancer, an area of research earlier brought to Pauling's attention by the work of Max Gerson and, more recently, by the diet-and-wheat grass therapy advanced by Eydie Mae Hunsberger, writing about her own case, and researcher Ann Wigmore.

Robinson believes Pauling wished to downplay the importance of diet overall in order to strengthen the overriding role of vitamin C. Dr. Pauling told me he had not wished to publish the dietary aspects of the mouse studies at the time "because we need tests carried out in a more reliable manner."

In the various aspects of the vitamin C movement, the dispute centers on the *therapeutic* value of megadoses of vitamin C versus the *prevention* and life-extension aspects. It is an argument not far removed from the championing of the vitamin B[17] prevention theory versus reliance on megadoses of laetrile as a "magic bullet" against cancer.

It is now obvious that vitamin C will come into its own, not only as a cancer fighter, but for a wide variety of uses that spell good health. And as this vindication is achieved, it will constitute the happy end to a story of vitamins and deficiency diseases that began 400 years ago—and which stands as one of the early, if classic, examples of how orthodoxy can be so often wrong, and so often blind.

For although Szent-Gyorgyi did indeed isolate the vitamin in 1937, its presence as the missing element in scurvy is directly attributable to explorers in the sixteenth, seventeenth, and eighteenth centuries. In 1653, Sir Richard Hawkins of England reported that 10,000 men under his command died from scurvy—and that feeding sailors a lemon or orange each day prevented the disease. Earlier, most of the members of French explorer Jacques Cartier's expedition had become ill with the disease while camping along the Saint Lawrence River. It was an Indian chief who showed Cartier how to make a tea from pine needles that restored the scorbutics to good health in as little as eight days' time. In 1604-06, while forty-seven of the seventy-nine colonists at the Acadian colony founded by the French on the Bay of Fundy were dying of scurvy, their Indian neighbors remained free of disease by drinking pine-needle tea and eating deer adrenals.

In the eighteenth century, James Lind, a doctor in the British navy, spent most of his life fighting scurvy. Despite Sir Richard Hawkins' report of a century and a half before, nothing had been done to stop scurvy, and the dread disease was killing more sailors than ever died in battle. It was in 1753 that Lind "cured" six seamen on the verge of death from scurvy by feeding them an orange a day.

When Lind proposed that an orange or a lime a day would keep scurvy away, English medical orthodoxy turned on him as a heretic. The glory of his ultimate vindication, of course, has been forever enshrined in the popular tag for British sailors, "limeys." Lind died without seeing his point of view established, even though a year later a British fleet made a twenty-three-week voyage stocked with lemons and limes and reported not a single case of scurvy. But almost a century passed before it became mandatory for British sailors to eat a lime a day.

Indeed, by the beginning of the twentieth century, it was still the view of Western orthodox medicine that scurvy was somehow an infectious disease. Its vitamin-deficiency nature was not accepted until the 1920s. That is to say, hundreds of years—whole centuries —had passed before the actual nature of scurvy, and the role of specific foodstuffs in preventing it, were accepted.

The Promise Of Vitamin E

In 1974, the interested American could take his pick of points of view about vitamin E. If he read the 1974 edition of *The Medicine Show,* a publication of Consumers Union supposedly reporting the latest "facts" in medicine, he would have read, "[Consumers Union's] medical consultants discourage, as a waste of money, the use of Vitamin E as a dietary supplement or as a medication for common ailments....For now, CU's medical consultants conclude, there is no convincing evidence that human beings need more vitamin E than they obtain in their ordinary diets, or that Vitamin E is useful in the treatment of any but a few rare diseases."

Or, he could have read that same year in the British medical journal *Lancet* that vitamin E—another free radical scavenger—is important in protecting cell-membrane integrity and is also useful in "intermittent claudication" (leg pain induced by lowered arterial flow). He might also have mulled over some laboratory reports suggesting the rejuvenating elements of vitamin E.

The vitamin was discovered by Drs. Herbert M. Evans and Katherine S. Bishop following earlier leads from other researchers. In 1936 Dr. Evans identified a factor in lettuce leaves that seemed to prevent sterility in rats as tocopherol. The early work on sterility prevention and vitamin E necessarily gave rise to the assumption that it must enhance fertility, and indeed there is some anecdotal evidence for this.

But the result that has most disturbed orthodoxy has been the indication that vitamin E is useful in combating heart disease, at least some manifestations of it, and may to a certain extent prevent it. This work is almost entirely that carried out since 1948 by the brothers Evan and Wilfred Shute in London, Ontario, with results tabulated on some 40,000 vascular disease patients.

Indeed, it was a reading of the Shutes' major book on the subject in the late 1960s that interested me in the entire field of vitamins. I found that a daily administration of vitamin E of from 600 to 800 IUs (International Units) apparently checked a raging skin problem I had suffered with intermittently for five years and which had stumped several dermatologists. As this is another of those nonlaboratory "anecdotes," my favorite dermatologist would not accept that vitamin E had anything to do with the sudden disappearance of my symptoms (where cortisone, salves, even special gloves had failed), but he was open-minded enough to ponder the possibility. This unexpected result from ingesting vitamin E (I had started popping the tablets out of interest in the thousands of cases the Shutes reported on concerning *heart* patients) was enough to convince this nonscientist journalist that the vitamin theory of preventive disease had at least *something* going for it.

The Shute Foundation for Medical Research has detailed the advent of their ground-breaking work in vitamin E therapy, and it should sound familiar by now:

> One would have thought it [alpha tocopherol, the primary vitamin E considered of therapeutic use would have been welcome, since its rivals [in coronary heart disease treatment] were so dangerous or so inadequate....[But] at the time so little was known of the accessory biochemical and physiological properties of alpha tocopherol that the proposal seemed doubly ludicrous. It met with a storm of rejection and is only now recovering from its harsh reception. Had its vascular properties been recognized first...it would have eased into cardiology as gently and persuasively as heparin and dicumarol.
>
> There should have been much preparatory animal work. Unfortunately we had no animals, and we made our observations as opportunity to came to us, not in the "scientific order" generally followed and increasingly insisted on. A wealth of support has accrued to us since, from every corner of the globe....
>
> Suffice it to say...that alpha tocopherol often relieves angina and reduces the need for nitroglycerine. It is almost as useful for thrombosis in the coronary system as elsewhere in the vascular tree. It is the safest and simplest prophylactic agent against the dreaded recurrent assault....It has

sent many a coronary derelict back to his job and reduced mortality, probably—for it is next to impossible to find in the literature an acceptable norm with which to compare its salvage. It has no serious rivals, for it is safe, simple, cheap and requires little or no hospital care—certainly no laboratory guidance.

Consumers Union, again in 1974, noted that "claims made for vitamin E by Drs. Shute, Shute and [Albert] Vogelsang were not based on double-blind or even on simple-blind trials. CU has seen no evidence that they were even based on trials comparing patients with controls."

The Shutes admit most of this, of course. They are among researchers who did not believe that sufferers from severe degenerative disease should be divided into two groups—one receiving something the Shutes *knew* to be of benefit, the others receiving a placebo. There is the gravest kind of ethical question raised in "double-blinds," anyway, particularly if a control group is getting no treatment at all. So the vitamin E researchers have tended to plead guilty to a lack of double-blind tests on humans and to a paucity of animal work, the obsession with which is one of the many reasons necessary substances do not reach the *human* market in the United States.

Luckily, vitamin E has been around without specific claims being made for it, and was more or less accepted as a vitamin before much of the controversy over its use arose. To the best of my knowledge, the FDA has yet to stake out a physician about to receive a load of hot alpha tocopherol and rush in with brandished badges.

The Shutes claim that vitamin E acts as an antithrombin—that is, it helps prevent the formation of blood clots in the circulatory system, helps dissolve blood clots already formed, increases the blood's oxygen transportation, and utilization capabilities, and decreases the heart muscle's need for oxygen. Vitamin E is a general antioxidant—that is, it protects cell membranes and other tissues against negative oxygen reactions. It is probably an immune system stimulator. It protects vitamin A and C against oxidation in the body and protects red blood cells from premature breakdown.

Biochemist Richard Passwater has shown that vitamin E controls the synthesis of prostaglandins (hormonelike compounds) that repair blood platelets. Its functions make it a natural aid in extending the life span of cells, and its detoxification of free radicals and transporting of oxygen make it useful for all-around metabolic health. It is apparently useful in heart disease, aging, senility, arthritis, asthma, muscular dystrophy, glaucoma, burns, emphysema, and a few other degenerative states and disease conditions, and has a role to play in cancer prevention and cancer therapy. It is so useful that it has been called an "elixir" in the tabloid press and from time to time given the same kind of press treatment vitamin B[15]—which it seems to complement—has received.

Metabolic/nutritional therapists frequently give vitamin E in the total therapy of cancer. In 1977 it was reported that it seemed to protect normal tissue from the ravages of the toxic chemotherapy drug adriamycin without lessening the drug's activity against cancer cells.

Dr. Passwater summarizes that the antioxidant vitamins—A, C, E—together with the mineral selenium protect the body against cancer by helping defend cell membranes against carcinogens, protecting the genetic material (DNA) of the cells, stimulating immune responses, and protecting against radiation. Famed surgeon Alton Ochsner used vitamin E with major surgery for twenty years on 15,000 operative cases, without a single patient suffering death from postsurgery embolism.

Going into this decade, there were more research lines than ever to help back up what Wilfrid E. Shute had proclaimed decades ago—that vitamin E is "the greatest discovery in medicine in this century."

By now, far more than 40,000 patients have been treated with vitamin E at the Shute Institute for Clinical and Laboratory Medicine in London, Ontario, Canada, and Dr. Shute was quoted in 1981 as saying:

"We have had patients who have exhibited no trace of heart disability as long as twenty-four years after severe heart attacks. Others, virtually on their death beds, have been placed on the road to recovery and extended life spans. Doses of vitamin E have, in some cases, even eliminated the need for heart surgery."

Dr. Richard Mavis, University of Rochester School of Medicine biochemist, has stated that vitamin E helps protect the linings of veins and arteries against plaque buildup, the primary cause of atherosclerosis, which in turn sets the stage for a wide range of cardiovascular diseases. "I am definitely excited about the possibilities of vitamin E in a protective role," he said.

Dr. Theodore Tyberg, cardiology instructor at Cornell University Medical Center, has also noted that "the basic research findings coming in support the concept that vitamin E helps prevent heart attacks and strokes." Clinical cardiologist Dr. Roger Palmer has also said that although the vitamin E heart attack prevention theory "has been around for years, now basic research is coming in to show that it is correct."

The record continues to develop in favor of vitamin E. And, while it has tended to move within the Club's semantics from quackery to unproven, it has still essentially received a cold shoulder from orthodox medicine. "You get all the vitamin E you need in your diet, so buying capsules is a waste of money," we're told. It's true that we get vitamin E in fresh vegetables, leafy greens, and whole grains. But how many vegetables do we eat, how many of them are fresh, and when was the last time *you* ate whole grains?

Vitamin A and Cancer

While the Club has continued to batter the concept of metabolic/nutritional approaches in cancer management, it has been forced to give way to the new medicine in at least two areas—the concept of stimulating the body's own natural defense system (immunotherapy) to help fight cancer, and the grudging acceptance of the role of vitamin A and its synthetic "cousins" in cancer therapy.

Both concessions can be claimed as victories for the new medicine, as well as the undeniable effect European research has had on American oncology. The metabolic/nutritional therapists can make the claim that more than half the therapies they advance in cancer *are* immune-stimulating substances, and that to say immunotherapy is, in a considerable way, to say metabolic/nutritional or holistic medicine, much to the chagrin of major propaganda pontiffs of the Club medicine whose careers have largely been shaped by denouncing the "nutrition cultists" and the "quackery" of treating cancer with food factors.

For the past several years, even the American Cancer Society has taken note of the undeniable evidence that *retinoids,* synthetic "cousins" of natural vitamin A, prevent bladder and breast cancer in mice and rats and "may" work against cancers of the lung, esophagus and pancreas in humans.

In 1981, researchers from four major scientific institutions in the United States reported in the British medical journal *Lancet* that vitamin A and vitamin A precursor significantly reduce lung cancer levels even in cigarette smokers. They also reported on significant new research in Great Britain showing the preventive and delaying aspects of vitamin A in female rats administered carcinogenic nitrosamines.

British and Norwegian research likewise has pointed to the cancer-prevention aspects of vitamin A in humans. Dr. Nicholas J. Wald reported in a study of 16,000 men at Oxford University that vitamin A levels were lower before and after cancer develops, and that the blood of lung cancer victims had the lowest vitamin A levels of all. Men with skin, kidney and G.I. tract cancer also had low vitamin A levels, according to this study, which bolstered findings by Dr. Erik Bjelke of the University of Bergen, Norway, that eating more carrots and fish liver, prime sources of vitamin A, may protect against cancer.

The new American research from Rush-Presbyterian-St. Luke's Medical Center in Chicago and the medical schools of Harvard, Northwestern and Michigan universities, shows that the consumption of high quantities of carrots, peaches, tomatoes, spinach and other deep red, green or yellow fruits and vegetables help prevent lung cancer, the most common form of malignany in America. All these foods are rich either in vitamin A or in carotene, a natural substance the body converts to vitamin A.

A nineteen year study of 1,954 Chicago men, all employees of Western Electic Company, found far less lung cancer than expected, even among smokers, whose diets were high in carotene. Among those who had smoked cigarettes for thirty years or more, those who consumed the least carotene had eight times the risk than those who consumed the most carotene.

Club scientists are still cautioning against vitamin A pills and capsules *per se* because of the known toxicity effects from extremely high doses of A and because it is thought that some pills contain a chemical which can cause liver damage in excess amounts.

Metabolic/nutritional therapists have been giving megadoses of vitamin A for years up to toxic levels and note that side effects taper off as dosages are reduced.

At least one researcher, Dr. Charles A. Parry of Virginia, has argued that alleged toxic levels of vitamin A, or levels at which side effects are observable, are actually associated with the stimulation of powerful defense mechanisms and are *desirable* conditions in therapy.

Before a meeting of the American Academy of Medical Preventics (AAMP) in 1981, the veteran vitamin A researcher argued that vitamin E substantially enhances the action of vitamin A and that the two, in proper amounts, may actually give rise to an entirely new vitamin—"vitamin I"—which, he suggested, might be *the* ideal antineoplastic vitamin, as evidenced by vitamin A's success against cancer alone.

Despite the Club's condemnation of the Manner studies at Loyola on prevention of cancer in test animals with laetrile, vitamin A and proteolytic enzymes, it is clear that vitamin A played a key role throughout.

Dr. Parry believes that his vitamin I, in combination with other necessary or complementary nutrients, may be able to lock into place genetic expression, so that cellular replication proceeds despite the stimulus of cancer-causing agents. This line of research also suggests resisting deterioration in the aging process.

Hence, both through the route of medical orthodoxy and a number of lines of research from those outside the Club, it is clear that vitamin A and its analogues will continue to increase in importance in cancer prevention and treatment.

The utility of vitamin A in cancer prevention and treatment is not the only good news about the food factor. In 1981, researchers correlated the decrease in heart disease in Israel to an increased consumption of vitamin A-containing foods.

Commenting on the results of twenty-eight years of data on that country's eating habits, Aviva Palgi, Ph. D., who first worked on the study as assistant professor of nutrition at Jerusalem's Hebrew University, said: "The study indicates that increased consumption of vitamin A will reduce mortality from heart disease."

Scientists at Rutgers Medical School have argued that appropriate amounts of vitamin A will lower cholesterol and that some 40 million Americans have a very low consumption of the vitamin.

Chapter Ten
The Fight for Chelation

By the end of the year, upwards of one million Americans will have died of cardiovascular—"heart"—disease. It will have caused 51 percent of all deaths, a little more than one out of every two. It was estimated in 1980 that 650,000 of these came from heart attacks, and that about 1.5 million such attacks would have occurred during the year.

The American Heart Association estimated in 1980 that more than 40 million Americans were suffering from some form of heart and circulatory disease, including the 1,750,000 sufferers of stroke of whom 172,000 die every year. Coronary heart disease was estimated to afflict 4,300,000 Americans and rheumatic heart disease another 1,880,000. Hypertension affects at least 35 million Americans, but the majority of them are not aware of it.

The *annual* cost of cardiovascular disease is now estimated at in excess of $39 billion simply in *direct* expenses-hospitalization, surgery, rehabilitation, and drugs. Indirect costs undoubtedly far bypass the overall figure of $46.2 billion estimated in 1980. The numbers, both of human fatalities and costs, make "CV," or heart disease, the major killer degenerative disease, even though cancer is rapidly gaining on it.

Despite a decline in actual heart disease mortality since 1970, the disease, or group of diseases, is far from under control. Indeed, a round of heart disease, and ultimate death from it, are virtually expected and accepted parts of the American way of life (and death) and are, in the popular mind, connected with aging, even though 25 percent of all people killed by heart disease are *under* sixty-five.

Heart disease statistics in terms of incidence are spreading both because of population increases and, ironically enough, the success of drug-based therapy in terms of keeping people alive. Since none of the recognized therapies actually *prevents* heart disease or initial heart attacks and strokes, the great successes parroted by American medical orthodoxy are in keeping heart disease patients alive after they have already undergone their initial attacks.

This situation has brought vast new industries into the field. As of 1982, reported the American Heart Association, Americans were spending more than $3.5 billion a year on heart drugs alone (compared to about $400 million ten years before). Hospital and nursing-home costs zoomed from $2.2 billion to $28.7 billion in the same period. The national fetish on coronary-bypass surgery had turned that cutting novelty into a $3.5-billion-per-year industry, with some surgeons who specialize in it earning up to a million dollars a year. Too, reported *U.S. News & World Report,* heart specialists by 1982 were making $7 billion annually for their services, compared to $1 billion a decade before.

New classes of heart drugs, particularly the "beta blockers" and "calcium blockers," are turning in enormous profits for the drug industry and, truth to tell, are of demonstrable benefit in helping stop *second* heart attacks. Propranolol, the first FDA-approved beta blocker, now brings in $171 million a year and as such is the number two prescription drug in America. The projected future for calcium blockers is likewise rosy: $225 million a year.

Despite the new classes of drugs and the rediscovered use of bypass surgery, the major "treatment" of heart disease goes by the unofficial and mellifluous tag of "expectant obvservation"—simply waiting for the patient to die. True, there are many medicines that orthodoxy provides to alleviate the symptoms and pain, the difficulty in breathing, the problems in climbing the steps, but for all intents and purposes, simply waiting for the patient to die is the normal "management" of the interlocking disease states known as heart disease.

Heart patients usually face the alternatives of surgery and/or expensive medicines during the expectant observation phase, which may stretch on for months and years. They are given no choice at all when a condition ultimately results in tissue-destroying gangrene— toes, feet, legs must go. In some cities, the onset of heart-disease-suggesting chest pains may have the patient whisked into an operating room and ready for surgery before he has had a chance to ponder the ramifications.

Physicians prescribe the specific drugs and surgery in the huge world of heart and circulatory disease because they don't know any better; drugs and scalpel are the "state of the art" in American medicine. Potential heart disease sufferers seldom hear about any other therapy.

And yet, in terms of grappling with the problem before and after its onset, there are two alternative approaches to heart disease, and as you might suspect, both of them have not found favor with the Club.

First, since the links between nutrition and heart disease are far more accepted among rank-and-file physicians than are those between nutrition and cancer, the theory that proper eating habits may head off serious circulatory problems was not as wild-sounding at the beginning of this decade as it was just a decade ago. But the insistence on megavitamins and special nutrition in preventive roles is still looked at with considerable suspicion, as we have seen in the case of vitamin E.

Such forward-looking scientists as Richard Passwater have argued that strategic, supplemented eating habits—"supernutrition"—are the answer for healthy hearts and well-functioning circulatory systems. In the light of the growing evidence in favor of metabolic/nutritional therapy, this can hardly be doubted. The effort *should* be made, as in the case of cancer, to *prevent* the disease conditions in the first place, and the nutritional approach is the central element in such prevention, together with exercise and a positive mental attitude.

As we have seen, the same general dietary habits that seem to account for lower to marginal rates of cancer in specific populations around the planet also seem to account for less cardiovascular, and degenerative, disease in general.

In this country, Dr. Ernst Wynder, president of the American Health Foundation in New York, years ago challenged the American Cancer Society to stress the link between nutrition and heart disease. He told the ACS that the world-wide evidence of diet and cancer was "related largely to specific deficiencies or excess of nutritional intake—an area which we may call 'malnutrition of the affluent,' already shown to be involved in cardiovascular diseases." He had already argued for a "prudent diet" to head off heart problems—reducing the intake of fat calories by 35 to 43 percent, reducing cholesterol intake from 600 to 300 milligrams a day, eating no more than four eggs per week and red meat no more than four times a week.

Metabolically-oriented physicians would say that following a more vegetarian diet, deemphasizing animal fats and proteins, and supplementing the diet with vitamin E would be an even better way to cut the chances of heart disease.

But, as in the case of cancer, the money is to be made in treating an existing disease, not preventing it. This is not an evil capitalist conspiracy but an outgrowth of drug-based medicine and attitudes in Western medicine that over the centuries developed into placing more emphasis on treating conditions than on preventing them. But, as in cancer, the interlocking vested interests that spur this lemminglike march to the sea of degenerative disease pandemicity certainly include the profit motive and the sacrosanct status of the surgical craft.

What if, even in *treatment*, there was an essentially nontoxic, nonsurgical way to arrest the horrors of most forms of heart and circulatory disease and even to have a palliative effect on arthritis and many other conditions, including "senility," when linked to heart problems and other conditions? What if such information on this treatment was actually abundant in world medical literature but virtually unknown to American medicine?

The fantastic reality is that there *is* such a suppressed treatment. While it is now becoming known to American medicine due to the medical revolution now underway by a minority of physicians, the dearth of information on it is still astounding—and appalling.

The treatment in question is chelation—a designation based on the Greek word for "claw." It is a process of "clawing out" toxic metals and other minerals from the circulatory system. Agents that can accomplish this are called chelates, or chelating agents. Vitamin C and the amino acids perform some chelating actions themselves, but generally are not strong enough to work alone in the therapeutic management of vascular disease, in which more drastic measures are called for.

The chelation controversy has arisen around the use of ethylene-diamene-tetraacetic acid, or disodium edetate, or other salts of this compound (EDTA), a synthetic chelating agent of choice, or similar compounds. Such agents claw out toxic mineral deposits in the circulatory system by chemically binding them so that they become soluble and can be excreted. The total effect on patients has been nothing short of astounding, leading to some rejuvenating aspects and victory over mental senility as well as multiple "heart disease" complaints.

Few American physicians are aware that in 1972 Czechoslovakian research concluded the EDTA was the treatment of choice for vascular disease-producing "claudication," and that chelation is a fairly common therapeutic tool in the mangement of cardiovascular disease in Iron Curtain countries. It has also been available for three decades in this country, where it ran into a wall of bureaucratic snarls and attacks roughly on a par with the Club's assault on unproven cancer remedies.

Dr. Harold Harper of California, with whom I authored *How You Can Beat the Killer Diseases* in 1977, is a veteran of the chelation wars and a foremost exponent and practitioner of this form of therapy. He has reported that there are twenty-one different demonstrated or postulated effects of EDTA within the body, that the known toxicity of EDTA is far less than that of aspirin, and that the scientific literature on chelation therapy is extensive, with 1,700 articles having been printed on the subject in English alone. Yet, he was astounded to learn, few American M.D.'s know anything about it, and most of those who do blindly accept the established line that there is no real evidence for EDTA's effects.

Indeed, Donald G. Carpenter, Ph.D., reported in a 1980 journal of the International Association on the Artificial Prolongation of the Human Specific Lifespan that "to date, approximately 600 medical and osteopathic physicians have used chelation therapy to treat in the neighborhood of 250,000 patients." Moreover, his statistical reviews of treatments and life extension led him to conclude that "the optimistic median and mean lifespan increases anticipated from widespread use of present chelation therapy on males are approximately 18 and 16.9 years; for females, 20 and 16 years." Assuming he is somewhere near the mark, the implications of chelation therapy life extension have awesome health—and economic—implications.

The fight to authorize EDTA use outside the area for which it was originally approved—against lead poisoning—was led in California by the nationwide American Academy of Medical Preventics (AAMP), originally founded by Harper, among others, and whose former president, Garry F. Gordon, M.D., is one of the nation's major chelation proponents. It was Ray Evans, M.D., who won a federal court decision that not only scored a major breakthrough for chelation but for the right of physicians to use medicines for purposes other than those described in their "package inserts" (see chapter three).

The 28 June 1978 decision by U.S. District Court Judge Robert E. Varner that "Congress did not intend to empower the FDA to interfere with medical practice by limiting the ability of physicians to prescribe according to their best judgment" had been echoed months before by California Attorney General Evelle Younger after state authorities began moving against all physicians who dared to use EDTA in the treatment of cardiovascular disease or anything else which might be construed as an "unlicensed new drug."

Dr. Evers has used chelating substances for twelve years, and in 1978 reviewed eight years of chelation therapy on 10,000 patients in a summary that I excerpt here:

> Historically, chelation by EDTA, its analogues and other chelating agents has been used for a wide range of disorders including lead and mercury poisoning, radioactive metal toxicity, porphyria, scleroderma, snake venom toxicity, and many types of calcinosis.... Like all new concepts in therapy, especially when there are results in patients who are usually considered as progressively deteriorating cases, a good deal of questioning, doubt, and frank denial has been leveled at chelation therapy.
>
> Concurrently, biophysicists are becoming intrigued with the wide range of physiological metal chelation that occurs at the microcellular level of

enzymatic chemistry.... It can be recognized that much of the future in medicine may well center around the chelation phenomena in all of its aspects along with enzymes and electronic therapy. It opens a large vista of insight into a wide range of disorders for which both etiology and therapy have been vague or undermined. This includes the psychotic disorders, the so-called collagenous diseases, many of the disorders of metabolism and enzyme deficiencies, and the vascular atheromatous disorders (all types of calcinosis)....

In arteriosclerotic *obliteran* cases [there has been] definite improvement of pedal artery pulsation, gain in color, return of normal temperature and improvement in tissue quality of the feet. We find that 90% of these problems in the lower extremities make significant gains, including regaining ability to walk long distances comfortably, freedom of claudication and evidence of improved distal circulation....

Those whose cerebral vascular system is severely damaged by arteriosclerosis and/or microcirculation thrombosis, suffering from amnesia, confusion, aphasias, and motor coordination have improved. There has been a notable improvement in coronary circulation in all cases of angina, characterized by the patient having no need for vasodilators after the fifth infusion.

An interesting, but not predictable, dividend in some cases consists of improved renal function, reduction of prostatic obstruction by calcucli, decrease in the degree of insulin required by the diabetic, almost normal breathing in emphysematous patients, great improvement in arthritic patients, and even in Parkinson's Disease sufferers.

Dr. Evers also detailed 467 cases in which patients responded partially to dramatically with chelation therapy for various forms of arthritis. He also had impressive responses in diabetic gangrene, and says of calcinosis (calcium poisoning leading to arteriosclerosis, atherosclerosis, etc.), "From our experience in treating these approximately 3,000 patients with varying degrees of calcinosis, we will unequivocally state that it is our opinion that every patient with this disease in any part of the body should be given a therapeutic trial before any type of vascular surgery is performed." The Food and Drug Administration twice went to court in Alabama to attempt to prevent Evers from using chelating agents. In the meantime, his grateful patients initiated a class action suit against the FDA to allow them to continue to receive the treatments.

At root—bureaucratically—was, as usual, the Food, Drug and Cosmetic Act as amended in 1962. Though EDTA had already been cleared for use in heavy metal toxicity, when Abbott Laboratories—which had marketed the drug since 1959—listed "vascular occlusive" disease as an indication for its use it ran afoul of the amended act, which mandated that all substances not only must be demonstrated to be safe but *effective* as well—an extremely time-consuming and costly procedure that can take years. Abbott dropped the claims because the potential cost of proving EDTA's "vascular occlusive" efficacy was simply too high to recover in the remaining years before the patent rights were to expire. In the FDA's eyes, this meant that EDTA's use in anything other than heavy metal—particularly lead—poisoning would be "illegal" and of course this provided a convenient loophole whereby opponents of nontoxic, non surgical, total-body heart disease therapy could bar EDTA.

In a general summary of chelation therapy and literature for *Osteopathic Annals,* Drs. Garry Gordon and Robert Vance pointed out that both the inconvenience of EDTA administration (ten to forty intravenous infusions over hours-long intervals) and lack of general information and understanding of chelating agents had contributed to "a serious delay in the widespread utilization of chelation therapy in medical practice."

EDTA was synthesized about 1930 and patented in 1949. Its first use in medicine was for the treatment of lead poisoning in 1941. In the 1950s clinical research was undertaken by Norman Clarke, M.D., director of research at Providence Hospital in Detroit, who speculated that since EDTA has been found effective in removing diffused—or metastatic—calcium deposits from the human body, it might also be useful in helping to disintegrate the "plaque" of arteriosclerosis and hence improve circulation.

Dr. Clarke—who, like Ernst T. Krebs, Jr., and vitamin B^{15} to some degree—is something of a prophet without honor in his own country. Few American physicians are aware of his pioneering work in the chelation areas, even while he has been hailed as a chelation pioneer in the Soviet Union, where chelation therapy is a relatively common form of treatment for arteriosclerotic vascular disease. Part of his work showed that nine out of ten patients treated with chelation therapy for angina pain—the terrific chest pain many heart disease sufferers have to cope with—underwent relief, and that after up to three months of the therapy mineral deposits continued to be excreted from the body.

To this day, coronary bypass surgery is touted as the answer to angina pain, and is staunchly defended by the medical Establishment. Yet by September 1977 an assessment of this surgical procedure—transplanting a portion of the leg veins into the chest cavity—showed that while the expensive technique, with an average cost of over $27,000, does indeed relieve severe chest pains, it contributes nothing toward getting heart patients back to work.

Glenda K. Barnes, R.N., and colleagues at the Medical Center of the University of Birmingham, Alabama, reported in the 19 September 1977 *Journal of the American Medical Association* that in a group of 350 patients who had had the operation "overall, there was no improvement in return to work or hours worked after surgery." Forty-four percent decreased their hours worked, 24 percent kept the same schedule, and 32 percent increased their work time—for no net improvement. This study cast into doubt the long-range benefits from an operation that 110,000 Americans undergo annually.

Earlier, Dr. Edgar Berman, who poked brutal fun at his medical colleagues in *The Solid Gold Stethoscope,* dispensed with the technique this way:

> The new answer to one of the biggest killers in medical history may yet become the biggest killing in medical economics. Though the "bypass" for coronary heart disease is similar to the one discarded twenty years ago, it's now back by popular demand and doing a landoffice business. It has not been conclusively proved yet, but neither has aspirin—and billions of dollars worth of that little moneymaker have already been sold. If tens of thousands of patients believe and are waiting—who among those altruistic, reticent, selfless cardiac surgeons is going to disillusion them?

In 1981, a Harvard School of Public Health study dropped a major bombshell into the growing coronary bypass industry by announcing that a medical team had determined that most people with clogged arteries can be treated successfully with medication and do not need the bypass operation—a procedure which as of 1981 was used annually on 110,000 Americans who had spent $1.6 million a year. (By 1982 the estimated cost was $3.5 billion a year.)

There has been plenty of dirty work at the crossroads in barring American access to chelation therapy, as such researchers as Gordon and Harper point out.

For example, the government's position against chelation therapy has failed to distinguish between *coronary* and *peripheral vascular* disease—that is, disease conditions in the extremities. As early as March 15, 1963, Kitchell and Meltzer, while reporting in the Club's *Medical World News* their disappointment with EDTA chelation therapy in coronary disease, saw great utility and promise for it in *peripheral vascular* disease.

Too, Gordon and the AAMP have noted, the federal side has

failed to acknowledge vital research by Doolin and Schwartz on the *lack* of kidney toxicity from EDTA. This is essential since the Club's major attack on EDTA and its analogues, aside from claiming insufficient data to indicate positive effect, is kidney toxicity. The true benefit-risk ratio of the chemical, hence, has never been adequately expostulated in this country.

Dr. Harper has observed, with chagrin, that as late as January 1970 the Food and Drug Administration had admitted that the use of EDTA was "possibly effective in occlusive vascular disorders and the treatment of pathologic conditions to which calcium tissue deposits or hypercalcemia may contribute...." That is, before such groups as the chelation-espousing American Academy of Medical Preventics were formed, the FDA had already agreed that EDTA might be useful for something other than lead poisoning! It was to forget this while seeking injunctions against Dr. Evers and pushing state government minions to go after chelation therapists in California and elsewhere.

"When this acceptance and quasi recommendation was withdrawn, chelation was 'wished away' and in some states 'legislated away,'" Dr. Harper noted. "There is simply no economic advantage to hospitals, thoracic surgeons, anesthesiologists, or the pharmaceutical and medical industry in chelation therapy programs." The current cost of the program is $2,500 to $5,000, far less than that charged for "standard" cardiovascular management.

Soviet medical literature has reported the use of the chelating agent Unithol with multivitamins in the successful management of coronary arteriosclerosis, and Soviet physicians recommend and use this treatment in the prevention of hardening of the arteries in aging. They have also reported on successful effects of EDTA on cerebral, coronary, and peripheral circulation in all patients studied.

Dr. Harper won few friends in the medical fraternity by referring to chelation therapy as "the Roto-Rooter of the vascular system," but that illustrative phrase fairly well defines the actual action of EDTA. By coursing through the entire circulatory system, it is able to bond with toxic metals and minerals wherever they may be found in that system. Such substances as calcium, lead, mercury, and copper are deposited on a layer of fats or in the arterial walls, the end result of overconsumption of junk foods—refined carbohydrates, although other factors are involved in hardening of the arteries as well.

The heavy toxic minerals are "divalent"—that is, they have a positive charge of two. EDTA has the unique capacity of donating from each of its six carbon atoms an electron that binds a divalent mineral and holds it in place. Because of this unique property, Harper and his colleagues have styled EDTA "man's miracle molecule." Its binding action changes a harmful mineral from a solid to a liquid, allowing it to be passed through the kidneys. The cast off minerals may be measured in the urine.

As this mineral-metal sludge is removed from the body, the pressure of the bloodstream moving through the arteries helps break down molecules of fats, cholesterol, and phospholipids to wash them into that stream and thence into the liver, which then excretes them into the digestive tract. In this way the body is cleared of many of the accumulations of toxic minerals within its arterial system.

It has become known that another primary action of chelating agents is the removal of toxic minerals from the walls and membranes of cells, greatly enhancing cellular health and life. Also, EDTA binds free, or ionic, calcium in the bloodstream, which in turn releases the calcium from plaques and joints into the bloodstream. Opponents of the chelation therapy who believe that EDTA attacks calcium in the bones are simply not familiar with the metabolic processes of the "calicum pool," the chelating therapists point out. Instead of bone-thinning or calcium loss in elderly patients under chelation, there is actually an *increased* calcium deposit within the bones after EDTA treatment, chelation proponents argue. EDTA will not bind the "good," or protein-linked, calcium—the kind in bone tissue—so the attack on chelation as a calcium-depleting therapy has been found unwarranted.

Drs. Gordon and Vance wrote, "The beneficial effects of chelation in other chronic diseases—such as arthritis, porphyria, renolithiasis, and scleroderma—as well as subclinical heavy-metal toxicities in lead, cadmium or selenium, and benefits in hypertension are noteworthy in the literature. Even improvement or restoration of vision in macular degeneration of the retina has been observed."

The chelation therapists also point out that heart surgery is apt to be a once-and-only thing. But there is no known limit to how many chelation infusions a patient may undergo. Some have received over 500 in a ten-year period. As Gordon and Vance observe, "where the history had shown several strokes or myocardial infarctions before chelation therapy, they now have had no further events during the treatment time. This approach seems safe when one reviews all the information on toxicology and especially interesting when one notes, in the July, 1975, edition of *Journal of Gerontology,* that rotifers treated every day of their lives with EDTA lived 50 percent longer than controls." They added:

> This flexibility is in striking contrast to the surgicial approach which is usually abandoned after no more than two operations and the patient simply dies or lives with his limitations. Vascular surgery frequently offers only symptomatic relief in the area of the chief complaint and thus is generally recognized as only mitigating and temporary. There is little or no evidence to suggest that bypass

surgery is significantly extending life. The causes are not attacked, and recurrence is the rule.

There are strong vested interests that will feel threatened by chelation therapy.... If widespread use of chelation therapy developed, the need for certain specialties, hospital facilities and bypass equipment would be soon diminished. It has been suggested that there appears to be an excess of catheter-trained cardiologists disgorged into the health ranks each year as well as an undue proliferation of cardiovascular surgeons.

As in the cases of vitamin E and amygdalin, controlled double-blind studies, the variety of research that the FDA holds so necessary to establishing the validity of treatment, are wanting in the case of EDTA chelation therapy. But also as in the cases of vitamin E and laetrile, proponents question the ethics of having a control group of patients who receive no treatment at all, while another group or groups receive the controversial modalities. So chelationists have put together reams of evidence, much of which the Club has responded to the same way it reacts to human success with laetrile: "It's anecdotal." Dr. Gordon has pointed out that double-blind studies were never run on coronary bypass surgery, either.

The case for EDTA grows stronger every year. One of its primary proponents in America is toxicologist and cancer researcher Bruce Halstead. He told the *Medical Tribune* in March 1978:

> Crude clinical data based on the experience of hundreds of physicians over two decades involving hundreds of thousands of treatments indicate that good to excellent results [with EDTA chelation therapy] occur in 75 percent of cases: and an additional 5 percent show mild improvement. Give me any group of patients with coronary artery disease—even the best cardiologist's most refractory patients—and I'll have four or five responding well to chelation therapy.

Metabolic/nutritional therapists are now using chelation therapy together with vitamin and mineral supplementation, diet management, exercise, and even "biofeedback" training as part of a holistic management program.

Richard E. Welch, M.D., then sixty, told of what this total approach meant to him when, in 1974, he "arose, shaved, showered, and collapsed on the bathroom floor" with symptoms that suggested the onset of a severe cerebral vascular crisis. In 1976 he wrote in *Let's Live:*

> I recently took a course of chelation with two friends. Together the three of us felt improvement in our blood circulation by the time the course of treatment was over. These two men were brilliant contributors to their respective professions, their minds were still keen, but the attrition of age was beginning to tell perceptibly. One of the men mentioned that for the first time in years his extremities felt warm. The other man, a diabetic with one limb amputated, was able to reduce his insulin substantially.
>
> It was not until I received chelation therapy that my blood pressure reached a normal level, even though I was on strong hypertensive drugs. The dividends were more energy, alertness, no headache, less nocturia, and reactivation of the libido. . . .
>
> The combination of controlled and judicious fasting, proper diet, vitamin and mineral supplementation, a graduated regimen for exercise, can indeed reverse this process [arteriosclerosis] and add years of effective life for many. . . . There is no magic pill to reverse the process of aging, but there is a program, scientific, safe, and relatively inexpensive, that is bringing hope, happiness, and health to thousands of people. Instead of finishing life as rusting hulks on some barren reef, we can find that our latter decades can be golden years filled with satisfaction, happiness and achievement.

A Swiss study and its followup—in 1976 and 1981, respectively—have provided chelation therapists with evidence that chelating agents, particularly EDTA, help cut the chances of developing cancer.

In the earlier study, Dr. Walter Blumer's research on 59 patients who had received calcium EDTA treatments for low-level toxicity due to their proximity to heavy automobile traffic conclusively proved that cancer incidence was markedly enchanced by the breathing of leaded gas. The second study, reporting on eight-year followups to the initial series of calcium EDTA infusions, revealed both a 50 percent decrease in the incidence of cardiovascular disease *and* a 90 percent likelihood of developing cancer, as contrasted with persons in the study who had not received EDTA treatment.

The suggestion here was that chelation therapy exerted strong cancer-inhibitory and immune system-enhancing effects on the patients.

With the relatively abundant research on chelation and heart disease in existence, and the minimal but exciting evidence of chelation therapy's usefulness in other metabolic dysfunctions, it is doubly tragic that in America patients and physicians have had to go to court to secure this kind of treatment as their right.

By the late 1970s chelation therapy was making such waves in the treatment of cardiovascular disease that, once again, the Club had to do something.

Across the country, physicians who used chelation found themselves embroiled in various disputes with state and federal agencies, and often local medical boards as well. Whatever the alleged problem, it almost always boiled down to a simple solution—stop chelating patients, and we'll stop harassing you.

Between hearings in one celebrated case, the ebullient Dr. Gordon told me, "It's only natural. After all, with new studies indicating life-extension of 8 to 16 years with chelation, the damage we can do is just getting started." (Behind the joke was a reality, though—the life-extension of Americans, whose patriotic duty seems to be to retire at sixty-five and die a few years later, implies serious problems for the already bankrupt Social Security apparatus and the entire federal pension system!)

In Florida, the State Board of Medical Examiners put Robert J. Rogers, M.D., on probation for using therapy that is not "generally practiced in this country." But Dr. Rogers fought back. The First District Court of Appeals, and then the Florida Supreme Court, quashed this idiotic and arbitrary action.

In a 7-0 ruling in 1980, the Florida judges put Florida medical authorities on notice they cannot penalize unproven procedures or medicines unless they are proven to be fraudulent or harmful. At the time, Dr. Rogers said he had been seeing "consistently excellent results" in 80 to 85 percent of the 500 patients he had treated with chelation therapy over fifteen years.

Leo J. Bolles, M.D. founder of the Northwest Academy of Preventive Medicine, has also been a tough nut to crack. A practitioner of preventive and nutritional medicine for over fourteen years, he has been a thorn in the side of the King County (Seattle, Washington) Medical Society during all that time. Chelation therapy has been only one of the progressive modalities he has used on some 4,000 patients in the last six years.

The way orthodoxy found to "get at" Dr. Bolles, who refused to cease and desist from this general metabolic and nutritional therapies, was to exclude his patients from Medicare payments. Believing he would be disciplined by state medical authorities should he not have contested the charges made against him by the Health Care Financing Administration (HCFA), Dr. Bolles also fought back. The outcome was still undecided as this book went to press.

In hearings concerning Dr. Bolles' Medicare exclusion, it was revealed that the government had a list of physicians who would undergo "total holdout review." All were involved in chelation therapy. Dr. Bolles was vaguely accused of furnishing "services or supplies which are of a quality which fails to meet professionally recognized standards of health," but it became apparent that the real target was chelation.

This was also clear in allegations of "gross incompetency" and "unprofessional conduct" brought against Dr. Robert Vance in Salt Lake City by the local city-county medical board. Dr. Vance, as we have seen, is one of the nation's foremost and most outspoken chelation therapy practitioners and theorists.

Dr. Vance has long ruffled orthodox feathers by open espousal of chelation therapy. Championing statewide efforts to block fluoridation of Utah's drinking water earned him no Club favors, either.

In the Vance case, as in a number of others, the medical authorities claimed that "unproven" methods of diagnosis were used to detect nonexistent metabolic dysfunctions, which were then treated by "unproven" means. Sometimes, "ringers" were sent into a doctor's office to pose as patients with vague complaints. Such patients were provided with a host of diagnostic practices—"not generally accepted" by the AMA, of course—and then determined to be chronically deficient, then treated.

Far from being quackery, the diagnostics and treatments more often than not bore down on the reality which most astounds the Club and its thought-control process—most Americans *are* metabolically deficient, metabolically "sick," but not in a gross clinical way which provides them with a clear set of symptoms that an AMA-trained physician is equipped to detect. The young men this country sent to die in Korea and South Vietnam, and who on autopsy showed up with arteriosclerosis, had certainly not been aware that they had the disease. They were the "completely healthy" soldiers conscripted for service, end products of "three square meals a day" from a population said to be "the healthiest and best-fed on earth." Metabolic/nutritional therapists are involved in detecting deficiency states and metabolic conditions *before* they become the gross exhibitions which "crisis" medicine-trained doctors are able to recognize and treat. This practice is emphatically *not* quackery, but bureaucrats and administrators cerebrally scrubbed by the allopathic school of medicine may be excused for thinking so.

No matter how long and red-tape-befouled the chelation battles are, they too, will result in final freedom of choice in cardiovascular therapy. The world is not going to be made safe only for the coronary bypass industry and the drug cartel, the preventive medicine doctors are confident.

Chelation, as in the metabolic/nutritional management of cancer, is an idea which must go through the ideological grinder described by William James, "First a new theory is attacked as absurd. Then it is admitted to be true but insignificant. Finally it is seen to be so important that its adversaries claim that they themselves discovered it." The day the Club lays claim to "discovering" chelation therapy may be a long time away...but it is surely coming.

Chapter Eleven
The Challenge of Promotive Health

In 1971, six physicians met to set up the International Academy of Preventive Medicine, an organization that took the lead in beginning the reeducation of physicians away from "crisis" medicine and rerouting them toward concepts of preventive medicine. IAPM's membership now includes hundreds of M.D.'s.

IAPM served as the model for other breakaway groups of otherwise orthodox doctors who dared to question the pronouncements of the American Medical Association and its iron control over medical education in this country. Since then, such organizations as the American Academy of Medical Preventics, primarily stimulated by the fight to vindicate chelation therapy, the American Holistic Medical Association, the Northwest Academy of Preventive Medicine, the Orthomolecular Medical Society, and several orthomolecular medical groups have sprung up.

These professional organizations have been able to make common cause with such vintage lay-oriented groups as the National Health Federation and the cancer-and laetrile-oriented Committee for Freedom of Choice in Cancer Therapy, the Cancer Control Society, and others. Together, the professional and lay organizations are helping to mold a whole new consciousness about medicine and health.

They have been joined by a spinoff of the turbulent 1960s, the back-to-nature champions of holistic health and do-it-yourself medicine. Such a coalition of interests, ranging from suspicion of, to outright hostility toward, the Establishment, is at best a marriage of convenience. It is also fraught with peril, for there is in the antiestablishment tide now underway as much room for fads, both silly and dangerous, as there is for constructive new ideas.

Dr. Richard O. Brennan, who founded the IAPM and who has

more than a quarter-century of active involvement in preventive medicine, encompasses the moderate position in the medical revolution. "Doctors are good people," this medical doctor and osteopathic physician told me. "We have to realize they're imprisoned. We shouldn't throw rocks at them."

Dr. Brennan believes that building friendly "spheres of influence" within the medical community will do more to move organized medicine into prevention and nutritional therapy than will the heavy-handed rhetoric of blind opposition. The more moderate exponents of change in medicine agree with him.

His was an enlightened and reasoned voice that testified in 1974 before the Senate Labor and Public Welfare Committee's public health subcommittee: "Optimum nutrition is a basic and vital part of preventive medicine. The increasing incidence of chronic degenerative diseases and the accelerated cost of sick care must make us understand that it is imperative to focus upon the prevention of disease and maintenance of health."

And it was Brennan who testified the same year before the Senate Select Committee on Nutrition, "It is time that those who produce, sell, teach, serve, talk about and eat food be honest. Honesty is our only hope in this existing morass of misinformation about the quality of our foods, and it is later than we think."

What Brennan and his colleagues have underscored is the need for public awareness about the food disaster of Western civilization. Awareness of the problem will be followed by action—but awareness must come first. That is only part of the task, albeit a Herculean one, of the medical revolution.

In arguing for "a positive renewal" in the *Journal* of the IAPM, Brennan emphasized the second major task, the reform of medical education:

> The problems facing our organization are tremendous. We are fighting to change the entire emphasis of the practice of medicine. Statistics from every source show alarming increases in the incidence of "breakdown" or chronic degenerative diseases.... Oddly enough, in spite of growing lip service to "preventive medicine," the medical community itself must accept the blame for our long slide into sickness. Medical schools simply do not train doctors to keep patients healthy—their academically oriented instructors continually emphasize treatment of illness, not the urgently needed maintenance of health. The net result is that the young doctor entering practice after years of training emphasizing treatment of illness does not think in terms of helping his patients to maintain

their health....

Our present type of medical care and its delivery are teetering on the brink of collapse. The hour is late, but there is still time for all of us to become part of this gigantic prevention-oriented movement which is so necessary to insure the health and progress of our country.

I am indebted to California anthropologist Joan Koss for the term *promotive health*—a term, I believe, more illustrative of what the long-range goals of the medical revolution ought to be than is *preventive medicine*. Promotive health is the common heritage of the nonindustrialized world, which is the majority of humanity. Living that lifestyle, doing those things, that promote health and well-being are positive actions—not negative reactions to a malady that has already broken out.

There is room under the broad umbrella of promotive health for innovation in medicine, and even more room for individual responsibility, which must be the keystone of the movement. For the taking of individual responsibility for one's own health is the beginning of medical wisdom and spells the demise of the current passive-active patient-physician role now nurtured and encouraged by Establishment medicine ("I am the patient and I am ill: I place myself in your hands and you will cure me").

Unhappily, neither the solution to the food problem nor the restructuring of medical education can remain free from political action. Awareness of both means concerted effort in the legislative area, and in this regard the first order of business is the wholesale retooling of the Food and Drug Administration, whose bureaucratic abuses have done so much to advance suffering and death. Few observers believe that there is no role whatsoever for the FDA; most would agree that, whether we like it or not, some governmental monitoring agency to oversee safety in foods and medicines is a necessary inconvenience of modern times. But the use of FDA regulations to terrify physicians away from creative medicine—and adherence to the Hippocratic Oath—is an abomination that our relatively free society can no longer tolerate.

As these lines are written, there is active legislation in both houses of Congress to de-fang the FDA and place it back within its constitutional bounds. This is a first order of business and in some form will probably be achieved.

The political successes of the Committee for Freedom of Choice in Cancer Therapy were far more due to the earthy simplicity of its message than to the bright promise of laetrile. For the committee argued, and the medical revolution essentially *is* arguing, that there must be freedom of choice *with informed consent* for physician and patient in choosing medical treatment. The adoption of this simple concept and its enshrinement in law—something freedom-of-choicers believe was done, at least by inference, in the Constitution—would solve most of the problems in medical innovation.

There are those within the medical revolution who see the flaws and follies of the problem as it relates to the United States—a failure of capitalist-republican society—and hence argue that *more* governmental control and the socialization of medicine are called for. But Dr. Brennan exposes this fallacy: "In the midst of this dilemma our Federal Government is becoming increasingly involved in the practice and delivery of medicine in the United States. The Government would like us to believe that every American citizen will be taken care of from the womb to the tomb, but this is not so. All one has to do is examine the disease statistics from countries which have been involved in socialized medicine for many years. A quick look proves that socialized medicine and 'sick care' do not work."

Because the market system is at best flawed, monopolies have resulted. But no monopoly can flourish anywhere without its twin, monopoly government. The excesses of the international drug trust and monopoly medicine do *not* point to the need for government control of both, for the attempt to inject government into medicine has already resulted in a major part of our overall health problem. The answers lie far more in the restoration of *genuine* free markets in medicine and pharmaceuticals, with only limited, if necessary, government intervention.

Easier said than done? Absolutely. But freedom is not an easy commodity to store. History is weighted against it. Like a rare desert flower, it needs special conditions and attention simply to survive. Freedom with responsibility at the political level, the free market with morality at the economic and ethical ones, must be the guideposts of the medical revolution in America.

Selected Bibliography

Adams, Ruth, and Frank Murray. *Megavitamin Therapy*. New York: Larchmont Books, 1973.
Beall, Morris A. *Super Drug Story*. Washington, D.C.: Columbia Books, 1962.
Beard, John. *The Enzyme Treatment of Cancer and Its Scientific Basis*. London: Chato and Windus, 1911.
Berman, Edgar, M.D., *The Solid Gold Stethoscope*. New York: MacMillan, 1976.
Bradford, Robert W., and Mike Culbert, eds., with Henry W. Allen. *International Protocols in Cancer Management*. Los Altos, California: The Bradford Foundation, 1981.
――――――. *Now That You Have Cancer*. Los Altos, California: Choice Publications, 1977.
――――――. eds. *The Metabolic Management of Cancer*. Los Altos, California: The Bradford Foundation, 1979.
Brennan, R.O., M.D., with William Mulligan. *Nutrigenetics*. New York: M. Evans, 1975.
Burk, Dean, Ph.D. *A Brief on Foods and Vitamins*. Sausalito, California: McNaughton Foundation, 1975.
Cameron, Ewan, M.D., and Linus Pauling, Ph.D. *Vitamin C and Cancer*. Menlo Park, California: The Linus Pauling Institute of Science and Medicine, 1979.
Cheraskin, E., M.D., and W. M. Ringsdorf, Jr., M.D., with Arline Brecher. *New Hope for Incurable Diseases*. Hicksville, New York: Exposition Press, 1971.
――――――. *Psychodietetics*. New York: Bantam, 1974.
Culbert, Michael L. *Freedom From Cancer*. New York: Pocket Books, 1977: Seal Beach, California: '76 Press, 1976.
――――――. *Vitamin B^{17}: Forbidden Weapon Against Cancer*. New

Rochelle, New York: Arlington House, 1974.
Dufty, William. *Sugar Blues*. Radnor, Pennsylvania: Chilton, 1975.
Ferguson, Wilburn. *The Jivaro and His Drugs*. Quito, Ecuador: Editorial Casa de la Cultura Ecuatoriana, 1957.
Fredericks, Carlton, Ph.D., *Breast Cancer and the Nutritional Approach*. New York: Grosset and Dunlap, 1977.
————. *Eating Right for You*. New York: Grosset and Dunlap, 1972.
————. and Herman Goodman. *Low Blood Sugar and You*. New York: Grosset and Dunlap, 1969.
————. *PsychoNutrition*. New York: Grosset and Dunlap, 1976.
Fredman, Steven, and Robert Burger. *Forbidden Cures*. New York: Stein and Day, 1976.
Galton, Lawrence. *The Silent Disease: Hypertension*. New York: Crown, 1973.
Gerson, Max, M.D. *A Cancer Therapy*. New York: Whittier Books, 1958.
Gurchot, Charles, Ph.D. *Biology—Key to the Riddle of Cancer*. New York: Moore, 1949.
Halstead, Bruce, M.D. *Amygdalin (Laetrile) Therapy*. Los Altos, California: Choice Publications, 1978.
————. *Metabolic Cancer Therapy*. Colton, California: Golden Quill, 1978.
————. *The Scientific Basis of EDTA Chelation Therapy*. Colton, California: Golden Quill, 1979.
————. with Sylvia A. Youngberg, R.N. *The DMSO Handbook*. Colton, California: Golden Quill, 1981.
Harmer, Ruth Mulvey. *American Medical Avarice*. New York: Abelard-Schuman, 1975.
Harper, Harold, M.D., and Michael L. Culbert. *How You Can Beat the Killer Diseases*. New Rochelle: New York: Arlington House, 1977.
Heinerman, John. *The Treatment of Cancer with Herbs*. Orem, Utah: Biworld Publishers: 1980.
Hoxsey, Harry. *You Don't Have to Die*. 1956: reprinted by Nature Heals, Chapala, Mexico, 1977.
Hunsberger, Eydie Mae. *How I Conquered Cancer Naturally*. San Diego: Production House, 1975.
Hur, Robin. *Food Reform: Our Desperate Need*. Austin, Texas: Heidelberg, 1975.
Illich, Ivan. *Medical Nemesis*. New York: Random House, 1976.
Kittler, Glenn D. *Laetrile—Control for Cancer*. New York: Paperback Library, 1963.
————. *Laetrile—Nutritional Control for Cancer*. Denver: Royal Publications, 1978.
Kloss, Jethro. *Back to Eden*. Santa Barbara, California: Lifeline Books, 1974.
Koch, William Frederick, Ph.D., M.D. *The Survival Factor in*

Neoplastic and Viral Diseases. Detroit, Michigan: The Vanderkloot Press, Inc., 1961.
LaGarde, Philippe, M.D. *Ce Qu'on Vous Cache Sur Le Cancer.* Lausanne, Switzerland: Favre, 1981.
Livingston, Virginia, M.D. *Cancer: A New Breakthrough.* San Diego: Production House, 1972.
Lucas, Richard. *Nature's Medicines.* New York: Award Books, 1966.
Lucas, Scott. *The FDA.* Millbrae, California: Celestial Arts, 1978.
Manner, Harold W., Ph.D., Steven J. DiSanti, and Thomas L. Michalsen. *The Death of Cancer.* Evanston, Illinois: Advanced Century, 1978.
Martin, Wayne. *Medical Heroes and Heretics.* Old Greenwich, Connecticut: Devin-Adair, 1977.
Mendelsohn, Robert S., M.D. *Confessions of a Medical Heretic.* New York: Warner Books, 1979.
Millman, Marcia. *The Unkindest Cut.* New York: Morrow, 1977.
Mindell, Earl. *Earl Mindell's Vitamin Bible.* New York: Rawson, Wade, 1980.
Moss, Ralph W. *The Cancer Syndrome.* New York: Grove Press, Inc., 1980.
Passwater, Richard A., Ph.D. *Cancer and Its Nutritional Therapies.* New Canaan, Connecticut: Keats, 1978.
_____. *Selenium as Food and Medicine.* New Canaan, Connecticut: Keats, 1980.
_____. *Supernutrition.* New York: Dial, 1975.
_____. *Supernutrition for Healthy Hearts.* New York: Dial, 1977.
Richardson, John A., M.D. and Patricia Griffin. *Laetrile Case Histories.* New York: Bantam, 1977.
Rosenberg, Harold, M.D., with A. N. Feldzamen. *The Doctor's Book of Vitamin Therapy.* New York: Berkley Windhover, 1974.
Sattilaro, Anthony, M.D. *Recalled by Life.* Boston: Houghton Mifflin, 1982.
Schauss, Alexander. *Diet, Crime and Delinquency.* Berkeley, California: Parker House, 1980.
Shute, Wilfred, E., M.D. *Wilfred Shute's Complete Updated Vitamin E Book.* New Canaan, Connecticut: Keats, 1975.
Stefansson, Vilhjalmur. *Cancer: Disease of Civilization.* New York: Hill and Wang, 1960.
Taylor, Renee. *Hunza Health Secrets.* New York: Award, 1960.
Timms, Moira, and Zachariah Zar. *Natural Sources: Vitamin B^{17}/Laetrile.* Millbrae, California: Celestial Arts, 1978.
Wade, Carlson. *Nature's Cures.* New York: Award Books, 1972.
Walker, Morton, D.P.M. *Chelation Therapy.* Atlanta, Georgia: '76 Press, 1980.
_____. *Total Health.* New York: Everest House, 1979.
Webster, James. *Vitamin C, the Protective Vitamin.* New York: Award Books, 1971.

Williams, Roger J., Ph.D. *Nutrition Against Disease.* New York: Bantam, 1971.
_____. *Physicians' Handbook of Nutritional Science.* Springfield, Illinois: Charles C. Thomas, 1975.
Winters, Jason, *Killing Cancer.* London: Skilton and Shaw, 1980.
Yudkin, John, M.D. *Sweet and Dangerous.* New York: Bantam, 1972.

Index

A
A. Bakh Institute of
  Biochemistry 250
Abbott Laboratories 272
Abkhasians 94, 247
Abrams, Bernard 71
Abrams, Felice 71
abscissic acid 199
*A Cancer Therapy: Results of 50
  Cases* 189
Accardi, Amanda 25-26
Accardi, Katherine 25-26
Accardi, Michael 25-26
Acevedo, Herman F. 224
"active respiratory groups" 182
additives, chemical, in U.S. food
  supply 103
adrenal cortical extract (ACE) 76-77
Ain, Diantha 71
Albany Medical Center 27
Allegheny General Hospital 224
Allen, Henry W. 207
allopathy 69, 82, 122
Alper, Phil 57
Alperin, Irving 39
Alperin, Mimi 39
American Academy of Medical
  Preventics (AAMP) 68, 269, 275,
  279, 286
American Association for Cancer
  Research 166
American Association for the
  Advancement of Science
  (AAAS) 58
American Biologics 11, 50
American Biologics-Mexico
  Hospital 150, 206
American Cancer Society 32, 43, 58,
  124, 125, 127, 129, 132, 137-40, 141,
  142-47, 151, 155, 165, 216, 268
American Chemical Society 330
American College of Surgeons 66
American Enterprise Institute for
  Public Policy Research 63
American Health Foundation 273
American Heart Association 61,
  271, 272
American Holistic Medical
  Association 68, 286

American Journal of Surgery 207
American Medical Association
  (AMA) 32, 34, 47, 79-83, 88, 151,
  154, 155, 156-58, 159-61, 162, 286
American Medical News 115
American Osteopathic
  Association 81
American Society of Clinical
  Oncology 54, 129
amygdalin, defined 10
  distinguished from
    "laetrile" 210-11
amygdalin (laetrile)
  as free radical scavenger 206,
    217-18
  Food, Drug and Cosmetic Act
    and 58
  NCI animal tests of 168-69
  NCI "retrospective analysis"
    of 48-50
  NCI-SRI tests of 168-59
  research in China 194
  Sloan-Kettering tests and 110-23
  technical specifications of 210
  toxicity of 177
  University of California-Davis
    and 174-76
Anatomy of a Coverup 116
antineoplaston 165
apricot kernels, seizures of 171
Aprikern 38, 171
Armstrong, Robert 126
arteriosclerosis 58, 99
arthritis 61
Ashbaugh, John 189
Atkins, Robert 249, 252
Austin, Donald F. 127, 134
"autogenous vaccines" 199
Aviva, Palgi 270

B
"B17 orotate" 241
bacillus Calmette-Guerin (BCG) 198
Bailar, John III 138
"balanced diet" 88, 107
Banting, Frederick 181
Barnes, Glenda K. 278
Beall, Morris A. 162
Beard, John 151, 222-23

294

Index

Bee Seventeen 38, 171
Benefits of Human Nutrition, Reserach 89
Benoit, Michael 27-28
benzaldehyde 229-30
Berenson, Gerald S. 91
Berman, Edgar 68, 278
Bernal, J. D. 123
Bestways 237
"beta blockers" 272
bethanidine 72
Binzel, Philip, Jr. 35, 237
Bishop, Katherine S. 264
Bjelke, Erik 268
"black and yellow" salves 192-93
Blewett Cancer Research Foundation 164
Block, Matthew 135
Blumer, Walter 287
Bobst, Elmer 146
Bogalusa Heart Study 91
Bolen blood test for cancer 207-09
Bolen, H. Leonard 207
Bolles, Leo J. 283
Boston Collaborative Drug Study 65
Boston University Medical Center 234
Bradford Research Institute 150, 206, 208, 230, 244
Bradford, Robert W. 48, 50, 51, 115, 165, 181, 206-09, 210, 229
Brain Bio-Center 352
Breast Cancer Detection Demonstration Program 138
"breast cancer screening project" of ACS 137-40
Brennan, Richard O. 89, 97, 286, 287, 289
Bricker, John 162
British Columbia Cancer Research Center 253
Broghamer, W. L. 200
Bross, Irwin 124, 125, 135-36, 140
Brown, Loren N. 15, 19
Brusch, Charles 191
Bull, W. T. 151
Burk, Dean 18, 106, 130, 155, 168, 169, 176-77, 181, 182-84, 210, 212, 256

Burton, Lawrence 20, 196-98
Burzynski, Stanislaw 165
Butler, Lawton J. 164
Buttons, Alycia 11, 29
Buttons, Red 11

C

Cabbat, Felicitas S. 217
Caisse, Rene 190-92
"calcium blockers" 272
California Board of Medical Examiners 131
Calvin, Helen 35, 237
Cameron, Ewan 253, 258
cancer: costs of 61
  statistics of 58-59
Cancer Commission (Canada) 154
Cancer Commission of the California Medical Association 167
Cancer Control Merit Review Committee 146
Cancer Control Society 36, 286
Cancer Facts and Figures (1980) 137
Cancer Facts and Figures (1982) 58, 126
Cancer Research Institute 151
carbenoxolone 72
carbohydrates 99
Carcalon 160
Carey, Hugh 15
Carpenter, Donald G. 275
Cartier, Jacques 262
Cason, James 220
Catholic Medical Center 113, 120
CDBA compound 230
Cedars/Sinai Hospital 10
cellular ("live cell") therapy 233-34
Center for Prisoner of War Studies 92
Center for Science in the Public Interest 109
chaparral tea 193
Chapman, Nathaniel 82
chelation therapy 271-83
chemotherapy, in cancer 133-34
chenodeoxycholic acid 72
Children's Hospital (Los Angeles) 25
chiropractic: AMA and 82-83
  suit concerning 82

295

Index

chlorambucil 135
chlorination 106
Chowka, Peter Barry 143, 146
chymopapain 71, 86
Cisarua Sanatorium 239
City of Hope Medical Center 169
Clarke, Norman 277
Clinica del Mar 236
Cohen, Jesse 28
Cohen, Arthur F. 18
Coley, William Bradford 151
"Coley's fluid"/"Coley's toxins" 151
Colombia 67
Committee for Freedom of Choice in Cancer Therapy, Inc. 10, 12, 16, 33, 35, 36, 39, 47, 48, 49, 50, 115, 118, 166, 206
Confessions of a Medical Heretic 66
Congressional Record 73, 160
Connecticut State Medical Society 81
Conquest of Cancer Program 112, 124, 126, 147
Consumer Reports 61, 136
Consumers Union 63, 264, 266
Contreras, Ernesto 22, 26, 178, 236, 237
Cornell University 148
Cornell University Medical Center 267
coronary bypass surgery 272
cortisone 76
Cott, Alan 252
Couch, Leslie 18
Cox, Kimberley 72
Creagan, Edward T. 261
Cree Indians 214
Crout, Richard 64, 75
Crown Zellerbach Co. 204
"CSS Syndrome" 256
cyclamates 76, 104-05
Cydel Clinic 35, 236
cystic fibrosis 61
CytoPharma de Mexico 52

D
Davison, Jacquie 189
Deaken, Tom 152
Decker, Nikki 27

dehydroepiandrosterone (DHEA) 235
Del Mar Clinic 35
Del Mar Hospital 26
Del Mar Medical Center 23
DeMarco, Peter 69, 159, 184-88
Detroit Medical College 153
DeVita, Vincent 128, 147-48, 261
diabetes 97
diazoxide 72
dichloroacetate 252
diet, American 90-91
Dietary Goals for the United States 87
diethylstilbestrol (DES) 103-04
diisopropylammonium dichloroacetate (DIPA) 252
Dilling, Kirkpatrick 18
dimethyl sulfoxide (DMSO) 202-05, 208
Dougherty, Ralph 106
Doyen, Louis Eugene 152
drug industry, U.S. 63
"drug lag", U.S. 72
Duncan, Robert M. 78
Dunn, Carol M. 177
Durovic, Stevan 159

E
East-West Journal 143
EDTA (ethylene-diamene-tetraacetic acid) 78, 274-75, 277, 279-82
Eijkman, Christian 181
Ellison, Neil 49
Ellestad, Melvyn 72
Endicott, Kenneth M. 183
Enright, William B. 131
Enstrom, James E. 126, 134
Environmental Defense Fund 116
Environmental Protection Agency (EPA) 106
Eskimos 214
Essiac 190-92
Evans, Herbert M. 264
Evers, Ray 68, 78, 275-76
Ewing, James 152
Executive Health 260

F
Fairfield Medical Center 14, 71

Index

Fall River General Hospital 207
fat, U.S. consumption of 96
Federal Trade Commission (FTC) 79-82
Feeding at the Company Trough 109
Fehleisen, Friedrich 151
Feldman, Michael 133
Ferguson, Wilburn 163-64, 192
Filipinos, vitamin B[17] and 214
Fishbein, Morris 156
Fisher, Bernard 140
Fitzgerald, Benedict F., Jr. 157-58, 160-62
Fleming, Sir Alexander 181
Florida State Board of Medical Examiners 283
Florida State University 106
Florida Supreme Court 283
flour industry 99-100
fluoride 105
fluoridation 105-06
Food and Drug Administration (FDA) 32, 35, 43, 44, 72, 74, 76-77, 103, 154, 162, 167, 186, 202-03, 248-49, 277, 279
Food and Nutrition Board, National Research Countil 108
Food, Drug and Cosmetic Act 35, 73, 84-85, 160, 277
food processing 93-94
Fountain, L. D. 124
Freedom from Cancer 33
"free-form" amino acids 244
free radicals 200, 205-06
Friedman, Milton 79
Fritz, Norman 188
Frost, Douglas V. 200

G

Garippa, Marc 27-28
Gazette Medicale de Paris 221
Gerarde, John 221
General Accounting Office (GAO) 74, 146
General Foods 108
Gerson, Max 153, 155, 188
Gerson therapy 188-90
glucose metabolism dysfunction (GMD) 98

Glyoxylide 34, 153-55
Godfrey, Forbes 154
Goenawan, Mas 230, 239
Gold, Joseph 184
Goldberger, Joseph 181
Good Samaritan Hospital (Phoenix) 28
Goodman, Eric 188-89
Gordon, Garry F. 275, 277, 278, 280, 281
Gore, Albert 103
Gori, Gio B. 94-95
Great Herbal of China 221
Green, Chad 13, 21-24
Green, Diana 21-24
Green, Gerald 21-24
Greenberg, Daniel 126, 130, 138, 139-40, 144
Gregory, Dick 249
Gruner, O. C. 207
Gurchot, Charles 223
Gutierrez, Carmen 30, 238

H

Halstead, Bruce 18, 48, 50, 172, 205, 220, 221, 281
Hames, Curtis 208
Hammond, G. Denman 135
Hankin, Elizabeth 172
Hankin, Mr. and Mrs. Dale 172
Hansen, R. Gaurth 102
Harman, Denham 205
Harper, Harold 60, 91, 274, 279
Harris, Louis 43
Harris, Malcolm 157
Harris Poll 43, 96
Harris, Robert 106
Hartwell, Jonathan 194
Hatch, Orrin 147
Harvard Medical School 16
Harvard School of Public Health 67, 108, 278
Hawkins, Paula 147
Hawkins, Sir Richard 263
Health Care Financing Administration (HCFA) 283
Health Research Group 81, 129
"heart disease," statistics of 58-59, 271

297

Index

Heaton, Gary 188
Hebrew University 270
Hegsted, Mark 89
Heinerman, John 193, 221
Heinsohn, Douglas 69, 171
Heitan, Henri 207
Heitan-LaGarde Color Microphotographic Test 208
Helms, Jesse 82
Herbert, Victor 18
herbs, in cancer 192-96
Herschler, Robert 204
Hezekiah 230
Hippocratic Oath 134
Hixson, Joseph 111
HLB Test 208
Hofbauer, John 13, 14, 20-21
Hofbauer, Joseph (Joey) 13-21
Hofbauer, Mary 13, 16
Hoffman-LaRoche 64
holistic medicine 69
homeopathy 82
Horton, John 18
House Government Operations Committee 124, 144
House Select Committee on Aging 203
House Subcommittee on Environment, energy and Natural Resources 105
Houston, Robert 153
How You Can Beat the Killer Diseases 60, 91, 274
Hoxsey, Harry 156-58
Hoxsey herbals 34, 156-58
Hoxsey, John 156
Huks 100
human chorionic gonadotrophin (HCG) 223-24
Hunsberger, Eydie Mae 263
Hunza 213
Hunzakuts 94, 247
hydrazine sulfate 184, 244
hypertension 60, 102
hypoglycemia 60, 91, 97

I
"iatrogenic" disease 65

Ichijo-Kai Hospital and Kochi Tumor Center 230
"IIMP" (individualized, integrated metabolic programs) 235
Illich, Ivan 64, 85
"immuno-augmentative" therapy in cancer 197
Immunological Research Foundation 197
immunotherapy in cancer 129, 144-45
Ingelfinger, Franz 45-46
Institute of Child Behavioral Research 252
insulin 181
interferon 129
International Association of Cancer Victims and Friends (IACVF) 26
International Association of Preventive Medicine (IAMP) 68, 286
International Association on the Artificial Prolongation of the Human Specific Lifespan 275
"international laetrile smuggling ring" 48
International Sugar Foundation 109
Israel, Lucien 132
Issahary, Myron 241
Ivy, Andrew 153, 159

J
Jacob, Stanley 202, 04, 208
Jacobson, Michael 109
James, William 284
Jansson, Erik 106-07
Japanese diet, salt and 102
Japanese Health and Welfare Ministry 198
Jivaro Indians 163, 192
John Beard Memorial Foundation 210
John Birch Society 34
Jones, Hardin B. 131-32
Jones, June 204
Jones, Stewart 204
Josephson, Emanuel M. 162-63
Journal of Applied Nutrition 214
Journal of Clinical Oncology 118

Index

Journal of Orthomolecular Psychiatry 256
Journal of the American Medical Association (JAMA) 64, 139, 174, 186, 278
Journal of the International Association of Preventive Medicine 287
Journal of the National Cancer Institute 138

K
Kark, Robert M. 102
Kaye, Greg 39-41
Keikkila, Richard E. 217
Kelley, William 12, 235
Kellogg Foods 108
Kelsey, John T. 114
Kennedy, Donald 125, 142
Kennedy, Edward 48, 183
Kenton, Barnard 169
King, Stephen 251
Klenner, Frederich 195-96, 258
Koch, William F. 153-55
Kochi, Mitsuyuki 230
Koss, Joan 288
Krebiozen 34, 153, 159-60
Krebs, Ernst T., Jr. 48, 116, 153, 210-18, 212, 222-27, 248-53
Krebs, Ernst T., Sr. 153, 222, 231, 248-53
Kuhn, Thomas 70
Kuhnau, Wolfram 234

L
laetrile, defined, distinguished from amygdalin 10, 210-11
Laetrile Case Histories 39, 237
"laetrile clinical trial" 5, 50-57
Laetrile (trademark) 10
LaGarde, Philippe 208
Lamonica, Daryle 204
Lancet 264, 268
Langer, Stephen E. 90
Langer, William E. 157
Lasker, Albert 145
Lasker, Mary 145
Laytner, Ron 192
Leaf, Alexander 66

Leek, Colleen 196
Leonard, George 69
Let's Live 281
Librium 64
Life Sciences 217
Lind, James 263-64
Lisi, Peter 119
Livingston, Virginia 199, 259
Loma Linda University 214
Louisiana State University 91
Loyola University 120, 239

M
MA-7 15
macrobiotic diet in cancer 242-43
MacMurray, Fred 11, 29
Maimonides Hospital 247
Makerere College Medical School 247
mammography 137-41
Markle, Gerald E. 58
Martin, Daniel 18, 113, 118, 120
Martin, Wayne 152,. 247
Maruyama, Chisato 11, 198
Maruyama vaccine 9, 198-99
Massachusetts General Hospital 21, 148
Massachusetts Supreme Court 22
Mavis, Richard 267
Max Planck Institute for Cell Physiology 182
Mayo Clinic 47, 261
McCormick, Pat 118
McDivitt, Robert A. 138
McDonald, Larry 35, 39
McGill University ???
McGovern, George 87
McGrady, Pat, Sr. 146
McNaughton, Andrew R. L. 34, 112, 210
McNaughton Foundation 48, 112, 168, 210
McQueen, Steve 9-13
McQueens-Williams, Morvyth 153
Medical College of Georgia 107
Medical Heroes and Heretics 152
Medical Tribune 224, 256, 281
Medical World News 23, 115, 135, 278

299

Index

Medina, Daniel 201
Mendelsohn, Robert E. 66
Merck Index 211
Methodist Hospital
 (Philadelphia) 242
Meyer, Alfred 141
Meyer, Theodore 193
Michaelis, Steven 69, 78-79
microwave hypothermia 244
Midnight Globe 196
"minimum daily requirement" 108
minoxodil 72
Moertel, Charles 46-47, 54-55, 262
Moore, J. J. 161
Mormons 94, 214
Morris, Nat 153, 156
Morse, Bill, Jr. 195
Moscow Clinical Hospital No. 60 250
Moscow News 249-50
Moss, Ralph 119, 182
Moulin, C. Mansell 151
Muhammad Ali 252
multiple sclerosis 61, 195-96
muscular dystrophy 61

N
Nabisco 108
Nader, Ralph 81
Natarajan, Nachimuthu 135
National Academy of Sciences
 205, 255
National Cancer Institute (NCI) 5,
 47, 48-50, 87, 94, 111, 121, 124,
 127-28, 132, 144, 146-47, 155,
 164-65, 183, 194, 236, 253, 261
National Center for Health Statistics
 58, 126
National Center for Toxicological
 Research 104
National Commission on Marijuana
 and Drug Abuse 63
National Enquirer 143
National Health Federation (NHF)
 18, 34, 36, 84, 240
National Information Bureau 143
National Nutrition Board 108
natural foods industry, U.S. 96
Nauts, Helen Coley 151

Navarro, Manuel D. 30, 128, 214,
 223-24, 237
Nelson, Gaylord 64
Nestor, John O. 75
*New England Journal of
 Medicine* 45, 52, 252, 261
New Haven County Medical
 Association 81
Newsweek 71, 130
Newton-Wellesley Hospital 101
New Times 127
New West 66
New York County Medical
 Society 155
New York Health Insurance
 Plan 139
New York Magazine 249
New York State Assembly
 Committee on Health 136
New York State Health
 Department 15
New York Times 45, 46
New York Supreme Court 16
Nieper, Hans 29, 228, 241
"nitrilosides" 211
nitrogen mustard 235
Nixon, Richard 112
N, N-dimethylglycine 249
nordihydroguaiaretic acid 193
Norman, N. Philip 207
Northwest Academy of Preventive
 Medicine 283, 286
Northwestern University
 Hospital 191
Now That You Have Cancer 55
Null, Gary 165
Nutrigenetics 97
nutrition, human health and 95

O
Obey, David 147
Ochsner, Alton 268
Oden, Clifford 30
Oke, L. K. 216
Old, Lloyd J. 112, 152
Oncolopgy 223, 256
Ontario Cancer Treatment and
 Research Foundation 192
Osteopathic Annals 277

300

Index

Oxford University 268

P
Page, Lot 101
Palmer, Roger 267
Panel of New Drug Regulations 75
Pani, K. C. 208
"Pap smear" 181
Parry, Charles A. 269
Passwater, Richard 120, 252, 266, 267, 273
Pasteur, Louis 181
pau d'arco 192
Pauling Institute of Science and Medicine 262
Pauling, Linus 182, 253-64
penicillin 181
Pepper, Claude 156
Pesce, Helen 187
Peters, M. Vera 141
Peterson, James C. 58
Pfeiffer, Carl C. 252
Pharmaceutical Manufacturers Association 72
phenylalanine mustard (L-PAM) 135
Philadel Labs 186
Philip Morris Co. 82
Philippines, longevity in 86
Philippine Cancer Society 30
Pills that Don't Work 65
Pitard, Cecil 148-49
Plag; John A. 72
Plaza Santa Maria General Hospital 9
pollutants, U.S. 105
Porcher, Francis 221
Powell, Deana 190
Prats Ruiz 193
President's Biomedical Research Panel 73
Princess Margaret Rose Hospital 141
Private Practice 80
Privitera, James 35, 237
procaine PVP 158, 185-88
procarbazine 135
Proceedings (National Academy of Sciences) 255
Progenitor cryptocides 199

Providence Hospital 27
Public Citizens Health Research Group 65

R
Raasch, Frank 24
radiation, dangers of,
  in cancer 133-34, 135
Randal, Judith 139-40
RaMar Clinic 78
Rauscher, Frank J. 130
"reactive oxygen toxic species" (ROTS) 207-08
"recommended daily allowances" 108
Red Dye No. 2 104, 143
Reed, Barbara 92
Relman, Arnold S. 252
Resperin Corporation 190
retinoids 268
Richardson Center 39
Richardson, John A. 32, 35, 39, 48, 237
Rimland, Bernard 252
R. J. Reynolds Co. 82
RN 66
Roberts, Tom 18
Robinson, Arthur 262-263
Robinson, Della 189
Rochester School of Medicine
Rodriguez, Rodrigo 11, 206
Roemer, Milton 67
Rogers, Robert J. 283
Roper, Burns 43
Roper poll 43
Rork, Mary Lee 189-90
Rosenbaum, Ruth 127
Rosenthal, Benjamin 109
Roswell Park Memorial Institute for Cancer Research 124
Rothblatt, Henry 15
Rubin, David 237, 241
Rush-Presbyterian-St. Luke's Medical Center 268
Rutgers Medical School 270
Rutgers University 206
Rutgers University College of Medicine 217
Rutherford, Glen 29, 38, 238

Index

S
Saccoman, William J. 259
saccharine 75-76
Salaman, J. Franklin 115
Salisbury State College 215
Salk, Jonas 180
Salk vaccine 180
salt (sodium) 101-03
Sattilaro, Anthony 242-43
Saturday Evening Post 242
Saytzeff, Alexander M. 204
Schachter, Michael 15-21, 252-53
Schmid, Franz 114, 116, 188
Schmidt, Alexander 104
Schmidt, Benno 112, 114
Schmidt, Eric S. 174
Schneiderman, Marvin A. 128
Schrauzer, Gerhard 200
Schweitzer, Albert 153, 155
Science 125
Science and Government 126
Second Opinion 116, 117, 119, 120, 123, 152
selenium 199-201
Semmelweiss, Ignasz 181
Senate Health Subcommittee 64
Senate Interstate Commerce Committee on the "Need for the Investigation of Cancer Research Organizations" 160
Senate Labor and Public Welfare Committee 287
Senate Select Committee on Nutrition and Human Needs 87, 94, 287
Senate Select Committee on Small Business 64
Seventh-Day Adventists 94, 214
Shires, G. Thomas 66
Shpirt, Yakov 250
Shute, Evan 265, 266
Shute Foundation for Medical Research 265
Shute Institute for Clinical and Laboratory Medicine 267
Shute, Wilfred 265, 266, 267
Simandjuntak, Todotua 239
Simonton, O. Carl 201-02
Slicher, Anna M. 207

Sloan-Kettering cancer research complex 50, 87, 111-23, 129, 151, 168, 225
Smith, Richard D. 120
sodium butyrate 149
sodium valproate 71
Soto de Leon, Mario 236
Southern Medical Journal 65
Southern Research Institute 169
Spallholz, J. E. 200
Spies, Thomas 181
SPP cassava 239
Stacpool, Peter W. 252
staphage lysate 149
St. Anne's Hospital 207
Stock, C. Chester 112, 114, 120
Stockert, Elizabeth 114
Stone, Irwin 253, 256, 259
St. Peter's Hospital (Albany) 13
Straus, Charlotte Gerson 155, 188
sugar 96-99
Sugar Association 108
sugar industry, cyclamates and 104
Sugiura, Kanematsu 110-23, 228
Summerlin, William 111
Super Drug Story 162
surgery, in cancer 132-33
Swanson, Marilyn 189
Swiss Medical Association 76
Symms, Steve 74, 82
Syracuse Cancer Research Institute 184
Szent-Gyorgyi, Albert 254, 257-58

T
tajibo tree 193
Tartaglia, Anthony 18
Taruc, Luis 100
"Technical Identification Specification for Amygdalin (Laetrile)" 210
Temin, Howard 125
Terman, Lewis 153
Test Laetrile Now Committee 112
Thank God I Have Cancer 30
thalidomide 73
The Cancer Blackout 153
The Cancer Syndrome 119
The Choice 16, 41

Index

The Death of Cancer 240
The Healing Factor 256
The Hopeful Side of Cancer 127
The Medicine Show 264
The Patchwork Mouse 111
"The Prime Cause and Prevention of Cancer" 183
The Sciences 120
The Social Function of Science 123
The Solid Gold Stethoscope 278
The Structure of Scientific Revolutions 70
thiocyanate 217
Thomas, Lewis 225
Time 101
Tobey, Charles 158, 160
Travis Air Force Base 201
trophoblastic theory of cancer 222-26
Trousseau, Armand 181
Truman, Harry 82
Truman, John 22
Tufts College Medical School 208
Tyberg, Theodore 267

U
UNESCO 213
University of Arkansas 107
University of Bergen 268
University of Birmingham Medical Center 278
University of California-Berkeley 205, 220
University of California-Davis 174-75, 219
University of California-Los Angeles (UCLA) 50
University of California-San Diego 200
University of California School of Health and Tumor Registry 127
University of Colorado Medical Center 135
University of Houston 251
University of Illinois 159
University of Iowa 206
University of Michigan 153
University of Nebraska 205

University of Oregon Health Sciences Center 203
University of Southern California Medical Center 135
University of Utah College of Medicine 138
Upton, Arthur 50, 125
U.S. Department of Agriculture 89, 96, 102, 108
U.S. District Court, Western Oklahoma 68, 167, 210
U.S. News & World Report 272
U.S. Public Health Service 208
Utah State University 102

V
Vale of Leven Hospital 258
Valium 64
van Breemen, Vern E. 215-16
Vance, Robert 227, 280, 284
Varner, Robert E. 78, 275
verapimil 72
Verrett, Jacqueline 103-04
Vilcabamba Indians 94, 247
vincristine 135
vitamin A 268-70
vitamin B^{13} 183
vitamin B^{15} 248-53
"vitamin B^{17}," defined 10, 212
Vitamin B^{17}: Forbidden Weapon Against Cancer 33, 213
vitamin B^{17}, in world cancer epidemiology 213-14
vitamin B^{17} *see amygdalin*
vitamin C 253-64
Vitamin C and Cancer 254
Vitamin C and the Common Cold 257
vitamin E 264-68
"vitamin I" 269
vitamin industry, U.S. 64, 96
Vogelsang, Albert 226
Volterra, Guy 22
von Ardenne Research Institute 215
von Liebig, Justus 221
Vortex 220

W
Wald, Nicholas J. 268
Wallace, George 204

Index

Wallace, H. James 18
Wallach, Joel D. 200
Wallis, Ben A. 165
Warburg, Otto 181, 182-83
Washington Post 138, 139, 147
Water, pollution and 105
Wauld, David 192
Waxman, Henry 103
Wedel, E. Paul 35, 233, 237
Welch, Robert J. 283
Western Electric Co. 269
Western Michigan University 58
Weizmann Institute 133
White, Beverly H. 207
Whiting, Robert 253
"Why Are Cancer Patients 'Pregnant'?" 224

Wigmore, Ann 263
Wohler, Freiderich 221
Wolfe, Sidney 65, 81, 125
World Anti-Cancer Union 178
World Cancer Congress 178
World Congress on Vitamin C 257
Woronoff, Sydelle 39-42
Wrightman, K. J. R. 192
Wynder, Ernst 95, 273

Y

Yaccarino, Thomas 42
Yiamouyiannis, John 106
You Don't Have to Die 156
Young, John 128
Young, Robert 147
Younger, Evelle 275